37835

D1196091

BRAIN UNIT
ACTIVITY DURING
BEHAVIOR

BRAIN UNIT ACTIVITY DURING BEHAVIOR

Edited by

M. IAN PHILLIPS, Ph.D.

Department of Physiology & Biophysics
College of Medicine
University of Iowa

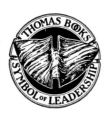

CHARLES C THOMAS · PUBLISHER

Springfield · Illinois · U.S.A.

WL 300
P561 B
1973

Published and Distributed Throughout the World by

CHARLES C THOMAS • PUBLISHER

Bannerstone House

301-327 East Lawrence Avenue, Springfield, Illinois, U.S.A.

This book is protected by copyright. No part of it
may be reproduced in any manner without written
permission from the publisher

© *1973, by* CHARLES C THOMAS • PUBLISHER

ISBN 0-398-02769-2

Library of Congress Catalog Card Number: 72-93225

*With THOMAS BOOKS careful attention is given to all details of
manufacturing and design. It is the Publisher's design to present books that
are satisfactory as to their physical qualities and artistic possibilities and
appropriate for their particular use. THOMAS BOOKS will be true to those
laws of quality that assure a good name and good will.*

LIBRARY
CORNELL UNIVERSITY
MEDICAL COLLEGE
NEW YORK CITY

OCT 1 5 1974

Printed in the United States of America

C-1

CONTRIBUTORS

BEST, PHILLIP J., Department of Psychology, Gilmer Hall, University of Virginia, Charlottesville, Virginia 22901

BROWN, KENNETH A., Departments of Physiology and Psychiatry, Brain Research Institute and Mental Retardation Center, U.C.L.A. Medical Center, Los Angeles, California 90024

BUCHWALD, JENNIFER S., Departments of Physiology and Psychiatry, Brain Research Institute and Mental Retardation Center, U.C.L.A. Medical Center, Los Angeles, California 90024

CASEY, KENNETH L., Department of Physiology, University of Michigan Medical School, Ann Arbor, Michigan 48104

DISTERHOFT, JOHN F., Division of Biology, California Institute of Technology, Pasadena, California 91109

FETZ, E., Department of Neurological Surgery, University of Washington, Seattle, Washington 98105

FINOCCHIO, DOM V., Department of Neurological Surgery, University of Washington, Seattle, Washington 98105

HARPER, RONALD M., Department of Anatomy, University of California, Los Angeles, California 20094

HIRSH, RICHARD, Division of Biology, California Institute of Technology, Pasadena, California 91109

JACOBS, BARRY L., Department of Psychology, Princeton University, Princeton, New Jersey 08540

KEENE, JAMES J., Department of Physiology, University of Michigan, Medical School, Ann Arbor, Michigan 48104

KORNBLITH, CAROL L., Division of Biology, California Institute of Technology, Pasadena, California 91109

JOHNSON, K., Division of Neurobiology, Department of Physiology and Biophysics, University of Iowa, Iowa City, Iowa 52240

LLINÁS, RODOLFO, Division of Neurobiology, Department of Physiology and Biophysics, University of Iowa, Iowa City, Iowa 52240

MAYS, LAWRENCE E., Department of Psychology, Gilmer Hall, University of Virginia, Charlottesville, Virginia 22901

McELLIGOTT, JAMES G., Department of Pharmacology, Temple

University School of Medicine, Philadelphia, Pennsylvania 19140

McGINTY, DENNIS J., Sepulveda Veterans Administration Hospital and Department of Psychology, U.C.L.A., U.C.L.A. Medical Center, Los Angeles, California 90024

NICHOLSON, J. CHARLES, Division of Neurobiology, Department of Physiology and Biophysics, University of Iowa, Iowa City, Iowa 52240

OLDS, JAMES, Division of Biology, California Institute of Technology, Pasadena, California 91109

OLMSTEAD, CHARLES E., Department of Psychology, Gilmer Hall, University of Virginia, Charlottesville, Virginia 22901

PHILLIPS, M. IAN, Department of Physiology and Biophysics, College of Medicine, University of Iowa, Iowa City, Iowa 52240

RANCK, JAMES B., JR., Department of Physiology, University of Michigan, Ann Arbor, Michigan 48104

SEGAL, MENAHEM, Division of Biology, California Institute of Technology, Pasadena, California 94109

SPARKS, D. L., Somolian Clinic, University of Alabama, Medical Center, 1700 Seventh Ave, So., Birmingham, Alabama 35233

THACH, W. THOMAS, Department of Physiology, Yale University, School of Medicine, New Haven, Connecticut 06510

TRAVIS, ROBERT P., Somolian Clinic, Medical Center, University of Alabama, Birmingham, Alabama 35233

WEBER, DAVID S., Departments of Physiology and Psychiatry, Brain Research Institute and Mental Retardation. Center, U.C.L.A. Medical Center, Los Angeles, California 90024

PREFACE

IT HAS BEEN generally true to say that the sciences have progressed at the same speed as new techniques have been developed. Advanced methods may not necessarily lead to more important discoveries, but such techniques are essential if certain fields of research are to be opened up at all. For many years there have been notable advances in our knowledge of the neurophysiology of the brain, but relating this knowledge to functional aspects of behavior has been limited because it has been necessary to use mostly anesthetized and otherwise drugged subjects, or subjects whose manifestations of consciousness are confined to the action of the first few nerves spared by spinal section. On the other hand, considerable advances have also been made in the study of behavior, but there is still a vast gap in our understanding of behavior and the brain mechanisms which function it is to control that behavior. To some extent the techniques of electroencephalogram (EEG) recording and evoked potential recording have shortened the gap. The EEG, however, is limited to detecting changes in the activity of a large, undefined number of cells which prevent us from precisely localizing the generators of the potentials. After forty years of research with the EEG it has to be admitted that, whereas its use in studies of sleep and drowsy states, brain lesions and epileptic foci have been fruitful, the correlates of EEG in spontaneously active, alert and freely moving subjects has been disappointing. This may not continue to be the case as the use of power spectra and computer averaging techniques become more universal than they are at present. Studies using evoked potentials have given more precision in research on fully conscious, unrestrained subjects, but with the drawback that the potentials do have to be evoked. Spontaneous changes in behavior and in neuron activity are not appropriately studied by evoking responses.

The chronic recording of unit activity—the recording of electrical activity of single cells in the brain of unanesthetized subjects—offers an alternative and relatively new approach to the

vii

electrophysiological analysis of brain behavior mechanisms. The approach has, potentially, a higher level of precision in localizing important neurons. Chronic unit recording opens to investigation neurophysiological correlates of behavior at a cellular level during the processes of sensory integration, memory formation, complex behavior, and motivational changes. Not only are these tantalizing phenomena becoming penetrable, but the behavior of the brain itself can be measured in intact subjects receiving drugs, hormones, brain stimulation, temperature or other homeostatic changes. Since the data of unit recording are based upon the premise that action potentials of a single neuron are being recorded, it is important to know the technique used to establish that this premise is true. There will be, therefore, some elaboration about the techniques which are being used.

Chronic unit recording began towards the end of 1950, but has only recently become widely used. In 1958 Strumwasser introduced steel electrodes for long term unit recording in squirrels to study their hibernating patterns. In the same year Jasper presented a paper at the EEG meeting in Moscow of a study of unit activity during conditioned avoidance learning by monkeys. Hubel in 1959 described the use of tungsten electrodes for chronic recording in cats. Since that time the major pioneers in the development of the chronic unit recording technique have been Olds, whose first account of recording in rats appeared in 1961, Evarts, who developed techniques, published in 1960, for cats and monkeys, which have led to their considerable widespread use, Buchwald whose methods of multiple unit recording have also been used on cats, and more recently Travis who has worked with monkeys.

The question of what this approach costs in terms of accuracy of recording from a neurophysiological viewpoint and restrictions on movement from a behavioral point of view is one of the issues raised in this volume.

The book is based on a workshop entitled *Potentialities and Limitations of Chronic Unit Recording Techniques* held during the IVth Annual Winter Conference on Brain Research at Snowmass-at-Aspen in 1971. Questions that arose at that meeting have yielded some of the answers to be found in the papers collected here. Answers to such questions as to what can the activity of a single cell in the brain among millions of other neurons tell us? Is this information unique or just limited? When behavior is so variable, can any unit be categorically correlated to a given behavioral change? Is there a best recording technique to use? Is one recording axons or somata? To what problems is chronic unit recording being applied and how successful is its application?

We hope that this book will be helpful to the many users and potential users of these techniques, and to the teachers and their students for whom the results of these studies give new information for a better understanding of brain functions. The coverage is not exhaustive but the contributors represent users of the currently viable techniques. We feel that the book can usefully serve as both a *source* and a *sink*.

M. IAN PHILLIPS

ACKNOWLEDGMENTS

T HE EDITOR IS GRATEFUL to the American Association for the Advancement of Science and the American Physiological Society for their permission to reprint two of the articles included in this book. To the authors and publishers from whose work illustrations have been taken and to Elizabeth Bencken for her assistance with indexing, I give my sincere thanks. Linda Balhorn is thanked for her excellent editorial assistance.

CONTENTS

BRAIN UNIT
ACTIVITY DURING
BEHAVIOR

PART ONE

TECHNIQUES OF RECORDING

Chapter I

UNIT ACTIVITY RECORDING IN FREELY MOVING ANIMALS: SOME PRINCIPLES AND THEORY

M. I. PHILLIPS

RECORDING THE electrical activity of single cells in the brain during behavior has become a bridge between neurophysiology and the study of behavior. In this book the contributed chapters represent attacks on many different problems using the same approach, across this bridge. The methods described and applied, allow the recording of bioelectric activity of a few or single brain cells in conscious, intact animals without resorting to anesthetics, brain surgery, paralyzing drugs, and other restricting techniques of the acute experimental procedures.

It has not been feasible to make intracellular recordings in the chronic preparations, however, and recording via chronically implanted electrodes is extracellular. Action potentials, appearing as unitary spikes, are usually recorded and analyzed, the analysis generally being of the time order of the spikes in terms of frequency or probability of firing.

Extracellular recording, however, can yield a great deal of information directly which can only be inferred from intracellular recording. For example, the site of spike generation and synaptic inputs can be established by using a movable extracellular microelectrode and suitable laminar field analysis. Such techniques may be too advanced for present needs when recording in chronic behaving animals, but they are developing into very powerful analytical tools, and ultimately they may become accepted as standard procedures to complement the analysis of spike activity re-

It is a pleasure to thank Dr. J. C. Nicholson for reading Part I of this manuscript, for his helpful suggestions and providing Figure 6. Preparation of this article was supported by National Science Foundation Grant GB 27704.

corded in chronic preparations. They add a new dimension to recording, beyond simply the registration of unit activity. For the present discussion they are important because they help to clarify our understanding of what is being recorded. In the following pages we shall first review some of the theoretical considerations and secondly, give a brief analysis of spikes recorded experimentally.

SOME BASIC PRINCIPLES AND THEORETICAL CONSIDERATIONS

In recording extracellularly we would like to know what is going on in the neuron closest to the recording electrode. To analyze extracellular recordings it is important to realize that (1) we are dealing with a volume conductor and (2) to understand the relationship of extracellularly recorded potentials, which can be measured, to the distribution of current in the neuron, which is not so easily measured.

Volume Conductor Theory

Nerve cells are immersed in a low resistance conducting medium, the extracellular fluid. This conducting medium is known as a volume conductor. Extracellular recordings are recordings of potentials in the volume conductor between the recording electrode and a distant, indifferent electrode. For the purposes of simplicity in dealing with the complexities of such a system, the capacitive components of the extracellular fluid are ignored and only the resistance is taken into account, *i.e.*, the volume conductor is considered as purely ohmic. Also the volume conductor is assumed to be isotrophic, *i.e.*, it has uniform conductance.

From the studies of Lorente de Nó (29), Coombs et al. (7), Freygang and Frank (12) it seems reasonable to assume that extracellular recordings are derived from current density changes across the membrane. The measure is the potential recorded. The relationship of the potential to the sources and sinks on the membrane is shown in Figure 1.1. In the neuron, consisting of a soma and usually dendrites and an axon, when an action potential (ap) is generated there is longitudinal current (I_i) flowing along the membrane and transmembrane current (I_m) flowing across the membrane, which are derivatives of the membrane potential

(V_m). I_i is the first spatial derivative and I_m the second spatial derivative (see Fig. 1.2). This means that only if there is a flow of current can an extracellular recording be made and therefore the resting potential cannot be recorded extracellularly.

The current density has magnitude and direction and is thus a vector. By Ohm's Law, current density is equal to the electric field multiplied by the conductance of the external medium. Since the conductance of the extracellular fluid may be considered as a constant and the current can be either positive or negative it follows that the electric field can be either negative or positive. The difference in field potentials between two points such as when one records extracellularly, is equal to the negative integral of the electric field along any path between the two points. Thus we arrive at a concept related to Coulomb's Law and the notion of charges on the membrane. This relationship of sources and sinks of membrane current to current density, to electric fields, and to the field potentials, holds for quasi-electrostatic currents where capacitance and magnetic effects can be neglected. A characteristic of field potentials is that they summate algebraically. Thus, where there are several neurons oriented at different angles to one another, some potentials will summate, some will cancel out, and what is recorded is the average potential of the fields as current flows through the extracellular medium. The geometry of the recorded nerve cells has, therefore, to be taken into account.

Classic studies demonstrating an electric field in a low resistance medium when an action potential is generated in a neuron, were made by Lorente de Nó (29). He took a segment of a frog sciatic nerve, put one end in a pool of nonconducting oil where he stimulated the fiber, and surrounded the rest with a conducting fluid. Recordings were made by an electrode with a 40 μ tip. The indifferent electrode was placed several cms away in the conducting medium. Lorente de Nó mapped the polarity and amplitude of a potential field away from and along the stimulated fiber. Each of the recordings had to be made at the same time after stimulation as current flow is instantaneous. When points giving the same values were linked together he could visualize the extracellular potential field generated by the action potential for that

VOLUME CONDUCTOR THEORY

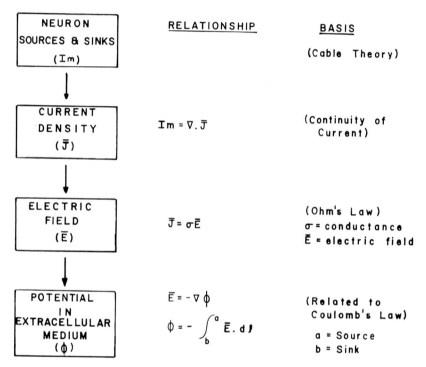

Figure 1.1. A summary of the relationships between what we want to know—the distribution of sources and sinks, and what is recorded—the extracellular potential in a volume conductor during extracellular recording.

Figure 1.2. Spatial representation of first and second derivatives of the action potential ($-V_e$) (29). The extracellular potential is proportional to the density of the transmembrane current and fits the negative of the second derivative of the intracellularly recorded ap. This may vary in practice where the electrodes are not recording from the surface, or where the impulse propagation is not a continuous process, such as at the IS-SD break. (Reproduced with permission from Lorente de Nó, *Studies from The Rockefeller Institute for Medical Research*, Vol. 132, 1947.)

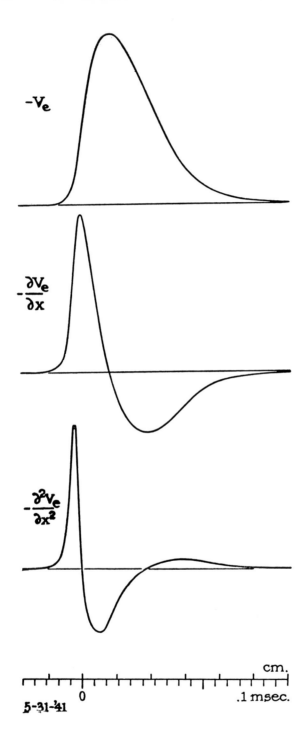

$-V_e$

$-\dfrac{\partial V_e}{\partial x}$

$-\dfrac{\partial^2 V_e}{\partial x^2}$

cm.

0

.1 msec.

5-31-41

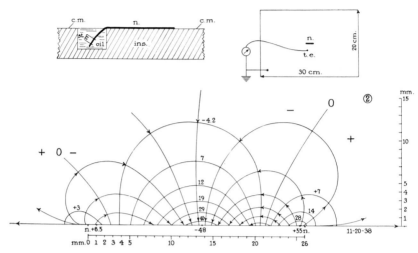

Figure 1.3. The experimental arrangement used by Lorente de Nó (29) (top). n = nerve, cm = conducting medium, ins = insulation, t.e. = recording electrode. Fields of current (arrows) are perpendicular to the fields of potential measured in the same instant in time. The units are arbitrary values but it can be seen that there is a sink of negativity in the middle and asymmetric sources (positivity) at either end with a stronger positivity value at the right. (Reproduced with permission, see reference 29.)

particular time segment (see Fig. 1.3). Lines drawn perpendicular to these isopotential contours show the current field. The current flow is shown by the arrows. Current density may be measured as the current per unit area (amps/cm²).

The potential fields are biphasic in polarity both at the beginning and end of the stimulated region of the nerve fiber, but are triphasic in the middle. At the stimulated end of the neuron, when the action potential (ap) is propagated down the nerve, the polarity is negative-positive (n-p), which indicates that the membrane there serves as a source of current supplying the activated region ahead with current. In the triphasic wave form, the potential is positive-negative-positive (p-n-p), which is interpreted as meaning that the membrane is behaving first as a current *source*, then as a *sink*, then as a source again. The sources supply current passive to the sink. The local currents are explained by the classical Hodgkin-Huxley analysis (17) which have shown that during depolarization where there is a current sink there is an inward current across the membrane and where there is a source there is an outward current flow. Inward current spreads longitudinally along the axoplasmic core of the nerve fiber and simultaneously leaks out across the membrane. The outward flow is seen as a positive polarity in the extracellular medium, and the inward current is detected as a negativity.

There are, therefore, two generalizations which can be made (with certain reservations) about the polarity of extracellular potentials in this simplest case of studying an isolated neuron in a volume conductor: (1) negativity usually indicates a sink of inward current and positivity a source of outward current; (2) negativity usually indicates an active site and positivity a passive site. *Active site* is actually in the core of the neuron and can be due to an action potential or an excitatory synapse. There are exceptions, for example, at an axon terminal the potential may be negative, but the membrane site is passive. This would happen where there is repolarization near the terminal causing a positivity which is big enough to make the terminal appear relatively negative even though it is passive. There are other factors which can mask these generalizations as is shown below.

More Complex Models

Lorente de Nó's model was a two dimensional one and the situation becomes much more complicated when a three dimensional picture is attempted. Clark and Plonsey (6) have investigated a three dimensional model of field potentials around a core conductor, demonstrating that current direction at any point results from both axial (*i.e.*, longitudinal) and radial currents compounded vectorially (since there is both magnitude and direction involved).

A further complicating factor in the real case of the neuron *in situ*, is the presence of dendrites. Dendrites alter the geometry of the field around a soma. Rall has calculated the theoretical extracellular fields of a relatively simple arrangement of dendrites (41). In his model, during the generation of an action potential on the soma, the soma is active and the dendrites are passive with appropriate positivity on their surface. The fields around the dendrites are, however, negative up to a certain distance (about eight dendrite radii) from the soma before they become zero. The reason for this can be seen in Figure 1.4, which shows that the potential distribution arising from inward current

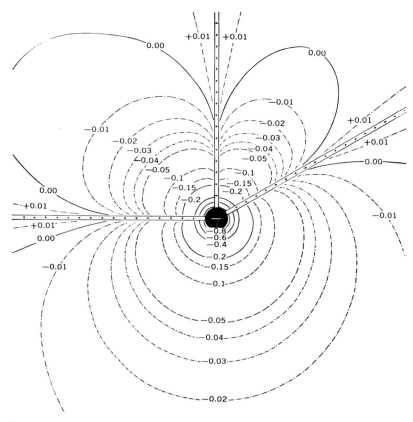

Figure 1.4. The potential field calculated by Rall (41) to occur at the peak of an action potential where the soma is activated in a theoretical model of a motoneuron. The soma is spherical and the dendrites are cylindrical and passive. The extracellular field is negative up to 8 soma radii from the soma. The solid line indicates the zero-isopotential contour. This means that an electrode near the dendrites on the negative side of this contour will record increasing negativity as the electrode is advanced towards the soma—a prediction borne out by the experimental evidence of Nelson and Frank (31). (Reproduced with permission, see reference 41.)

generated in the soma extends throughout the conducting medium and thereby envelopes much of the dendrites. The isopotentials which are shown in the figure attenuate with distance. It has been shown by Nelson and Frank (31) that extracellular microelectrodes can detect negative potentials 200-350 μ from the soma of motoneurons, giving support to this theoretical model. Rall's analysis is quite useful therefore in obtaining some insight into the nature of the extracellular potential. This is despite the simplistic shape assumed for the cell and the assumptions on which the calculations are based of a completely isotropic, homogenous and infinite extracellular medium.

Inevitably in the nervous system such assumptions do not hold. The extracellular space is finite, it has two limitations: (a) the channels between cells, and (b) the boundaries and interfaces of the brain, such as the pial-glial boundary for example. Nevertheless the theoretical treatment provides an approximation which is not unreasonably out of line with experimental evidence, at least for the motoneuron which has received the brunt of many recording studies and given most of the answers.

Branching Dendrites.

Other cells do not have the radial symmetry of their dendrites which the motoneuron does. In the olfactory bulb, for example, the dendritic tree of the mitral cell forms a relatively thick trunk growing out of the soma into narrower and narrower branches. Rall and Shepherd (42) have used the olfactory bulb to model a simple cortical system. They again simplified and idealized the neuron, but in this case the dendritic branching was considered as a branching symmetric pattern. The spatial aspect of this dendritic tree was reduced to an equivalent cylinder to give a single dimension of distance from the soma to the tips of the distal dendrites. This was shown mathematically by using the partial differential equations from cable theory for spatiotemporal distributions of membrane potential in membrane cylinders, which are assumed to be passive.

Each cylinder has a *characteristic length* (λ) based on the resistivity of the membrane. For branching dendrites the λ was calculated for each pair of daughter branches. When the actual length is divided by the characteristic length a value is given for the electrotonic length. This has proved important in understanding the properties of synaptic potentials (42). The equivalent cylinder concept while simplifying the electrotonic state of the neuron, cannot deal with nonuniformity of the membrane potentials. To overcome this, compartmental regions were introduced, each representing a uniform membrane potential within a given compartment, but not between compartments. For the passive system the compartments are dealt with mathematically as differential equations which are linear and of the first order. Figure 1.5 shows the schematics of these kinds of abstractions from cell to compartments. Of interest to the present discus-

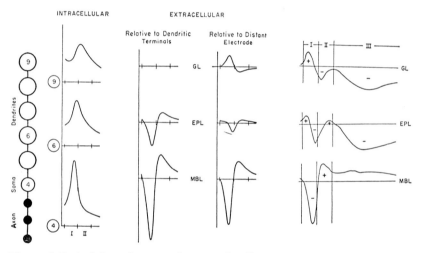

Figure 1.5. At left, reduction of a mitral cell to a theoretical cell of compartments by Rall and Shepherd (42). The predicted intracellular recording for three compartments at the soma—4, mid-dendrite—6, and terminal dendrite—9, when an ap was initiated in compartment four and propagated through the soma-dendritic complex. Next, the extracellular potentials computed first relative to the dendritic terminals and secondly with reference to a distant electrode. It can be seen that the potential divider effect (at the reference electrode) has reduced the amplitude in compartments four and six, but an amplitude is recorded at the dendrite terminal since it is not being used as the reference point. Right, experimentally obtained records showing the close resemblance to the predicted transients in the same time periods I and II. (Modified from Rall and Shepherd with permission, see reference 42.)

sion is that such an abstraction gives a greater understanding of extracellular recording in a group of cells, particularly a population of neurons which is symmetrically arranged. Rall chose the olfactory bulb to demonstrate the computation of field potentials but the results are applicable to other anatomically *cortical* systems such as the hippocampus, neocortex, cerebellum, prepyriform cortex and the retina, although not to the spinal, brain stem nor thalamic nuclei.

If one thinks of the olfactory bulb as a perfect sphere containing radially arranged mitral cells each generating equal amounts of extracellular current, the current will be held within the sphere because the structure would be symmetrical. The symmetry of the structure is equivalent to the *closed-field* which Lorente de Nó (29) described. This holds for either the case where there is a soma or where there are somata in the center and dendrites arranged radially in the periphery, such as is found in the olfactory bulb and the motoneuron pools of the III (oculomotor) and IV (trochlear) nerves, or where the dendrites are in the center and the somata are arranged radially in the periphery, such as in the superior olivary nucleus. The important characteristic of closed fields for the present interest is that recordings of activity from cells in such a field can only be made when the microelectrode is inside the field or very close to the peripheral surface. (The inferior olivary nucleus incidentally behaves as a closed field without having the apparent symmetry.)

The olfactory bulb, however, does not behave as an ideal closed field. Extracellular recording at the bulb surface can detect a transient potential during the antidromic (*i.e.*, artificial) synchronous firing of mitral cells. Since the potential is recorded with reference to a distant electrode, there is a flow of current away from the bulb. This current can return as a source of secondary current to the mitral cells, thereby completing the circuit. The bulb is *punctured*—it has the olfactory tract poking into it, providing a pathway to and from the rest of the brain. Because the reference electrode lies on the current pathway, it will also record a potential, which will sum algebraically with the microelectrode potential. This led Rall to postulate a potential divider effect at the reference electrode. The potential divider ratio is based on the resistance in the path to and from the indifferent electrode. One of the important factors in extracellular recording is therefore emphasized, namely that the reference electrode must be relatively distant from the recording electrode. In large animals the distance is usually of the order of centimeters but in small animals, such as rats, especially where multiple microelectrodes are used, the distance may only be a few millimeters which can lead to distortions of the recorded potential.

In Figure 1.5, we have put together Rall's predicted results for intracellular and extracellularly recorded potentials. It can be seen that the theoretical computations bear a reasonable resemblance to the recorded potentials.

Dendritic Spikes

Zucker (52) has used the same method of computation to calculate the field potential of Purkinje cells in the cerebellum. His analysis was stimulated by a controversy over the interpretation of potentials recorded from the cerebellum of alligator. This controversy was begun by Llinás et al. (27), who used volume conductor theory to analyze their cerebellar recordings of extracellular potentials and was taken up by Calvin and Hellerstein (5) who argued that a passive model based on cable theory predicts the recorded potentials without hypothesizing an active process of the spike generation by the dendrites. At the crux of the argument is the question: What can we tell from the extracellular recordings of field potentials in complicated neural tissue?

Calvin and Hellerstein applied the cable model by assuming that since the intracellular and extracellular regions are symmetrical in a large ensemble of oriented cells the potentials are proportional and that a group of synchronously firing cells can be treated on the same basis as an isolated one dimensional, cable-like neuron with synaptic excitation. The predicted action potential was a monophasic one. Zucker (52), however, pointed out that when two identical nerves are laid out parallel in a conducting medium separated by 2 cm, the potential recorded in the middle is a triphasic one as would be predicted from a volume conductor theory and therefore the cable model is not adequate alone. Llinás et al. discriminated the intracellular ap and EPSP that they recorded by use of volume conductory theory. This predicts that a spike propagating through the dendrites of a single open field type of neuron will be triphasic at all depths below the surface and nonreversible, while the EPSP on the other hand, will reverse in polarity as the electrode passes from sink to source. The *open-field* type of neuron or neuron ensemble has the neural elements arranged in a palisade—with the dendrites aligned together at one end of a volume conductor and somata aligned together at the other. This type of field is found in the cerebral cortex, the cerebellum and hippocampus. The important point here is that a recording electrode can pick up the field potentials from relatively far away. The field potential at a given point is proportional to the integral of membrane current divided by the distance to each membrane segment. When the electrode is very close to, or on, the membrane surface, the potential is nearly proportional to the membrane current at that point. This current can be calculated, as was noted earlier, since it is proportional to the second spatial derivative (see Fig. 2).

By treating the dendrites as a narrow leaky cable, Nicholson and Llinás (33) derived the transmembrane current for a single dendrite using cable theory. The extracellular potentials, however, are governed by quite different physical factors from the intracellular potentials, since the dendritic trees form a *jungle-like* matrix and are bound by the pial-glial surface. The simplifying model which they use for this matrix was to confine it to a volume in the form of a cylinder, comprised of the population of synaptically depolarized cells. The axis of the cylinder is defined by the trajectory of the recording electrode. The extracellular potential was represented by Poisson's equation (not to be confused with Poisson's distribution): $\Delta^2\phi = I_m/\sigma$, where σ is the conductivity of the extracellular fluid. Being able to apply Poisson's equation is important because much is known about it mathematically from its use in electrodynamics (22). Poisson's equation represents the current flow of the cylinder in a three dimensional resistive medium with a specified source density. The latter term was derived from a one dimensional cable equation for the transmembrane current of a dendrite by assuming that (a) I_m is confined to the cylinder and (b) I_m only changes with depth and does not vary on any given horizontal plane. Since recording electrodes are biased towards the potential at the tip, a weighting

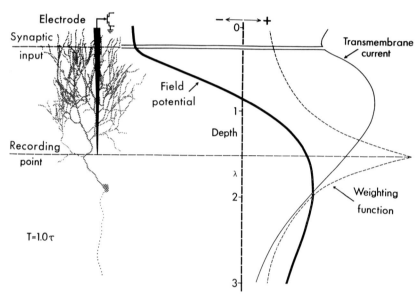

Figure 1.6. Model for deviation of field potentials from transmembrane currents in cerebellar cortex. Typical cerebellar Purkinje cell (alligator) outlined at left; this cell is one member of a discrete neuronal ensemble which receives synchronous synaptic input (from electrical stimulation) near superficial dendritic tips. This input produces transmembrane currents which are governed by the cable properties of the dendrites. These currents act as a set of current sources and sinks for the extracellular medium which results in current flow in this three dimensional resistive space, thus producing the field potentials. The potential is recorded by an electrode tip at the recording point. Theoretical analysis (Nicholson and Llinás (33), Nicholson (32), shows that the geometry of the neuronal population and resistive properties of the medium determine the *impor-tance* (weighting function) which the electrode assigns to current sources and sinks at different distances from the tip. The integrated product of the weighting junction and transmembrane current gives the field potential. Transmembrane current and field potential expressed in arbitrary units for time $T = \tau$ where τ is the time constant of the equivalent cylinder used to represent the dendritic tree. Instances measured in units of λ, the length constant of the equivalent cylinder. (Figure by C. Nicholson, 1973, by permission of *I.E.E.E. Trans. Bio. Med. Engr.*)

function was included in the equation (Fig. 1.6). By solving the equation with respect to cerebellar anatomy, the geometry of the recording and stimulating electrodes and the pial-glial boundaries, the model predicted that (1) a negative potential which does not reverse as the electrode penetrates deeper into the neural layer, indicates an active process of spike propagation and (2) a negative-positive potential which reverses with depth of recording indicates a passive process such as the presence of an EPSP. The model fitted well with the experimentally recorded potentials.

This cursory introduction to field potential analysis relates some of the techniques that can be used for a more sophisticated analysis of spike potentials than their time order of appearance alone. Such analyses depend on knowing the neuroanatomy and correctly applying the principles which govern current flow in volume conductor.

AXON OR SOMA?

When making extracellular recordings it is important to know whether the recording is from the axons or the somata-dendrites of the neurons. In studies of learning, memory, or habituation, for example, where the pathways involved are not clear, errors may be made by attributing the unit responses seen to a given nucleus in the brain where, in fact, an axon is being recorded. The recordings may only be of messages *en route* to other locations and not the arrivals or departures from that particular area.

The finding of some studies on intracellular and extracellular recording can give a degree of confidence in separating axon and soma spikes, but the degree depends on several limitations. The most important factor is a knowledge of the cytoarchitecture of the cells being recorded, not only the structure of the cell—the axon, soma and dendrite complex, but also the arrangement of the neighboring cells surrounding the recording electrode.

There have been several attempts to establish the nature of spikes from known structures. Lorente de Nó's study of the hypoglossus nucleus, published in the *Journal of Cellular and Comparative Physiology* in 1947 (29, 207-288) remains the classic in this field. Svaetichin (46) made recordings from ganglion cells while visualizing them under a microscope. Hild and Tasaki (16) also visualized neurons while recording and established some characteristics of soma surface potentials.

Nelson and Frank (31) took a different approach to the problem. They stimulated a single axon in the ventral root of the cat's spinal cord and proceeded to penetrate the motoneuron pool until they were by the soma of a neuron being thus antidromically stimulated. Their results showed that with an extracellular microelectrode of about 2 μtip diameter, the fields around a motoneuron were large and predominantly negative. As the site of the potential generation was approached, the amplitude became larger until its peak was reached.

Terzuolo and Araki (49) employed what they termed *parallel microelectrodes* with which they could record intracellular and extracellular potentials simultaneously. The tips of the electrodes were separated by 3-20 μ and, therefore, both types of recordings were in all probability from the same cell. Based on their work with voltage clamp techniques and the studies of Coombs et al. (7) on intracellular recording analysis, they were able to determine the location on a motoneuron of antidromically produced spikes. Their study is one of the few to include a clear analysis of the axon spike. Another study is that of Frank and Fuortes (11) who defined axon spikes by comparing recordings of primary sensory fibres, in the roots or in the cord, with those from the motoneuron areas. Their recordings were intracellular, but they found important time duration differences between axon and soma spikes which are pertinent and equally applicable to extracellular records. The main points of agreement from these and other studies are summarized below.

Axons

Extracellularly recorded spikes which suggest they are generated in axons have (1) a sharp rising phase, (2) a short duration and (3) a triphasic potential wave pattern. The triphasic pattern is positive-negative-positive (p-n-p), which would be predicted from an ap propagated in a volume conductor where the external current field is of the open type. Axon collaterals would not make any appreciable difference. The p-n-p characteristic

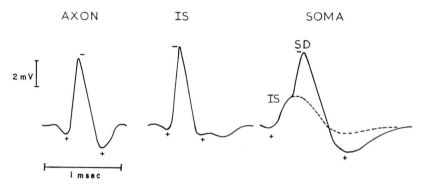

Figure 1.7. Wave form of extracellularly recorded spikes. Taken from records of antidromically stimulated motoneurons (49) independent evidence indicated that at left the electrode was close to an ap in an axon; center, the electrode was closer to the initial segment (IS) and right, the electrode was in the vicinity of the soma. For simultaneously recorded intracellular responses see reference (49). Triphasic activity is seen in the axon and IS, but a tetraphasic pattern is recorded when the soma-dendritic (SD) complex is activated. Failure of the ap to propagate into the SD complex is recorded as the spike outlined by the dotted line, by an electrode on the soma.

represents a source-sink-source on the membrane close to the electrode tip. This wave pattern is, of course, characteristic of other open field types which are not axons, but they usually have longer duration.

We have looked at spike duration from a population of units recorded from the hippocampus, reticular formation and hypothalamus of freely moving rats. Measurements were based on photographs and computer plotted pictures of spikes. The computer measured the wave pattern every 22.4 μsec for sixty-four successive locations (3). The total sweep was 1.4 msec. with a peak synchrony point at .7 msec. which limited the measurement of spikes over 1 msec. duration. Data were taken from units recorded from rats with implanted 62 μ nichrome wire electrodes. The rats were operated two to eight days prior to testing. Spikes were measured from the beginning of a detectable change from the baseline. The measured durations of these spikes were the case in the frequency histogram shown in Figure 1.8. It can be seen that there is a bimodal distribution with one peak at 0.7 msec. and an-

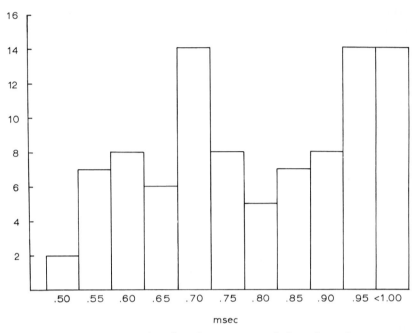

Figure 1.8. Histogram of spike duration recorded with nichrome wire (62 μ) electrodes. Measurements were made from photographs and computer averaged transients. Cells recorded from were in the hippocampus, midbrain reticular formation and hypothalamus. There is a bimodal distribution of long and shorter duration spikes, which would fit the duration times given for axon and soma recordings, but because the neuroanatomy of the structures is not known, this differentiation can not be made categorically. Very small cells might also yield short duration spikes.

other at 0.9->1.0 msec. All the spikes at 0.75 msec and below which had large amplitudes were triphasic. Spikes of longer duration included triphasic, biphasic and tetraphasic and most wave patterns had slower rising phases. This distribution suggests that in the population studied there were a number of axon spikes. The duration agrees well with Frank and Fuortes' measure of 0.6 $\pm$ 0.2 msec for motoneuron axon spikes. Tasaki et al. (47) recorded the duration of presynaptic axon spikes in the optic tract and lateral geniculate area as 1 msec. or less and felt that the distortion by the capacitance of the myelin sheath and of the recording electrode made more accurate determination difficult. Hippocampal pyramid cells are of the open field type and reticular formation cells probably have a mixed type of field configuration.

The sharp rising phase of the axon spike is to be expected because of the small size of the axon membrane. Compared to a larger soma membrane there are fewer *hot spots* which have to be activated so that activation occurs faster. The smaller size will also offer a higher resistance and when resistance is high the area fires more readily. Sometimes notches appear in the extracellularly recorded spike from fiber tracts. The notches occur after the initial rising phase. According to Tasaki et al. (47) these are the *nodal signs* of injured axons. They are associated with a resting potential, positive in sign and the notch represents a delay in the propagation of an ap between two portions of the neuron. Such responses do appear to be limited to axons and are not reported from somata or dendrites. The second, or late, positivity of the triphasic spike is longer than the first, because a larger area of membrane has to be repolarized after the spike peak has passed, than before the peak arrived.

Cell Body

Soma spikes are of longer duration, with slower rising phases than axons and the wave pattern of the potentials depends where on the soma the spike is recorded and the neuroanatomy of the neuron and the type of neuron, or neuron pool that the electrode is recording from. The type of current field—open, closed or open-closed types (see theoretical section) will greatly influence the polarity of the potentials recorded.

To understand the generation of the spike in the neuron it is also necessary to recall the results from intracellular recordings. The first component of an action potential (ap) recorded intracellularly in the antidromically stimulated soma of spinal motoneuron is the IS (or A) spike resulting from activity in the initial segment (i.e., the axon hillock and the adjacent unmyelinated portion of the axon). The subsequent component of the ap is the SD (or B) spike which occurs when there is electrotonic spread to the soma dendritic portion of the neuron. As an example of the closed field type of neuron, the antidromically stimulated motoneuron is given.

a. Initial Segment

The IS represents the area of transition from the open field state of the axon to the closed field of the soma and a recording electrode in the vicinity during ap propagation will record a triphasic potential (Fig. 1.7). The first positivity is due to the IS acting as a source for the axon potential, the negativity is recorded as the area becomes activated and the late positivity results from the repolarization of the IS, which becomes a source for the soma potential. In the case under consideration, however, where the electrode is close to the center of a closed field and there is a spread of current throughout the SD complex, the negativity of the center tends to obscure the late positivity and thus a reduction is seen compared to that of the axon potential (Fig. 7).

b. Soma

An electrode outside the soma of a neuron of the closed field type records a tetraphasic (p-n-n-p) wave pattern with a slower rising phase and longer duration than the axon spike.

The initial positivity of this extracellular recording may be interpreted as the soma acting briefly as a source for the IS spike. The first negativity indicates the dendrites have become the source for the IS. The second negativity occurs when the SD complex becomes the sink, still supplied by the dendrites as the main source of current, according to the closed field hypothesis. The whole SD complex is not uniform and does not fire instantaneously. The late positivity results when the soma repolarizes and becomes a source for activity in the dendritic part of the SD complex. Terzuolo and Araki showed that the SD spike recorded intracellularly coincided with the second negative potential. As additional evidence for the meaning of the two negative spikes, they showed that where the SD spike failed to materialize, only the first negative wave was recorded (Fig. 1.7).

The duration of the soma spike is variously measured as 1.5 $\pm$ 0.3 msec. (11), 1.5-3 msec. (47) and from our own data as 1.5 $\pm$

0.7 msec, although Betz cells apparently have spikes of a shorter
duration of approximately 1 msec (38). The evidence for this is
based on (a) the electrode showing blockade of antidromic invasion when two stimuli are given close together, which indicates
that the tip is at the soma or axon hillock (11), and (b) knowing that the electrode tip was in a cell layer region, such as the
motoneuron pool.

It is helpful when one can clearly recognize from the recording
that the electrode tip is in a cell layer. It appears that there are
areas where one can do this. In Figure 1.9 the characteristic spontaneous firing of hippocampal pyramid cells are shown. Here the
electrode tip was shown by histological examination to be in the
soma layer of CA1 cells. The initial large spike is followed by

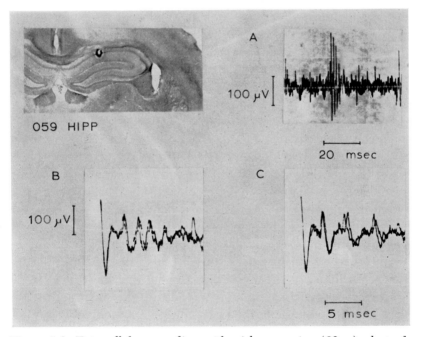

Figure 1.9. Extracellular recording with nichrome wire (62 μ) electrode
from hippocampus. The site of recording was in the soma layer of the CA1
area and the type of spike train seen is easily recognized by its patterned
spike train (A). It is also found in the CA2, CA3 and CA4 regions. The
number of spikes vary over time; between B and C ten minutes elapsed
but the original pattern recurs.

several spikes in descending amplitude probably as a result of depolarizing after potentials (24). The number of spikes following the initial spike vary and over a few minutes may fluctuate from six to two but the second potential remains faithful following the first and the entire wave pattern is restored over ten to thirty minutes so that this configuration of patterned spike activity is easy to recognize. Thach (48) has also described spikes which identify a cell. In the cerebellum *simple* spikes, he suggests, probably result from granule cell firing of Purkinje cells while *complex* spikes indicate climbing fiber responses of the same cells. Aghajanian et al. (1) report recognizing units of the raphé system by a diphasic (p-n) wave pattern and a slow regular rate of firing (1-2 spikes/sec), which distinguishes them from other midbrain areas where they find the rates to be either faster and/or irregular in rhythm. While the meaning of p-n spikes is not clear, the rate of discharge can be an important variable in recognizing cells.

Amplitude alone is a limited indicator of all location since it is related to (a) the distance of the recording electrode from the site of generation (in a volume conductor amplitude is proportional to the square of the distance), (b) the type of field, e.g., outside a closed current field the potential is virtually absent and (c) the current density. Fast background activity recorded when the multiple unit activity method technique is used, however, has been shown to have characteristic amplitudes for different brain areas (4). In the limbic system (amygdala, habenula and fornix) the amplitudes were of 10-20 μV. Extrapyramidal sites also had small amplitude characteristics (15-25 μV). Larger amplitudes were displayed by the medial geniculate and red nucleus (80-120 μV). The authors considered that these characteristics reflect extracellular spike potentials of different amplitude in these prescribed parts of the brain, and they concluded (13) that this was a function of cell size rather than any other variable.

Dendrites

An electrode on the surface of a dendrite records a diphasic potential (p-n) of long duration (15-20 msec) when the neuron is stimulated (47).

If the dendrites are the main source of current then an electrode on the dendrite surface will record a positive potential when the IS and soma are activated by an ap. When the ap invades the dendrites the wave pattern will change to negative. Since there will be no further reversal of the sink-source relationship there will be no positivity recorded after the negative potential. The diphasic characteristic (as opposed to a monophasic one) identifies an active process rather than an electrotonic spread. If the ap fails to invade the dendritic tree then only the initial positivity is recorded.

Soma of the Open-Field Type

Many neurons in the brain have the open-field type of arrangement, including some motoneurons. An extracellular electrode records a triphasic wave pattern (p-n-p) when the soma is antidromically stimulated (Fig. 1.10). The open-field motoneuron is envisioned as having dendrites mostly congregated at the end of the soma opposite to the axon. Simultaneous intracellular recording shows that the first positive potential of the extracel-

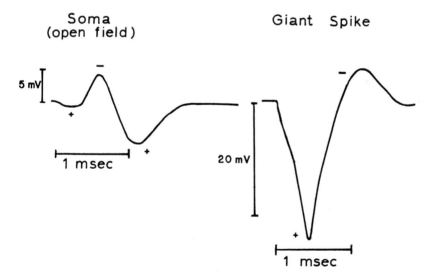

Figure 1.10. Left wave form of potential recorded from an electrode close to the soma of an open field type of neuron (49). Note the basic triphasic pattern. Right, a *giant extracellular spike* recorded when a microelectrode is pushing against the soma membrane during the propagation of an ap.

lular record occurs at the same time as the IS is activated and suggests that the soma is acting as a source. The negativity coincides with the start of the SD spike at which time the soma becomes a sink. The dendrites and the repolarizing IS become the sources. When the ap is propagated into the dendrites the electrode over the soma records positivity. This late positivity can be long lasting, because of the large membrane area which has to be repolarized after the spike has peaked.

Giant Extracellular Spikes

These spikes have a characteristically high amplitude (up to 25 mV), a long duration and are biphasic (p-n) spikes which differentiates them from the smaller, negative going spikes of the most frequently recorded extracellular spikes (39) (Figs. 1.10 and 1.11). They can be differentiated from injury spikes because they are long lasting. Injury spikes have some of the same characteristics such as a high amplitude, diphasicness (p-n) but are short lived (less than half an hour) and regular. The giant spikes follow closely the first derivative of the intracellular spike and their recording may be regarded as a poor intracellular recording rather than as an extracellular recording. Evidence for this is illustrated when the recording electrode is moved a few microns resulting in a dramatic change in amplitude and wave pattern to the more typical extracellularly recorded spike following the second derivative of the intracellular potential. This indicates that in the case of giant spikes the electrode is pushing against the membrane. It has been suggested that the pressure of the tip inactivates the membrane (12) and passive membrane current predominates. Llinás in reference (18) points out, however, that the dimpling of the membrane by the electrode could make the microelectrode capacity coupled to the inside of the cell and the spike is mainly due to capacitative current and very little ohmic current.

When such spikes can be held during an experiment with freely moving animals they offer an excellent signal to noise ratio and maximize the probability that the spikes are recorded from a single cell.

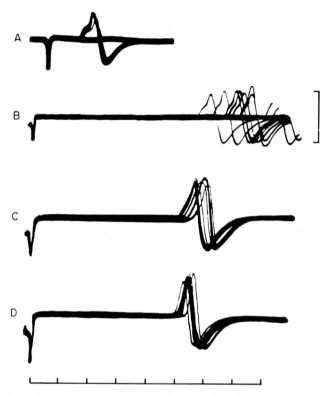

Figure 1.11. Example of a *giant spike* recorded by micropipette on the surface of a mitral cell in the olfactory bulb. A, the response to antidromic stimulation via the lateral olfactory tract. In B-D, responses to orthodromic stimulation by shocks to the olfactory nerve. The wave is positive-negative, about 25 mV peak to peak. Time in msec. From Shepherd (44). (Reproduced by permission of the author and publisher.)

Caveat Emptor

Although some of the principles of extracellular potential analysis have been outlined, it needs no emphasizing that the brain is so complex that ambiguous answers can and may be given to our relatively simple questions. For example, if an electrode is advanced into a neuroanatomically unknown region and a negative field is recorded in the spontaneous activity, what does this mean? It could mean that the tip is in the vicinity of a sink and indicates an ap, it could also mean that there is an EPSP generated by local synapses, or there is an IPSP at a distance, or that a quite unrelated field is generated in a remote region but is based on enough powerful current density to be picked up by the recording electrode. By understanding the underlying neuroanatomy a more definitive answer will be gained. Marking the site of extracellular recording is difficult because it involves some damage to the cell from which it was recorded. The most successful methods are suitable only for intracellular micropipettes where a dye, such as Procion yellow (28), can be injected into the cell.

TECHNIQUES OF RECORDING IN UNANESTHETIZED ANIMALS

The major problems posed by chronic unit recording include (a) the choice of an appropriate method of electrode implantation, (b) eliminating cardiovascular and respiratory movements on exposed brain and (c) minimizing movement artifact due to the movements of the animal.

a. Methods of electrode implantation

There are presently three types of techniques for recording from chronically prepared animals. The electrode is fixed in place, or the electrode is attached to a moveable micromanipulator or a multiple assembly of electrodes is implanted.

The method of Olds (34, 35) employs fixed electrodes. The electrodes used were first introduced by Strumwasser (45) for his studies of long term recording in hibernating squirrels. The electrodes are made of insulated steel or nichrome wire about 62 μ in diameter—a dimension so large compared to other commonly used microelectrodes that they might be called *macro-microelectrodes*. The advantage of these electrodes is that they require virtually no preparation—one can simply snip off the required length from a role of wire and the uninsulated cross sectional surface becomes the recording tip.

These macro-microelectrodes are sturdy enough for implantation without support of a guide sheath. The impedance values are of the order of 100 Kohm (of 100 Hz). This may increase, however, if the wire is crimped during snipping, because there is less surface area present.

It is widely assumed that in order to resolve unitary action potentials an electrode must have a tip diameter of 20 μ or less and the smaller the tip the greater the resolution. In view of the fact that good signal to noise ratios can be achieved in recording with the macro-microelectrodes (36, 40) it seems possible that they are biased towards recording from large cells. In a population of small cells these electrodes behave as a multiple unit activity detector where a smaller tip would differentiate the cellular activity. Since the current density of the membrane, *i.e.*, amps/cm², is measured, then the larger the surface the more likely there is to be a greater current density in populations of large cell surfaces. At small diameters, steel is not robust enough for recording which led to the introduction by Hubel (19) of the etched tungsten electrodes. The tips of such electrodes may be as small as 5 to 0.5 μ with an impedance of 75 Mohm (at 100 Hz) or 0.5 to 5 Mohm (at 5 to 10 Hz) and measurement during spike recording are reported as 2.5 to 10 Mohm. Tungsten electrodes have a shaft diameter of 125 μ and the tip is cone shaped with insulation coating to within 15-25 μ of the tip. The metal tissue surface area is difficult to determine because of the angle of taper. It has been noted that for very much smaller surface-to-tissue areas ($< 10 \; \mu^2$), electrodes are unstable enough to give spikes in dead animals (2).

Fixed microelectrodes are useful on small animal brains where there is not sufficient skull space to mount micromanipulators. The method permits several electrodes to be implanted for simultaneous recording. In Olds' technique the electrodes are implanted to the appropriate site in the brain stereotaxically and where a spike is recorded within that site the electrode is fixed in place and mounted to a ten contact electrode holder on the cranium. The disadvantage of this method is that the spike activity may not always be retained after surgery, although in practice a skilled investigator can regularly *fix* on several lasting units.

The first microelectrode manipulators began to appear in reports in the late 1950's (20, 25, 26, 43). A mechanical thread drive micro-manipulator was used by Ricci et al. (43) during a study of conditioning in monkeys. The rigidly implanted peg used by Ricci et al. was adapted by Hubel (20) in the design of an hydraulically driven manipulator, first used in unanesthetized, unrestrained cats. The tungsten wires described earlier were held in the cylinder part of the apparatus and driven when the piston part was moved. A nylon peg was screwed into a threaded hole in the skull. An adapter connected the cylinder to this peg, but by using an eccentric or concentric ring in the adapter the electrode could be guided to enter different parts of the brain within a 2 mm radius.

Evarts (9, 10) has modified this technique with great success. He introduced a stainless steel cylinder which is screwed into the skull thereby making a nylon peg redundant. His *tilted base* implant cylinder gave a greater degree of stereotaxic accuracy. His system also allows guide change to new brain areas for subsequent penetrations. On a large animal more than one cylinder can be implanted giving the dual advantages of simultaneous recording from different parts of the brain and manipulability with a movable microelectrode. In this book the technique is used by Fetz and Thach for studies of motor movement to which it is most appropriately applied. The use of a movable electrode has the huge advantage of permitting many cells to be recorded in one subject. One can look at a cell's response during a given movement and then go to another cell to test its response to the same behavioral movement. In conditioning experiments, however, the fixed electrode approach has an advantage because the conditioning procedure affects the state of the whole brain and provided the same cell is recorded, its response may be determined throughout the trials of the conditioning procedures. This type of information is unique. With a movable electrode it is possible to record a large sample of cells during the different phases of conditioning but one can only arrive at a statistical picture of the activity during the procedure, one cannot hope to view the same cells throughout the multiple probings. It remains, of course, to be seen whether the larger sample approach versus the more individual approach gives the same answers.

Other techniques using movable microelectrodes are the multiple assembly implants. Verzeano (50) offers such a system where several microelectrodes are moved downwards together by being connected to a bakelite piston, in a lucite cylinder, which is moved by a screw turn. A longitudinal slit in the wall of the cylinder allowed the microelectrode wires to move down with the piston and yet be connected to a plug so that connecting to the amplifiers did not alter the position of the electrodes. The inside of the assembly was filled with paraffin and the outside was mounted in acrylic cement to the skull. John and Morgades (23), Davis and Tollow (8) and McGinty in this volume also describe multiple assembly procedures for varying numbers of microelectrodes. Maclean (30) and Hayward et al. (15) have introduced a different feature where a perforated plate is mounted over the skull as a platform and electrodes are introduced through the guide and holes in the perforations. This allows several electrodes to be placed stereotaxically and fixed in place or advanced by micro-manipulators.

The technique of Humphrey (21) seems to offer the *best of all worlds*. It is a system which permits multiple microelectrodes (up to five) being implanted close to each other but they can each be independently controlled. Five microdrives are incorporated and set at a slight angle so that as the electrodes are lowered the tips converge into smaller and smaller areas of the brain. The eccentric disc concept, used by Hubel and Evarts is also used here so that successive sets of penetration can be made in different parts of the brain. Because of the size of the assembly, the technique is appropriate for larger experimental animals.

The technique of multiple unit activity recording with large electrodes has been successfully pursued by Buchwald and her method of recording in a way that yields EEG, multiple unit activity and simple unit activity recordings is presented in this volume.

b. Brain movements

Exposed brain may move as much as 200 μ or more with each pulse and respiratory cycle. For chronic recording it is therefore necessary to minimize the amount of brain tissue exposed to the atmosphere. Generally this is achieved by making holes in the dura small enough to be filled by the microelectrode and sealing the electrode to the skull, or where a guide shaft is used, sealing any gaps between the electrode and microdrive system by tight fitting instrumentation threading the bone, and bone wax.

c. Movement artifact

The problem with movement artifact is that unwanted spikes may be picked up by the amplifiers and included in the recordings. It is, therefore, important that the distance between the electrodes and the preamplifiers be short and/or well shielded, and that the connections be tight. In Wall's technique (51) for recording chronically from the spinal cord of rats, it was found to be necessary to have a field effect transistor and transistor amplifier mounted directly on the manipulator. In Olds' technique, the electrode holder affixed to the skull is connected to preamplifiers by a short low noise cable for each electrode. In addition, a movement detecting device is used which consists of a high noise cable attached loosely to the head holder jack. Any movement is picked up by the cable, amplified and digitized at the same time as the unitary spikes are amplified and digitized. Thus if movement is present it is revealed in the analysis of the spike data, which serves as a criterion for accepting or rejecting the data and distinguishing movement related unit activity.

In addition the animal's head can be restrained, for example, by mounting brackets on the skull which can be used to bolt the animal's head rigidly in place during experimentation. Adaptation to this restraint is necessary to avoid isometric effects. Giving low doses of tranquilizers or sedatives would seem to defeat the purpose of chronic recording but has been used where the drug is not critical to the experiment. New methods of avoiding movement artifact are possibly to be found in the telemetry systems such as McElligott described in this book. Gualtierotti and Bailey's (14) novel method uses the concept of floating electrode holder by attaching the electrode to an air filled capsule which has the same density as the surrounding tissue and is suspended in agar. This method has been used on frogs to study their vestibular activity during a flight into space and recordings were successfully made for more than twelve hours (F. Bracchi, personal communication).

In recording extracellularly, the electrodes may be AC coupled to the amplifying system rather than directly coupled as is the case for intracellular recordings. The signal can be passed through an amplifier that will filter out slow waves below 300 H$_z$ and high frequencies above 10,000 H$_z$. The choice of electrodes is somewhat arbitrary given a reasonably robust, low impedance probe with a tip diameter of something less than 70 μ. Since extracellular potentials are recorded in a volume conductor they may be recorded at some distance from their sites of generation. Large tip electrodes have the disadvantage of recording a lot of the activity in an active area, requiring single units to be discriminated out by wave form detectors. Small tip electrodes in such an active pool of generators tend to be more exclusive in recording. Both types of electrodes record the biggest potentials, which are usually from active cells near the recording surface. The potentials could be, however, produced by the activity of a cell; or cells, some distance from the electrode, or, theoretically, by two or more cells positioned equidistant from the electrode tip and firing synchronously, so that the potential recorded is the summated activity of this group. Thus there is always some uncertainty about the true uniqueness of the source of recording unless the electrode is clearly on the surface of a neuron as is the case when a *giant spike* is recorded. This can be made by either large or small tipped electrodes (Fig. 1.12). Apart from the giant spikes, most spikes are predominantly negative, and initial positivity is indicative of injury potential. Injury spikes are commonly seen as having a rapid rate of firing, which diminishes until a few seconds later when there is no more electrical response. In some cases, however, the initial activation subsides to a lower, more stable rate indicating that no fatal damage has been done, but there is no way of knowing whether the activity is normal or abnormal.

Nevertheless, chronic unit recording gives a method of reporting the news from discrete populations of participating cells in the brain during behavioral events. The message may need editing and translating but as in all experiments the answer we get depends on the way we phrase the question. For chronic unit

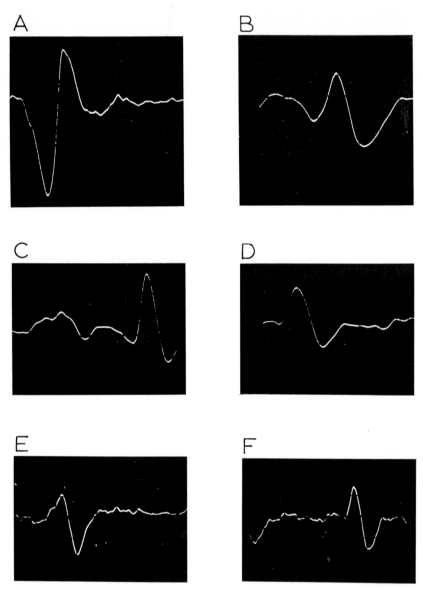

Figure 1.12. Unitary spikes recorded with 62 μ tip diameter nichrome wire extracellular microelectrodes, from the spontaneous activity of neurons in the rat brain. In each photograph the spike is shown with negativity up and no resting potential is recorded. A. *Giant extracellular spike* with high amplitude (6 μV peak-to-peak) initially positive of 1.7

recording, there are sufficiently reliable techniques to give the answers, the onus is on designing the behavior that can appropriately pose the question.

REFERENCES

1. Aghajanian, G. K., W. E. Foote, and M. H. Sheard. Lysergic acid diethylamide: Sensitive neuronal units in the midbrain raphe. *Science,* 161:706-708, 1968.
2. Amassian, V. Evoked single cortical unit activity in the somatic sensory areas. *Electroenceph. Clin. Neurophysiol.,* 5:415-438, 1953.
3. Best, P. J. An on-line computer technique for display and analysis of single cell activity. In: *Brain Unit Activity During Behavior.* M. I. Phillips (Ed.). Thomas, Springfield, Ill. 67-75, 1973.
4. Buchwald, J. S. and F. Grover. Amplitudes of background fast activity characteristic of specific brain sites. *J. Neurophys.,* 33:148-159, 1970.
5. Calvin, W. H. and D. Hellerstein. Dendritic spikes vs. cable properties. *Science,* 163:96-97, 1969.
6. Clark, J. and R. Plonsey. A mathematical evaluation of the core conductor model. *Biophys. J.,* 6:95-112, 1966.
7. Coombs, J. S., D. R. Curtis, and J. C. Eccles. The interpretation of spike potential of motoneurones. *J. Physiol.,* 139:198-231, 1957.
8. Davis, R. and A. S. Tollow. Adjustable stimulating and recording electrodes in brain of the unrestrained animal. A study of red nucleus. *Electroenceph. Clin. Neurophysiol.,* 21:196-200, 1966.
9. Evarts, E. V. Methods for recording activity of individual neurons in moving animals. In: *Methods in Medical Research.* R. F. Rushmer (Ed.). Year Book Medical Publishers, Chicago, Ill., 241-250, 1966.
10. Evarts, E. V. A technique for recording activity of subcortical neurons in moving animals. *Electroenceph. Clin. Neurophysiol.,* 24:83-86, 1968.

---

msec. duration recorded in the reticular formation. B. A triphasic spike (p-n-p) of lower amplitude (200 μV) and shorter duration (1.3 msec.) recorded in the reticular formation, presumably from a soma in an open field pool of neurons. C. and D. Shorter duration spikes (0.68 msec and 0.65 msec respectively) with a p-n-p wave pattern and fast rising negativity, suggesting that the possibility of their being recorded from axons cannot be ruled out. Amplitude of C. is 100 μV and D. 120 μV. Both recorded in the hypothalamus. E. Spike recorded from the oculomotor nucleus showing slow rise in negativity with a break suggestive of a recording from a soma-dendritic complex in a closed-field neuron pool. Amplitude 180 μV, duration 1.8 msec. F. Biphasic spike (n-p) recorded from the preoptic nucleus, amplitude 200 μV, duration 1.1 msec.

11. Frank, K. and H. G. F. Fuortes. Potentials recorded from the spinal cord with microelectrodes. *J. Physiol.*, 130:625-654, 1955.

12. Freygang, W. H. and K. Frank. Extracellular potentials from single spinal motoneurons. *J. Gen. Physiol.*, 42:749-760, 1959.

13. Grover, F. S. and J. S. Buchwald. Correlation of cell size with amplitude of background fast activity in specific brain nuclei. *J. Neurophys.*, 33:160-171, 1970.

14. Gualtierotti, T. and P. Bailey. A neutral bouyancy microelectrode for prolonged recording from single nerve units. *Electroenceph. Clin. Neurophysiol.*, 25:77-81, 1968.

15. Hayward, J. N., M. D. Fairchild, D. G. Stuart, and J. A. Deemer. A stereotaxic platform for microelectrode studies in chronic animals. *Electroenceph. Clin. Neurophysiol.*, 16:522-524, 1964.

16. Hild, W. and I. Tasaki. Morphological and physiological properties of neurons and glial cells in tissue culture. *J. Neurophysiol.*, 25: 277-304, 1962.

17. Hodgkin, A. L. and A. F. Huxley. A quantitative description of membrane current and its application to conduction and excitation in nerve. *J. Physiol.*, 117:500-544, 1952.

18. Hubbard, J. I., R. Llinás, and D. M. J. Quastel. *Electrophysiological Analysis of Synaptic Transmission.* E. Arnold (publishers) Ltd., London, p. 283, 1969.

19. Hubel, D. H. Tungsten microelectrode for recording from single units. *Science*, 125:549-550, 1957.

20. Hubel, D. H. Single unit activity in striate cortex of unrestrained cats. *J. Physiol.*, 147:549-555, 1957.

21. Humphrey, D. R. A chronically implantable multiple microelectrode system with independent control of electrode positions. *Electroenceph. Clin. Neurophysiol.*, 29:616-620, 1970.

22. Jackson, J. D. *Classical Electrodynamics.* John Wiley, New York, 1962.

23. John, E. R. and P. P. Morgades. A technique for the chronic implantation of multiple movable micro-electrodes. *Electroenceph. Clin. Neurophysiol.*, 27:205-208, 1969.

24. Kandel, E. R., W. A. Spencer, and F. J. Brinley. Electrophysiology of hippocampal neurons. I. Sequential invasion and synaptic organization. *J. Neurophysiol.*, 24:225-242, 1961.

25. Katsuki, J., K. Murata, N. Suga, and T. Takenaka. Electrical activity of cortical auditory neurons of unanesthetized and unrestrained cat. *Proc. Jap. Acad.*, 35:571-574, 1959.

26. Kogan, A. B. A method of electrode implantation in unrestrained animals. *Electroenceph. Clin. Neurophysiol.*, 11:812-813, 1959.

27. Llinás, R., C. Nicholson, J. A. Freeman, and D. E. Hillman. Dendritic spikes and their inhibition in alligator Purkinje cells. *Science*, 160: 1132-1135, 1968.

28. Llinás, R. and C. Nicholson. Electrophysiological properties of dendrites and somata in alligator Purkinje cells. *J. Neurophysiol.*, 34: 532-549, 1971.
29. Lorente de Nó, R. A study of nerve physiology. *Studies from the Rockefeller Institute*, Vol. 132, Chap. 16, 1947.
30. MacLean, P. D. A chronically fixed sterotaxic device for intracerebral exploration with macro- and micro-electrodes. *Electroenceph. Clin. Neurophysiol.*, 22:180-182, 1967.
31. Nelson, P. G. and K. Frank. Extracellular potential fields of single spinal motoneurons. *J. Neurophysiol.*, 27:913-927, 1964.
32. Nicholson, J. C. Theoretical analysis of field potentials in anisotropic ensembles of neuronal elements. *I.E.E.E. Trans. Biomed. Eng.* (in press).
33. Nicholson, C. and R. Llinás. Potentials in the alligator cerebellum and theory of their relationship to Purkinje cell dendritic spikes. *J. Neurophysiol.*, 34:509-531, 1971.
34. Olds, J. The limbic system and behavioral reinforcement. In: *Progress in Brain Research* (Structure and function of the limbic system). W. R. Adey and T. Tokizane (Eds.). Vol. 27. Amsterdam, Elsevier, 1967.
35. Olds, J. Operant conditioning of single unit responses. Excerpta Medica International Congress Series No. 87. *Proceedings of XIII International Congress of Physiological Sciences*, Tokyo, 372-380, 1965.
36. Olds, J., J. Disterhof, M. Segal, C. L. Kornblith, and R. Hirsh. Learning centers of rat brain mapped by measuring latencies of conditioned unit responses. *J. Neurophysiol.*, 35:202-219, 1972.
37. Oomura, Y., H. Ooyama, F. Naka, and T. Yamamoto. Microelectrode positioners for chronic animals. *Physiol. Behav.*, 2:89-91, 1967.
38. Phillips, C. G. Intracellular records of Betz cells in the cat. *Quart. J. Exper. Physiol.*, 41:58-69, 1956.
39. Phillips, C. G. Actions of antidromic pyramidal volleys on single Betz cells in the cat. *Quart. J. Exper. Physiol.*, 44:1-25, 1959.
40. Phillips, M. I. and J. Olds. Unit activity: motivation-dependent responses from midbrain neurons. *Science*, 165:1269-1271, 1969.
41. Rall, W. Electrophysiology of a dendritic model. *Biophys. J.*, 2:145, 1962.
42. Rall, W. and G. M. Shepherd. Theoretical reconstruction of field potentials and dendrodendritic synaptic interaction in olfactory bulb. *J. Neurophysiol.*, 31:884-915, 1968.
43. Ricci, G., B. Doane, and H. H. Jasper. Microelectrode studies of conditioning technique and preliminary results. *1st Congress Int. Sci. Neurol. Réunions plénières*, 401-415, 1957.

44. Shepherd, G. M. Responses of mitral cells to olfactory nerve volleys in the rabbit. *J. Physiol.*, 168:89-100, 1963.

45. Strumwasser, F. Long term recording from single neurons in brain of unrestrained mammals. *Science*, 127:468-470, 1958.

46. Svaetichin, Gunnar. Analysis of action potentials from single spinal ganglion cells. *Acta Physiologica Scandinavia*, Supplements 83-88: 23, 1956.

47. Tasaki, I., E. H. Polley, and F. Orrego. Action potentials from individual elements in cat geniculate and striate cortex. *J. of Neurophysiol.*, 17:454-474, 1954.

48. Thach, W. T. Natural functions of cerebellar circuits. In: *Brain Unit Activity During Behavior*. M. I. Phillips (Ed.). Thomas, Springfield, Ill. 179-196, 1973.

49. Terzuolo, C. A. and T. Araki. An analysis of intra- versus extra-cellular potential changes associated with activity of single spinal motoneurones. *Am. N.Y. Acad.*, 94:547-558, 1961.

50. Verzeano, M. Evoked responses and network dynamics. In: *The Neural Control of Behavior*. Whalen et al. (Eds.). Academic Press, New York, 27-53, 1970.

51. Wall, P. D., J. Freeman, and D. Major. Dorsal horn cells in spinal and freely moving rats. *Exp. Neurol.*, 19:519-529, 1967.

52. Zucker, R. S. Field potentials generated by dendritic spikes and synaptic potentials. *Science*, 165:409-413, 1969.

Chapter II

CHRONIC RECORDING AND QUANTIFICATION OF SUBCORTICAL SINGLE AND MULTIPLE UNITS

KENNETH A. BROWN, DAVID S. WEBER, and
JENNIFER S. BUCHWALD

THE INCREASING VARIETY of recording techniques available for investigating brain function has become a problem *per se* for the experimenter. Different techniques provide different kinds of information about the brain, and while each technique has certain advantages, each also has corresponding disadvantages. Multiple unit activity (MUA), for example, provides a useful summary of activity levels at the recording site, but individual unit firing patterns are lost. Thus, behaviorally divergent cells within a recorded population may not be observed. Single cell recording, on the other hand, does reveal firing patterns, but practical considerations limit the number of units sampled in a given region, and it may be difficult to arrive at general conclusions from experiments based on relatively small, perhaps biased, samples. Similarly, although the EEG has been the most commonly applied measure of subcortical brain activity, it is not necessarily always the most appropriate, since it is thought to be primarily a measure of graded synaptic events or after potentials (1, 10, 11, 13, 17, 23) rather than a summary of propagated action potential discharge at the recording site. In some cases, levels of MUA and the EEG show parallel variation (3, 20, 28), but other studies have indicated that subcortical MUA is more sensitive to certain experimental variables than is the EEG and may show changes without any apparent alterations in the concurrent slow wave activity (2, 6, 7). The experimenter's choice of weapons, though influenced by many factors, is eventually reduced to that which provides the most appropriate, meaningful data with the smallest possible investment of time. We feel that an approach which combines the advantages of several techniques, allowing maximum flexibility with a variety of simultaneous measures of brain activity, is of great value. This paper describes a method for recording subcortical EEG, MUA, and single unit activity concurrently in chronic subjects. A convenient and relatively inexpensive device for preliminary analysis of either MUA or single unit data is also described.

Electrode Construction and Implantation

Recording from subcortical cell *populations* in chronic preparations is relatively simple, and MUA and the EEG have been used as measures of regional brain activity levels for many years. In contrast, *single-unit* recording from deep structures in chronic subjects has been technically difficult until recently. Recordings of single cells have been maintained for relatively short durations in chronic subjects with stereotaxically implanted, rigid microelectrodes (e.g. 13, 14, 20), but a major problem with this technique is that pulsations of the brain cause individual cells to move in relation to a rigid microelectrode, so that the activity of a given cell can rarely be recorded over an extended period of time. Since electrode rigidity is essential for accurate subcortical stereotaxic implantation, single unit studies have largely been restricted to cortical or easily accessible brain regions in acute animals, where brain movement can be mechanically controlled and delicate electrodes can be used. To overcome this limitation, in the early fifties flexible microelectrodes made of fine wires were lowered into the brains of acute subjects with tweezers and used for cortical and subsurface recording (4, 5, 27). A loop of the wire above the brain allowed the microelectrode tip to *float,* or move with the brain, and thus to maintain its position relative to a particular cell. Later, flexible microelectrodes made from larger diameter wires were implanted by hand for extended subcortical recordings in chronic subjects (19, 22). O'Keefe and Bouma (18), modifying these and other techniques, were able to implant small diameter, flexible microelectrodes subcortically with stereotaxic control. Thus, individual cells in deep structures could be recorded for several hours or days at specific sites in chronic preparations while a number of experimental procedures were performed. Variations of this method are now used in several laboratories (e.g. 16), and we have developed modifications which allow simultaneous recording of EEG, MUA, and single unit activity from the same site, as will be described.

Rigidity for stereotaxic implantation is provided by a standard EEG-MUA macroelectrode made of an insulated insect pin (monopolar electrode), stainless steel tubing and core wire (concentric electrode), or a pair of 34 gauge insulated stainless steel wires twisted together (bipolar electrode). The flexible microelectrodes, made of insulated, stainless steel 25 μ or 62.5 μ wires (Wilbur B. Driver Co., *Tophet-C*), are temporarily fixed to the macroelectrode by dipping them together in melted *Carbowax* polyethylene glycol (M.W. 6000, Union Carbide). When the Carbowax cools and solidifies, the microelectrode wires are bonded to the macroelectrode and are then cut approximately flush

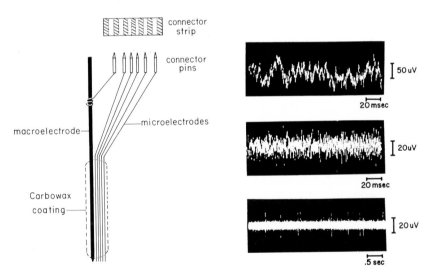

Figure 2.1. Diagram of assembled electrode array with examples of electrical activity recorded from such an array implanted in the amygdala of a cat. The top trace, unfiltered MUA dominated by EEG activity, and the middle trace, MUA with slow components filtered out, were obtained concurrently from the macroelectrode. The bottom trace, single-unit activity at the same site, was recorded from one of the 25 μ microelectrodes in the array.

with the macroelectrode tip. All electrode leads may be soldered or crimped to connector pins (Amphenol #220-P02), which are then inserted into a connector strip (Amphenol #221-1260). The final electrode array is shown in Figure 2.1. Alternatively, the wires may be attached directly to the pins of a prefabricated miniature connector (e.g., Amphenol #222-12N31). Typically, we combine five microelectrodes with a macroelectrode in each array. The impedance of a 25 μ microelectrode is about 200K; that of a 62.5 μ microelectrode is about 80K.

For implantation, an electrode array is fixed in a stereotaxic holder and positioned within the brain by the usual methods. The Carbowax bonding coat which holds the microelectrode wires to the macroelectrode will dissolve within a thirty second to five minute period, depending upon the number of bonding coats applied to the array. Time limits for electrode positioning within the brain can be estimated by pretesting the waxed arrays in saline warmed to body temperature. The electrodes and connectors are fastened to the skull with dental cement. As the Carbowax dissolves, the microelectrode wires separate from the macroelectrode and are free to *float* in the brain, cemented to the macroelectrode only at the skull surface.

We have held single units for one to two weeks with both microelectrode sizes, though three or four days is more typical. It is usual to obtain units from only one or two of the microelectrodes in a given array, the others showing either no activity or multiple unit activity from which single cells may be difficult to discriminate. An amplitude discriminator or signal *window,* however, often permits extraction of a single unit in the latter case. When a unit is lost from a microelectrode, other units may appear on other leads from the same array or another unit may be obtained from the same lead after a few days. It is quite rare to find no activity from any of the electrodes in an array; when no isolated units appear, multiple unit records can be obtained from either the microelectrodes or the macroelectrode.

An important aspect of the technique described here is that the experimenter does not manipulate the position of the microelectrode wires after implantation, and this feature may be advantageous in certain experimental situations. The usual procedure of lowering a microelectrode and isolating an active cell before an experiment is initiated inevitably biases the sample of units taken from a population. Thus, the lower the average spontaneous firing rate of a cell population, the more uncharacteristic is the sample obtained by such a procedure. Individual cell firing rates can be very low in some brain regions, notably in the hypothala-

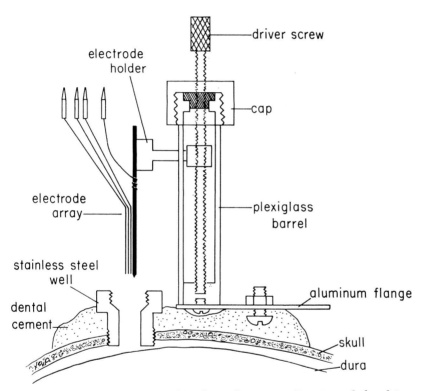

Figure 2.2. Diagram of moveable electrode carrier. Rotation of the driver bolt moves the threaded portion of the electrode holder vertically inside the plexiglass barrel of the carrier. The arm of the electrode holder protrudes through a vertical slot extending to the top of the carrier barrel, which permits quick removal and replacement of the driver bolt-holder, electrode assembly. Adjustment of electrode position in a horizontal plane is accomplished either by loosening the nut on the headplug bolt, which frees the slotted aluminum baseplate of the carrier, or by loosening the bolt attaching baseplate to carrier, which permits rotation of the carrier barrel. Between experimental sessions, the skull well is closed with a threaded nylon plug (Mechanical Development Co., #3-0554).

mus (12), and, in our experience, the amygdala. Implanted, flexible microelectrodes, on the other hand, provide a more impartial selection of units. A relatively inactive cell is as likely to be isolated as a more spontaneously active cell; furthermore, phasic responses of such *silent* cells are perhaps more likely to be recorded, since each electrode may be tested repeatedly for unit activity during various experimental procedures.

In cases where a large sample of units is required from the same animal, it is possible to modify the flexible microelectrode technique for use with a movable electrode carrier. Several investigators have used variations of such a method with rigid electrodes (14, 21, 24, 25). Our own version consists of bolting a simple electrode holder to a screw fixed in the subject's headplug (Fig. 2.2). The subject is restrained or paralyzed and respired (9), and the electrode array is positioned in the holder and lowered through a stainless steel well (Mechanical Developments Co., #3-0553) implanted in the skull over the target area. Penetration depth is estimated from the dura or brain surface. When a cell is isolated, experimental procedures are carried out and then a 50 μA, ten second current is passed through the microelectrode to facilitate later histological identification of the recording site, utilizing the Prussian blue reaction. The array may then be moved and the experimental process repeated. The 62.5 μ wires are preferred for this procedure because of their greater rigidity; they can be shifted within the brain without damage even after the Carbowax coating has dissolved. The procedure may be easily refined to provide more stereotaxic accuracy, if desired, and can be carried out day after day in a single subject.

Analytical Techniques

Both single and multiple unit data present the experimenter with problems of quantification and analysis. The data may eventually be handled in several ways, but we feel it advisable in all cases to tape the units directly. If the activity is fed into preliminary circuits and only a pulse output derivative is taped, it may subsequently be difficult to discriminate misleading artifacts in the record.

A Schmidt trigger, or amplitude discriminator, provides a

means for selecting a signal amplitude above which all taped units are analyzed. Thus, each unit signal above a selected voltage level is converted into a standard pulse regardless of its initial size or shape. Amplitude discrimination levels can easily be calibrated by applying standard signals of known amplitudes to the recording amplifier input and lowering the Schmidt trigger reference voltage level until an output from the Schmidt trigger is first observed. The converted data may then be fed to analyzing circuits.

In the case of MUA, analysis of converted potentials by frequency integration (7) as opposed to a simple resistor capacitor (R-C) integration of the data (26) allows quantitative, day to day comparisons of activity levels at a recording site. Such quan-

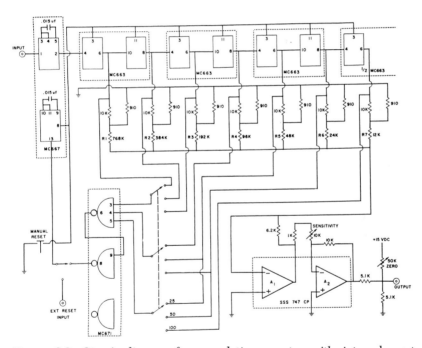

Figure 2.3. Circuit diagram for cumulative counter with internal reset gates wired for twenty-five, fifty, and one hundred counts. The integrated circuits included are: four Motorola type MC 663 dual J-K flip-flop, one Motorola type MC 667 dual monostable multi-vibrator, one Motorola type MC 671 triple three input and gate, and one Precision Monolithics type SSS747P dual operational amplifier. The power supply requirements (not shown) are ± 15 VDC @ 25 ma and + 15 VDC @ 100 ma.

tification is expedited by gating the integrator and displaying its output on a digital voltmeter, thus producing a decimal number that is related to the frequency of discharge of the discriminated unit activity during each gated period.

We have recently devised another method which is especially convenient for on-line or preliminary analysis of single unit data, as well as MUA, using a cumulative counting circuit in place of either simple R-C integration or frequency integration. This circuit requires a pulse at the input; therefore the unit activity must first be amplitude-discriminated as previously described. The discriminated pulse is fed, via a monostable multivibrator, into a series of flip flops wired in toggle configuration with a binary output (Fig. 2.3). The summing resistors, R1-R7, in conjunction with amplifier A1, convert the binary count into an analog or stepping pattern with the slope indicating the rate of unit discharge, *i.e.*, the steeper the slope, the higher the frequency. The output of this circuit will respond immediately to any change at the input, producing a very accurate measure of discharge frequency.

The circuit provides two modes for resetting, the first of which is an automatic reset after a preselected number of counts. Figure 2.3 shows wiring at the reset gate inputs for twenty-five, fifty, or one hundred counts, with Figure 2.4a showing an example of the output when reset occurs at twenty-five counts. This output constitutes a cumulative record of neural activity, and any preselected number of counts can easily be wired into the reset gate. Either the slope or the reset frequency of the output provides a rapid visual summary of the data, which can easily be quantified. The second mode for resetting utilizes an external reset input; a pulse at this input will cause immediate reset to zero. By using the external reset mode, one can synchronize the counter to an external pulse source generated by some experimental condition. Also, the external reset provides a means for sampling over any practical period of time, either continuously or at intervals imposed by a pulse generator. An obvious application of this option is to obtain a frequency *histogram* of unit activity by causing the counter to reset at a fixed interval (Fig. 2.4b). Furthermore, if the unit activity to be analyzed is of relatively low ongoing fre-

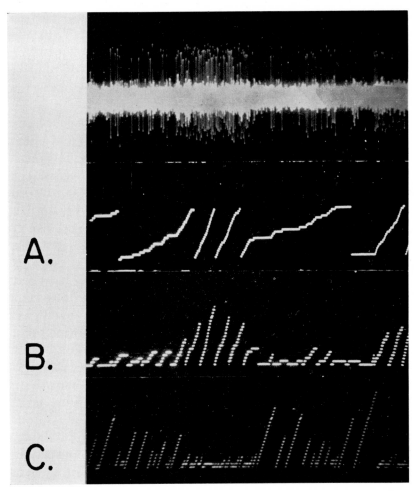

Figure 2.4. Cumulative counting circuit outputs derived from a common MUA input (top trace). The MUA was recorded from the ventral hippocampus of a paralyzed cat with implanted 62.5 μ wire electrodes. A: cumulative record with automatic reset at twenty-five counts. B: frequency histogram obtained by externally resetting counter at two hundred msec intervals. C: inter-spike interval histogram obtained by applying a constant-frequency input to the counter with the discriminated units used to reset the counter externally.

quency, the cumulative counting circuit can also be used to display the interspike interval rather than spike frequency. This can be accomplished by using the discriminated unit activity to reset the counter externally while applying a constant frequency from a pulse generator to the counter input (Fig. 2.4c).

SUMMARY

By combining EEG, MUA and single unit recording from the same electrode array in chronic subjects, it is possible to obtain simultaneously both a summary of activity levels and a view of individual unit firing patterns at a given site. This variety of measures not only extends the range of activity observed at a recording site but also provides useful information about the relations between different measures of brain activity and the relative effects of experimental variables upon them. Such flexibility may be particularly important to an experimental program directed to problems in which various measures of brain activity have been taken in the past with differing results. Furthermore, the single unit recording technique described here enables the investigator to observe the activity of individual cells for relatively long periods of time, in some cases over days.

The cumulative counting circuit, used with either single or multiple unit inputs, can provide an immediate, on-line picture of the experimental data and is a convenient screening device prior to more expensive and time consuming analyses. Outputs resembling frequency histograms or inter-spike interval histograms may be obtained from amplitude-discriminated data and can be synchronized to experimental events via an external reset control.

REFERENCES

1. Ajmone-Marsan, C. Electrical activity of the brain: slow wave and neuronal activity. *Israel J. Med. Sci.*, 1, 104-117, 1965.
2. Alcarez, M., C. Guzman-Flores, M. Salas, and C. Beyer. Effect of estrogen on the responsivity of hypothalamic and mesencephalic neurons in the female cat. *Brain Res.*, 15, 439-446, 1969.
3. Balzano, E., and M. Jeannerod. Activite multi-unitaire de structures sous-corticales pendant le cycle veillesommeil chez le chat. *Electroenceph. clin. Neurophysiol.*, 28, 136-145, 1970.
4. Brookhart, J. M., G. Moruzzi, and R. S. Snider. Spike discharges of

single units in the cerebellar cortex. *J. Neurophysiol.*, 13, 465-486, 1950.

5. Brookhart, J. M., G. Moruzzi, and R. S. Snider. Origin of cerebellar waves. *J. Neurophysiol.*, 14, 181-190, 1951.
6. Brown, K. A., and R. Melzack. Effects of glucose on multi-unit activity in the hypothalamus. *Exp. Neurol.*, 24, 363-373, 1969.
7. Buchwald, J. S., E. S. Halas, and S. Schramm. Comparison of multiple unit and electroencephalogram activity recorded from the same brain sites during behavioral conditioning. *Nature*, 205, 1012-1014, 1965.
8. Buchwald, J. S., D. S. Weber, S. B. Holstein, F. S. Grover, and J. A. Schwafel. Quantified unit background activity in the waking cat during paralysis, anesthesia, and cochlear destruction. *Brain Res.*, 15, 465-482, 1969.
9. Buchwald, J. S., S. B. Holstein, and D. S. Weber. Techniques, Interpretation and Application of Multiple Unit Recording. In *Methods in Physiological Psychology Vol. I. Recordings of Bioelectric Activity*, R. F. Thompson and M. M. Patterson, Eds., Academic Press, New York. (In press)
10. Caspers, H. Über die Beziehungen zwischen Dendritenpotential und Gleichspannung an der Hirnrinde. *Pflügers Arch. ges. Physiol.*, 269, 157-181, 1959.
11. Clare, M. H., and G. H. Bishop. Potential wave mechanisms in cat cortex. *Electroenceph. clin. Neurophysiol.*, 8, 583-602, 1959.
12. Cross, B. A., and I. A. Silver. Electrophysiological studies on the hypothalamus. *Brit. med. Bull.*, 22, 254-260, 1966.
13. Fromm, G. N., and H. W. Bond. Slow changes in the electrocorticogram and the activity of cortical neurons. *Electroenceph. clin. Neurophysiol.*, 17, 520-523, 1964.
14. Fuster, J. M., and A. A. Uyeda. Reactivity of limbic neurons of the monkey to appetitive and aversive signals. *Electroenceph. clin. Neurophysiol.*, 30, 281-293, 1971.
15. Hubel, D. H. Cortical unit responses to visual stimuli in nonanesthetized cats. *Am. J. Ophthal.*, 46, 110-121, 1958.
16. Jacobs, B. L., R. M. Harper, and D. J. McGinty. Neuronal coding of motivational level during sleep. *Physiol. Behav.*, 5, 1139-1143, 1970.
17. Motokizawa, F., and B. Fujimori. Fast activities and DC potential changes of the cerebral cortex during EEG arousal response. *Electroenceph. clin. Neurophysiol.*, 17, 630-637, 1964.
18. O'Keefe, J., and H. Bouma. Complex sensory properties of certain amygdala units in the freely moving cat. *Exp. Neurol.*, 23, 384-398, 1969.
19. Olds, J. Operant conditioning of single unit responses. *Proc. XXIII Intern. Congr. Physiol. Union*, 4, 372-380, 1965.

20. Podvoll, E. G., and S. J. Goodman. Average neural electrical activity and arousal. *Science,* 155, 223-225, 1967.

21. Sawa, M., and J. Delgado. Amygdala unitary activity in the unrestrained cat. *Electroenceph. clin. Neurophysiol.,* 15, 637-650, 1963.

22. Strumwasser, F. Long term recording from single neurons in brain of unrestrained mammals. *Science,* 127, 469-470, 1958.

23. Verzeano, M., and I. Calma. Unit activity in spindle bursts. *J. Neurophysiol.,* 17, 417-428, 1954.

24. Vinogradova, O. S. Dynamic classification of the reactions of hippocampal neurons to sensory stimuli. *Fed. Proc. Trans. Supp.,* 25, T397-T403, 1966.

25. Vinogradova, O. S. Registration of information and the limbic system. In *Short-term Changes in Neural Activity and Behaviors.* G. Horn and R. A. Hinde (Eds.) Cambridge Univ. Press, N.Y., 1970, pp. 95-140.

26. Weber, D., and J. S. Buchwald. A technique for recording and integrating multiple unit activity simultaneously with the EEG in chronic animals. *Electroenceph. clin. Neurophysiol.,* 19, 190-192, 1965.

27. Whitlock, D. G., A. Arduini, and G. Moruzzi. Microelectrode analysis of pyramidal system during transition from sleep to wakefulness. *J. Neurophysiol.,* 16, 414-429, 1953.

28. Winters, W. D., K. Mori, C. E. Spencer, and R. T. Kado. Correlation of reticular and cochlear multiple unit activity with auditory evoked responses during wakefulness and sleep. I. *Electroenceph. clin. Neurophysiol.,* 23, 539-545, 1967.

Chapter III

A TELEMETRY SYSTEM FOR THE TRANSMISSION OF SINGLE AND MULTIPLE CHANNEL DATA FROM INDIVIDUAL NEURONS IN THE BRAIN

JAMES G. McELLIGOTT

TELEMETRY, BROADLY DEFINED, consists of the transmission of information from a distance. There are myriad ways of accomplishing this. However, common and everyday usage of the term implies that the transmission is carried out by means of electromagnetic radiation. Thus, the term radiotelemetry is a more precise one. In the field of biotelemetry, data or information about an organism is transmitted. This includes all the electrical signals that emanate from the body, such as the electromyogram (EMG), the electrocardiogram (EKG) and the various forms of central nervous system electrical activity. Also, information about bodily pressures, temperature, respiration and pH have been transmitted. Telemetry has been used to record almost all of the parameters that have been measured by more conventional means. In spite of this, biotelemetry, although gaining in popularity, is not widely used. This is probably due to the lack of appropriate commercially available devices and a general lack of familiarity with the techniques involved. At this point it may be

It is a pleasure to thank Dr. W. Ross Adey for his support. I would also like to thank Paul Kaminsky for design and construction of a number of the telemetry units, Rod Zweizig for his many helpful suggestions, Jackie Payne for preparation of the figures, and Moya Flaxman for typing the manuscript.

This work was carried out at Space Biology Laboratory of the Brain Research Institute and the Department of Anatomy at University of California at Los Angeles. Support was obtained from NASA Grant NGR 05-007-195 and United States Air Force Grant F 44620-70-C-0017 to the Space Biology Laboratory.

appropriate to paraphrase statements made by MacKay in his book on biotelemetry (2). In the introductory chapter he states that the use of telemetry methods adds nothing but extra complication and sometimes unreliability. Thus, the uncritical application of telemetry to a study will add little benefit to an experiment and could provide some extra technical difficulties. Nevertheless, there are many situations in which its use makes an otherwise impossible experiment feasible. These methods prove important particularly in those situations where it is desirable to leave the subject in a relatively normal physiological or psychological state by interfering with his normal pattern of activities as little as possible.

In the central nervous system, the use of biotelemetry has gained some acceptance in measuring the electroencephalogram (EEG) from animals and humans. The other biopotential of the brain that is most frequently recorded is the action potential of an individual nerve cell. Until a few years ago, the application of telemetry to aid in recording the neural spike would have added little to the study. In most of these experiments the animal is anesthetized, paralyzed or otherwise physically restricted in a stereotaxic instrument. In part, this immobilization or restriction is necessary for stabilization purposes, since slight movements of the electrode with respect to the cell can cause the spike potential to be lost.

However, in recent years, it has been possible to record neural spikes in unanesthetized and unrestrained animals by means of flexible fine wire electrodes. Many examples are given in other chapters of this book. The activity of a particular neuron can be recorded over extended periods ranging from hours to days in the freely moving animal. In some situations, it is extremely desirable to have the animal free from the encumbrance of connecting wires. Thus, the use of telemetry is most advantageous and sometimes even mandatory.

The particular telemetry units that will be described in this chapter were designed for use in a study involving the relation of cerebellar neuronal firing to coordinated motor behavior in the cat (3). Presumably, the cerebellum serves as a negative feedback system in controlling such motor functions as posture, gait, balance and other finely coordinated motor activities. In one particular experiment, a cat was required to walk from one platform to another on two rows of pegs elevated above a trough of water (Fig. 3.1). Cats were readily trained to this task since they prefer to walk on the pegs rather than in the water. Food reinforcement or general encouragement from the experimenter induced the animal to walk back and forth. Thus the animal was required to make fine discrete paw placements and his particular gait was dictated by the position of the pegs. In as much as a great deal of balance and fine motor coordination is required, the presence of a long recording cable would have severely disturbed the cat's motor behavior. Thus, telemetry was an obvious solution to this and other problems. In a second experimental paradigm it

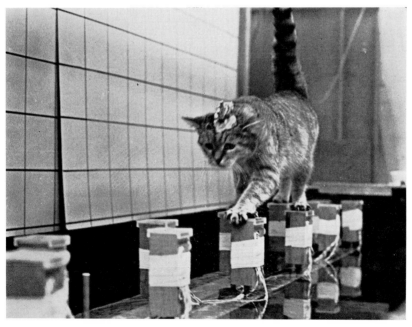

Figure 3.1. A cat is performing a motor coordination task while spike potentials of individual cerebellar neurons are telemetered and recorded. The animal is required to make discrete paw placements on a series of pegs elevated above a trough of water.

was necessary to handle the animal and manipulate various limbs and muscle groups while neural spikes were being recorded. Telemetry facilitates this procedure by eliminating connecting electrode cables and thus reduces various electrical artifacts such as cable noise. In addition, these manipulations can be carried out in a normal laboratory without the electrical shielding that is usually required. The 60 Hz pickup, sometimes present when cables are used, is absent in the telemetered signal. This is due to the fact that ground loops are eliminated and the animal is not capacitively coupled to ground.

The transmission and recording of neural spikes from flexible fine wire electrodes permanently implanted in the brain of a freely moving animal poses several unique problems and dictates the desirable characteristics of the telemetry device. In contrast to the EEG, the neural spike possesses relatively high frequency components. An upper band limit of 10 kHz is necessary to obtain a faithful picture of the spike potential. If the upper band is less than this there is considerable *rounding-off* of the spike with a subsequent decrease in its amplitude. This can be a serious problem in the situations where the amplitude of the spike is not that much greater than the background noise. In general, the amplitude of a neural spike recorded with a fine wire electrode, ranges from about 30 to 150 μV with signal to noise ratios of 2:1 to 10:1 for different neurons.

The tip of these fine wire electrodes (25 μ to 60 μ) is prepared by merely cutting the wire from the spool. There is no further electropolishing of the tip. Measurements that have been made in our lab indicate that these electrodes have impedances of not more than 500 kΩ. Thus, the transmitter must have an input of several megohms. Other considerations that enter into design of a telemetry device are the weight of the unit and the range or distance over which the signal is to be transmitted.

Telemetry Circuits for Transmission of Neural Spikes

A previously published report described an FM (frequency modulated) telemetry device used for recording neural spikes (4). The two circuits presented in Figure 3.2 are basically of the

SINGLE ENDED INPUT BIOTELEMETRY TRANSMITTER

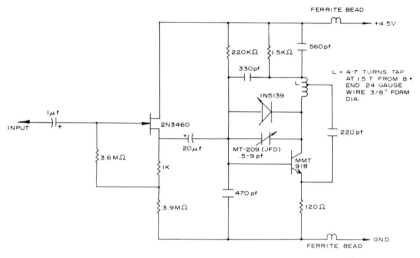

DIFFERENTIAL INPUT TELEMETRY TRANSMITTER

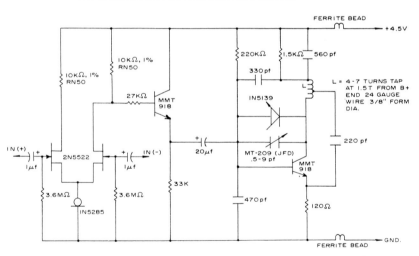

Figure 3.2. A. Circuit diagram for a high input impedance single ended transmitter. B. Circuit diagram for a high input impedance differential transmitter.

same general design, but with several improvements. This includes the development of a transmitter with a high impedance differential input (Fig. 3.2B). Furthermore, a dual channel telemetry system was developed that uses separate transmitters and operates off the same battery supply. In addition to these circuits, there are several others that have been used for recording single unit activity (1, 5).

Single Ended Telemeter

The circuit presented in Figure 3.2A is a single ended FM transmitter that can be easily and inexpensively constructed from discrete components. It consists of a cathode follower stage and a RF (radio frequency) oscillator stage which is sometimes referred to as a tank circuit. The cathode follower is a field effect transistor or FET (2N 3460) which was chosen for its high input impedance and low noise characteristics. The RF transistor (MMT 918) also has a low noise figure and operates at low current levels. This RF stage is a Hartley oscillator. Its resonant frequency is determined by the coil inductance (L) and the capacitance of the other components. One of these is a varactor or variable voltage capacitor (1N 5139) which translates voltage changes into capacitance changes. This capacitive shift results in a change in the resonant frequency of the tank circuit and thus frequency modulation is attained. There is also a small variable capacitor (MT 209) which is used to set the center frequency of the transmitter. The transmitter was designed to operate in or around the commercial FM band (88-108 MHz) because of the availability of inexpensive entertainment type FM receivers. It has been found that a coil of 4.5 turns (dia. ⅜″) wound from #24 gauge wire with a tap at one and one-half turns from the positive battery side will set the center frequency at about 90 MHz. In a number of cases after the construction and potting of the components the transmitter was found to occupy the same frequency as a commercial FM station. Thus, the small variable capacitor was added to allow easy adjustment of the center frequency in order to avoid this station interference.

Differential Telemeter

Figure 3.2B presents a second transmitter with a differential input that has also been used to transmit neural spikes. This is employed in cases where there are more than one fine wire electrode implanted in the brain. In this situation an electrode on which there is a spike potential is connected to the positive input side. One of the other fine wire electrodes, on which there are no spikes, is attached to the negative input side. This results in a significant reduction in the background noise level. Experience has shown that from an array of implanted electrodes some are better than others in reducing the noise level. The differential transmitter can also be operated as a single ended device by connecting the negative input to ground. This transmitter employs a matched pair of field effect transistors (2N 5522), that also have relatively high input impedances and low noise figures. Furthermore this transmitter has an additional gain stage. Table 3.1 provides a list of the components that were used in the construction of these two devices. The main advantages of the two transmitters presented is that they can be fabricated inexpensively from discrete components that are readily available. Furthermore, a number of these units have been constructed and used successfully in a number of experiments. The neural spikes recorded by these transmitters are comparable to those recorded by direct wire (Fig. 3.3).

TABLE 3.1

TRANSMITTER AND TELEMETRY ASSEMBLY COMPONENTS

Field Effect Transistors		
Single Ended	2N 3460	Amelco
Differential	2N 5522	Siliconix
R. F. Transistor	MMT 918	Motorola
Diode	1N 5285	Motorola
Varactor Diode	1N 5139	TRW Semiconductor
Variable Capacitor	MT 209	JFD Capacitors
Ferrite Bead	56-590-65/4B	Ferroxcube Corp.
Battery (Silveroxide)	S76E	Eveready
Male Connector Plug	SRE-34P-JT	Winchester
Female Connector Plug	SRE-34S-J	Winchester
All Resistors ⅛ Watt 5% except 10 KΩ @ 1%		

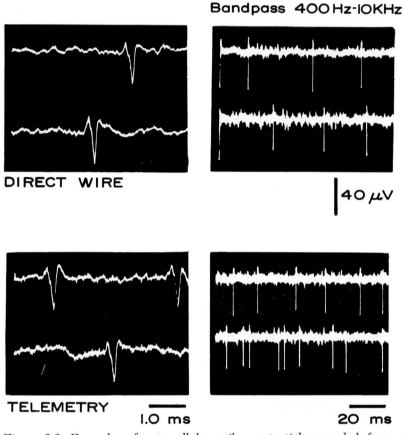

Figure 3.3. Examples of extracellular spikes potentials recorded from a neuron in the cerebellum. These recordings were made via direct wire (top) and telemetry (bottom). In both cases traces were obtained at two recording speeds (1 msec and 20 msec).

Specifications

The specifications for a typical differential transmitter are given in Table 3.2. The single ended transmitters have similar characteristics. The bandwidth of the units is wide (0.8 Hz to > 20 kHz) and more than covers the range required for neural spikes (400 Hz − 10 kHz). Other uses of the extra bandwidth will be presently considered. The input impedance of 3.6 MΩ has been found to be adequate for use with the fine wire electrodes. If a

TABLE 3.2

DIFFERENTIAL TRANSMITTER SPECIFICATIONS

Carrier Frequency	Approx. 90 MHz (Tunable ± 3 MHz)
Deviation	4 kHz/100 μV
Input Impedance	3.6 MΩ
Bandwidth	0.8 Hz to > 20 kHz
Input noise	4 μV rms
Common Mode Rejection	40 db
Maximum Input Signal	1.8 mV
DC Power Drain	1.5 mA @ 4.5V
Battery Life	100 hrs—1 transmitter
	50 hrs—2 transmitters
	(4.5 volts Eveready S76E)
Weight	3 gms (Transmitter alone)
	25 gms (2 Transmitters, Battery Supply and Male Connector Plug)

higher value is desired this can easily be accomplished by a simple modification. The D.C. current drain is relatively low (1.5 mA) and when the specified batteries (S76E) are used one transmitter can operate for more than one hundred hours. Generally this is more than adequate since the batteries are mounted externally and can be changed easily between experimental sessions. The weight of the transmitter connector plug and battery supply is light enough to be carried by the cat. If the transmitter is to be used on smaller animals a different connector and lighter battery supply can be substituted. The RF signal of the transmitter is sufficiently strong to be recorded within a laboratory room (20′ × 20′) without any significant loss of signal.

Dual Telemetry System

When multiple arrays of fine wire electrodes are implanted in one animal, it is often possible to record spike potentials on more than one electrode. Thus, it is desirable to have another channel to record a second spike potential. This can be accomplished in several ways. One of the most common methods is to multiplex by using subcarriers. Therefore one transmitter contains several channels of information that are later decoded by subcarrier discriminators. For our purposes, the simplest, and least expensive solution was to incorporate a second transmitter into the telemetry assembly and operate it off the same battery supply. A

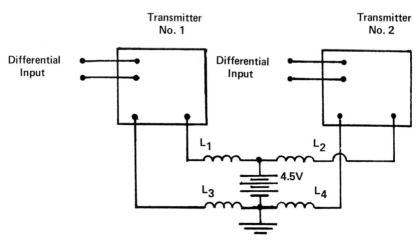

Figure 3.4. Schematic circuit diagram for operating two independent differential transmitters from the same battery supply (4.5 volts). Ferrite beads (L_1, L_2, L_3, L_4—#56-590-65/4B Ferroxcube Corp.) are placed over each of the leads that connect the transmitters to the battery supply. These act as low pass filters to eliminate cross talk between the two transmitters.

second receiver is tuned to that transmitter's frequency. A number of problems were encountered which dealt with cross talk or unwanted interaction between the two transmitters. However, it was found that this cross talk could be reduced to tolerable levels by placing ferrite beads over all the transmitter leads that went to the power supply (Fig. 3.4). These act as low pass filters. In addition, it was necessary to set the center frequencies of the two transmitters about 10 MHz apart. Therefore, for operation in and around the FM band, the first transmitter was set at 88 MHz and the second at 108 MHz.

Telemeter Assembly

In chronic brain implants the indwelling electrodes are soldered to a female connector plug. This plug is then attached to the skull by means of screws and dental cement. In our experiment a thirty-four pin female connector plug was used (SRE-34S-J, Winchester). The telemetry assembly consisted of two transmitters and a battery supply that were incorporated onto the complimentary male plug (SRE-34P-JT, Winchester). Figure 3.5 is a photo of this assembly with the various component parts indicated. This particular arrangement has several distinct advantages. The telemetry device is external to the animal and thus easy access is provided for battery replacement. One telemetry assembly can be used for several animals. In addition, the individual transmitter is brought as close as possible to the signal source, thereby improving the quality of the recording.

When many electrodes are implanted, there are several possible inputs for each transmitter. Thus some sort of switching arrangement is necessary. This is accomplished on the top side of the male connector plug. The electrodes are soldered to the pins in

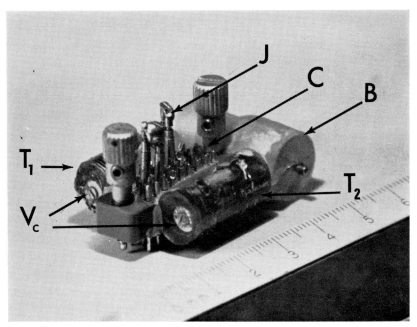

Figure 3.5. This photograph depicts the complete telemetry assembly. It consists of two independent transmitters (T_1 and T_2), common battery supply (B) and male connector plug (C). The top portion of this plug is used as a switching network where *jumpers* (J) connect the electrodes to the transmitters' inputs when the assembly is attached to the female plug on the animal. Also depicted are the variable capacitors (V_c) that are used to tune the transmitters.

one row on the female plug. The input to a transmitter occupies a second and adjacent row but on the male plug. Thus, when the telemetry assembly is attached to the animal, there is no direct connection between an electrode and the transmitter input. An electrode is connected to the input by making contact between the appropriate pin in the first row with one in the second row by means of a small *jumper*. The transmitters are only activated when the assembly is attached to the plug on the cat. This is accomplished by soldering together two pins on the female plug which serves as a battery switch.

The construction of the transmitter itself is done under a dissecting microscope. The various electronic components are packed tightly together one by one and the appropriate solder connections are made. Care must be taken not to destroy the components by too much heat from the soldering iron. The resistors, capacitors, transistors and coil are laid out so as to form a cylindrical module (10 mm dia. × 20 mm length), which weighs about three grams after potting in epoxy. The total weight of the entire telemetry assembly is about twenty-five grams.

Other Telemetry Considerations

Both the single ended and differential transmitters have a wide bandwidth (0.8 Hz to > 20 kHz) which is greater than that required for neural spikes (400 Hz − 10 kHz). It therefore is possible to carry additional information outside the range that is needed for the spikes. For example, the lower end of the band could be employed for transmitting the EEG or evoked response potentials that emanate from the same electrode as the neural spike. These slower components and the spike potentials can be separated from each other by appropriate high and low band pass filters placed after the telemetry receiver. Other uses of the excess bandwidth include transmission of the EMG or other relevant information pertaining to the experiment. This can be accomplished through the use of subcarriers.

Satisfactory recordings of neural spikes have been obtained from instrumentation type receivers (Astro Communication SR-201A) as well as from those of the entertainment variety. These include portable as well as secondhand monaural FM receivers. The use of these receivers requires several modifications though. They have a de-emphasis network which attenuates the high end of the frequency band that is broadcast by the FM stations. In the transmission of neural spike data this network should be bypassed. Secondly, if the EEG is to be transmitted, it is necessary to turn off or otherwise inhibit the automatic frequency control (AFC). Furthermore, the signal containing the biological information must be taken directly from the discriminator stage of the receiver. The normal output of these receivers will generally not pass frequencies below the audio range ($<$ 20 Hz) and so the EEG signal would not be detected.

In our experiments a wide variety of antennas have been used. These have included a string of randomly arranged jumper cables, a simple rod antenna and a horizontally mounted four foot diameter coil antenna. This coil when mounted in the center of a laboratory about a foot from the ceiling seemed to work the best of those we tried. There are many types of antennas that can be used but it is well to remember that for the choice and positioning of a particular antenna the transmission in a small laboratory room is near field transmission. The situation in which the dual system of two independent transmitters is used requires two receivers. Both receivers can be fed from the same antenna if a signal splitter is employed. This is the same apparatus that is used in the home to connect two television sets to a single external house antenna.

SUMMARY

Single ended and differential input transmitters are described which telemeter the activity of individual neurons from the awake and unrestrained animal. A dual channel device is also depicted which utilizes two independent FM transmitters that operate off the same battery supply. These transmitters have high input impedances and wide bandwidths. The transmitters and battery supply are incorporated onto a male connector plug that, in turn, fits on the complimentary female plug which is attached to the animal's head. The telemetry assembly can be constructed inexpensively from readily available components. These transmitters are designed to operate in the FM band (88-108 MHz).

REFERENCES

1. Beechey, P. and D. W. Lincoln. A miniature FM transmitter for the radio telemetry of unit activity. *J. Physiol.*, 203:5P-6P, 1969.
2. Mackay, R. S. *Bio-medical Telemetry.* J. Wiley & Sons, New York, 1968.
3. McElligott, J. G. Telemetry recordings of cerebellar neurons in the unrestrained cat during walking and striking motor behavior. *Proc. 2nd Ann. Winter Conf. on Brain Res.*, Snowmass, Colo., 119-120, 1969.
4. McElligott, J. G., R. T. Kado, and J. R. Zweizig. A miniaturized telemetry device for the transmission of the electrical activity of single nerve cells in the brain. *Proc. Nat'l Telemetering Conf.*, Washington, D.C., 207-210, 1969.
5. Skutt, H., R. G. Beschle, D. Moulton, and W. Koella. New subminiature amplifier transmitters for telemetering biopotentials. *Electroenceph. Clin. Neurophysiol.*, 22:275-277, 1967.

Chapter IV

AN ON-LINE COMPUTER TECHNIQUE
FOR DISPLAY AND ANALYSIS OF
SINGLE CELL ACTIVITY

PHILLIP J. BEST

THE SUCCESS OF single cell recording techniques in the behavioral laboratory is dependent in part on the ability of the experimenter to record from the same cell for long periods of time. In order to accomplish long term recording some investigators have used larger electrodes. The advantages gained by the use of large electrodes are offset by certain disadvantages. The signal from each neuron is much reduced and consequently there is a much lower signal to noise ratio than is found on smaller electrodes. Special purpose electronic devices have been developed in order to discriminate individual neural responses from background noise. One such discriminator device, designed by Olds (1965), consists basically of two voltage level detectors (Schmidt triggers) and two timing devices (one-shots). Any action potential appearing in the signal from an electrode can be discriminated from other activity by setting the triggers and timers such that the action potential reaches a peak between the two trigger levels and falls back to baseline between the two timer settings. Figure 4.1a illustrates the discriminator settings for a particular action potential. The convention used here is to plot the peak of the action potential as positive. All examples in this paper are taken from electrodes in the midbrain reticular formation of rats.

This paper describes two computer procedures that have been developed to assist in the analysis of cellular activity recorded from 67 μ nichrome electrodes (See Olds, 1965). The first procedure was developed to monitor and display the electrical signals that the discriminator circuits tagged as neural activity. The

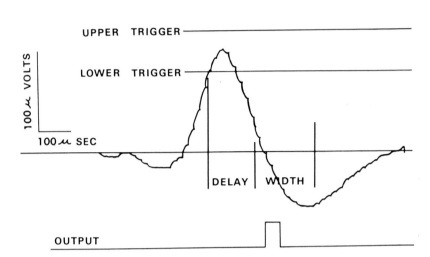

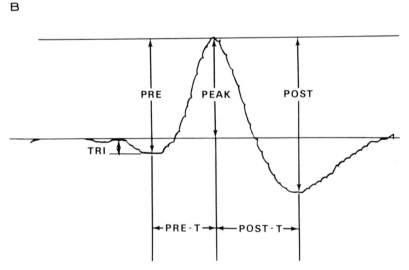

Figure 4.1. A typical action potential. (A) Appropriate timing and trigger level settings for discrimination of an action potential. Lower trace is the discriminator output. (B) Parameters of an action potential used in the computer programs.

second procedure was developed to allow the computer to serve as the discriminator. The purpose of this paper is to illustrate the general principles of the programs and not to present specific detail of coding for each variation of these two programs.

Computer System

The system used in the procedures includes a Digital Equipment Corp. PDP8 computer with 4096 core locations, an analog to digital (A-D) converter, a multiplexer for the A-D converter, a thirty-six bit digital input buffer, and a Huston Instrument Co. X-Y plotter. Both of the procedures could be accomplished on any comparable 4K machine with one channel A-D converter, one digital input line, and any XY or XT display.

The Computer as a Monitor

The central part of the program consists of a closed search loop in which A-D conversions are accomplished every twenty-five microseconds and stored in a data list. The size of the list is kept minimal by returning to the first position on the list after position number 128 (200 octal) has been used. The list therefore contains the digitalized heights of the signal for the last 3.2 milliseconds. During each pass through the search loop the program looks to see if a discriminator has fired. The discriminators in our situation fire after the peak of the action potential when the signal falls to the baseline (Fig. 4.1a). If the discriminator has fired in the last pass through the loop the computer now moves into another very similar loop which performs forty more conversions (*i.e.,* one more millisecond). The program then searches back over the list of signal heights to detect the peak of the action potential. From this point the program can calculate a variety of parameters of the action potential. The parameters that we found to be most reliable and useful are shown in Figure 4.1b. They are the peak of the action potential with respect to the baseline, the amplitude and time of the pre- and post-potentials with respect to the peak, and the relative size of the pre-potential. This last parameter, called Triphasicness, may imply that the recording is from an axon, or at least downstream from the point of generation of the action potential (Woodbury, 1962). The signal to noise ratio is also calculated. Any combination of the above parameters can be used to discriminate between action potentials from different cells. These parameters are stored and the program returns to the search loop looking for another action potential.

The program has been used to check the reliability of the discriminator circuits in two ways. First, when more than one cell is recorded on one electrode it is necessary to demonstrate that each discriminator is tagging one and only one cell. Figure 4.2 shows two different cells recorded from the same electrode simultaneously but tagged by different discriminators. The program analyzed one hundred occurrences of the action potential, displaying every tenth wave form, centered in time with respect to the peak. The average signal and one standard deviation above and below the average are plotted in the lower traces.

The second and more widely used application is to guarantee that during a long experiment, the same action potentials are tagged for the duration of the experiment (Phillips and Olds, 1969). Figure 4.3 illustrates samples of tagged activity from an electrode taken thirteen hours apart. No modification was made of amplifier or discriminator settings during the thirteen hour period.

In current use the program samples the activity from five discriminator channels on each of six animals simultaneously. Discriminator outputs are interfaced with the computer via a thirty-

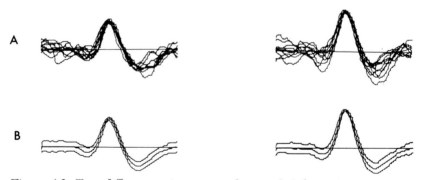

Figure 4.2. Two different action potentials recorded from the same electrode. (A) Ten overlapping traces of each action potential, (B) Mean and standard deviation of one hundred traces.

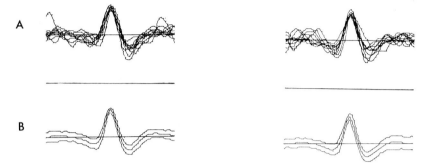

Figure 4.3. Two samples of the same action potential taken thirteen hours apart. (A) Ten traces, (B) Mean and standard deviation.

six bit input register. The program randomly searches for an animal from whom data are being collected and selects a channel (discriminator) on that animal. As long as data are being recorded the computer will sample cellular activity and store the list of signal heights until either no animal is being sampled from or there is no room left to store signals. The program will then plot the signals from its stored lists until there is room to store more and another sample is taken from one of the animals.

Computer as Discriminator

In the previous procedure the most important function, that of deciding which signals were cellular action potentials, was still being made by the special purpose discriminators. The present procedure was programmed to do away with the discriminators entirely and to pass all the work on to the computer. The use of the computer as the discriminator gives added flexibility in deciding which of the many parameters of the wave form are most appropriate in distinguishing between action potentials from different cells.

The program is constructed around the same basic loop as the previous program. The search loop is a little longer since besides A-D conversion and storage more complex decisions have to be made during each pass. Also there are quite a few search loops, all of identical length, but all asking a different type of question or performing a different type of function. For example: one loop continues sampling until the signal goes above a baseline. Control is then shifted to another which continues sampling during the rising edge of the wave form, until a peak in the wave form is detected. Appropriate time and height parameters are stored and another loop is entered which seeks the low point in the after potential. The program determines if the sample time has been exceeded and if not returns to the first loop.

Before accepting samples for data analysis the program must make a few passes over the analog signals to *get a feel* for the general characteristics of the signals. The first pass defines the baseline. During the next set of passes a histogram is made of the peak to post-potential heights. Every time a peak is encountered, the program finds the post-potential, calculates the peak to post-potential height and increments the bin in the histogram reflecting that height. After a fixed number of 1.6 second passes the histogram is plotted as in Figure 4.4. The experimenter then decides the range of peak heights that are appropriate for action

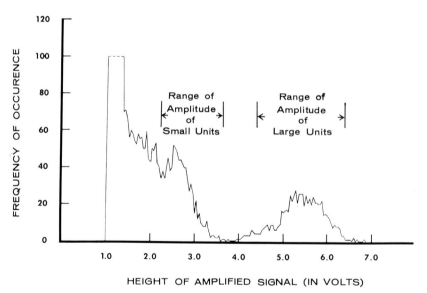

Figure 4.4. Histogram of frequency of occurrence of signals with different amplitudes (Peak to Post-potential height). The two peaks in the distribution are used to define single cell action potentials.

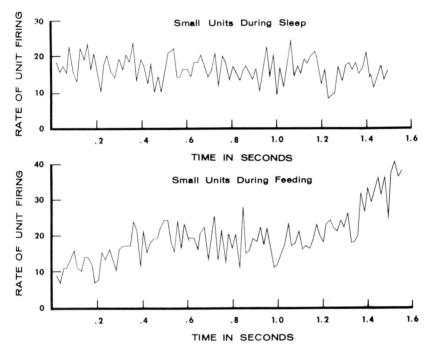

Figure 4.5 Rate of firing of the small cell during sleeping and during a lever holding response for food.

potentials and types these values into the computer. In the example given all amplitudes less than one volt were ignored by the program. The histogram reveals that anything under 2.0 volts is too close to the background to be discriminated. The peak in the distribution around 2.5 volts seemed to cover a small action potential, and the peak around 5.5 volts is indicative of a large action potential.

Following definition of the range of peak to post heights that are to be used as criteria for an action potential, the program analyzes samples of neural activity during two or three behavioral states. In the current example two states were defined: sleeping and holding a lever in a depressed position for food. Figures 4.5 and 4.6 show the rate of unit activity over the 1.6 second samples for each behavioral state for the small and large signal respectively. The rate of firing along the abscissa is in

arbitrary units and should just be considered as a relative measure. Note that during sleeping no systematic change is expected
in rate of firing since the activity is not synchronized to any
relevant event. However, the activity during lever pressing is synchronized to the initiation of the lever depression. Note that
during barpressing for food the two units show a slightly different
template of activity. The smaller unit shows sustained activity
during the lever press but a burst of activity just prior to food
delivery. The larger cell shows an increase in activity peaking at
about .6 seconds, decreasing to a lower level at around 1.0 second and increasing again just prior to food delivery.

After plotting the above histograms the program then plots
the inter spike interval histogram for each unit under each
condition. One such histogram is shown in Figure 4.7. By fitting a
Poisson distribution to such a histogram one can determine if the
units fire in a random or fixed manner, *i.e.*, bursting or pacing of

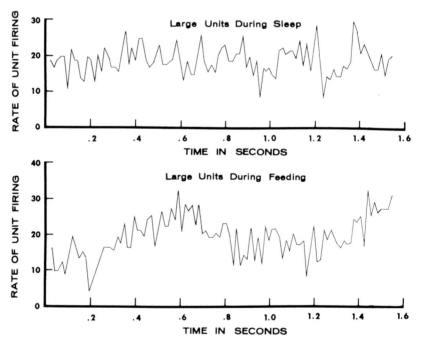

Figure 4.6. Rate of firing of the large cell during sleeping and during a
lever holding response for food.

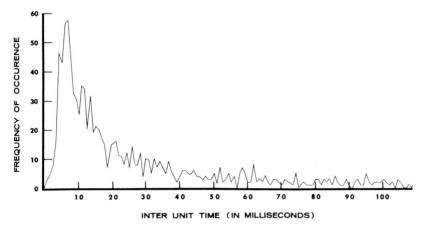

Figure 4.7. Histogram of the frequency of occurrences of different intervals between successive occurrences of the action potential from the larger cell.

firing would be revealed in systematic deviations from a Poisson distribution.

The above procedures are reported to illustrate that the small general purpose laboratory computer can be used to perform a number of functions in the laboratory that are typically done by special purpose computers and other electronic devices. The advantage gained is that many procedures can be performed simultaneously or at least sequentially, thus freeing valuable experimenter time and increasing the reliability of results. These types of procedures will become more important as the need for longer term recording in behavioral studies necessitates the move to larger electrodes and subsequently to more sophisticated methods for discriminating unit activity from background noise.

REFERENCES

Olds, J. Operant conditioning of single unit responses. *Proceedings of the XXIII International Congress of Physiological Sciences*, Excerpta Medica International Series No. 87, 1965, 372-380.

Phillips, M. I., and J. Olds. Unit activity: Motivation dependent responses from midbrain neurons. *Science*, 1969, 165, 1269-1271.

Woodbury, J. W. Potentials in a volume conductor. In Ruch, T. C., H. D. Patton, J. W. Woodbury and A. L. Towe. *Neurophysiology,* Saunders, Philadelphia, 1962, pp. 83-91.

Chapter V

A MOVABLE MICROELECTRODE FOR RECORDING FROM SINGLE NEURONS IN UNRESTRAINED RATS

JAMES B. RANCK, JR.

THIS MOVABLE MICROELECTRODE for recording from single neurons in unrestrained rats has been used successfully in this laboratory for a year and one-half. Action potentials can be recorded extracellularly from single cells for several hours, unaffected by motion of the rat, picking him up in my hand, hitting the electrode with a screw driver or banging the electrode against the side of the cage. The system has the advantage of being simple, reusable, lightweight, easy to build and repair as well as small (two of them are placed on a rat's head routinely).

Under pentobarbital anesthesia one or two 3 mm diameter holes are drilled in the skull without damaging the dura. A tungsten microelectrode, to be used as the indifferent electrode, which is identical to the movable one for recording from cells is fixed in place in each hole. The tip of the fixed microelectrode is within 1-2 mm of the intended recording positions of the movable electrode. The hole in the skull is filled with Silastic A-RTV (Dow Chemical Company).

One quarter-20 nylon nuts are placed in the skull over the holes in the skull. They are cut so that the electrode assembly which screws into the nut will be at the desired angle. They can be placed stereotaxically. A plug is screwed into the nut until recordings are made. Neocortical electrodes for recording of EEG, and electrodes for recording of eye movement (EOG) and EMG from the dorsal neck musculature are also implanted, and attached to an Amphenol connector implanted in the rat's skull. Three stainless steel sheet metal screws are screwed in the skull and all the attachments are imbedded in acrylic. The electrode

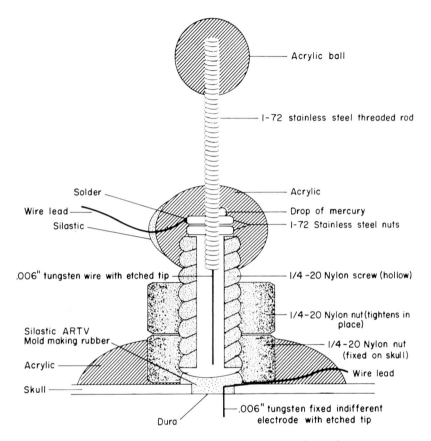

Figure 5.1. Details of the moveable microelectrode.

assembly is shown in Figure 5.1. It is screwed into the nylon nut when recording is to begin, usually one to three weeks after surgery. Before placement, the electrode assembly is sterilized in an iodine solution, washed with distilled water and dried in an air jet.

The microelectrode is .006″ (150 μ) tungsten with an etched tip, insulated to within 10 μ of the tip with Epoxylyte. The acrylic around the stainless steel screw determines how tightly the screw turns. If it is too tight, it is difficult to turn while the rat stands in the cage, and the turning is aversive to the rat. However, some acrylic can then be chipped off or the screw moved up and down a few times and the screw becomes loose. If the screw is too loose it may be difficult to hold neurons, but the screw can be tightened by adding more acrylic. After a few runs the screw does become loose, but it is an easy matter to control the tightness by changing the top layer of acrylic. The drop of mercury assures good electrical contact between screw and nut. The tungsten wire is attached to the stainless steel screw, by bending a loop on the end of the tungsten wire, and imbedding this loop in solder in a hole on the end of the screw. Since tungsten wire does not solder, this electrical and mechanical junction is simply from embedding the tungsten in the solder and must be made carefully. A single electrode can be used many times. Sometimes the tips must be re-etched or reinsulated (this time with an insulation not requiring much heat, e.g. Insulex).

The microelectrode is lowered while the rat is going about his business in his cage. He readily adapts to the situation and sometimes even sleeps while the microelectrode is moved. At the surface of dura, electrical contact is made, so by counting the number of turns below dural surface, the approximate depths of the microelectrode is known (363 μ/turn). Even with the rat moving the electrode can be advanced in stages of about one twentieth of a turn, *i.e.* in about 15 μ steps. I have seen no indication that the rotation of the electrode is a disadvantage. Cells can be recorded as the microelectrode is lowered and also when it is raised.

Initially, 50 μ tungsten wire was used to make the electrodes, following the suggestion of Olds that a flexible wire will move with the brain as the brain moves. More recently 150 μ wire has been used with no change in the ease of holding cells. With the stiffer wire the electrode can be aimed more accurately. There is about a 50 percent chance of being able to hold a cell with adequate isolation for three or four hours if I can hold the cell five minutes (and most cells can be held for five minutes). I have not tried to record from neurons for longer than four hours. The electrode tip is often left in the brain for weeks as many different cells are studied.

Recording is made differentially between the movable microelectrode and the fixed microelectrode on the same side. The reason for this is to cut down or eliminate the EMG recorded during chewing. This can be quite large in a rat, obscuring action potentials, because of his large jaw muscles being a comparatively small distance from any spot in brain. The wire from each electrode goes directly to a Field Effect Transistor (2N5459) on the connector which plugs on the connector on the rat's head. These wires must be stiff enough so that they do not wiggle with movement of the rat. This system is almost completely free of movement artifact. Both action potentials and slow waves of publishable quality record can be routinely obtained during the most vigorous movement I have seen in a rat. (Another serious source of movement artifact can be electrostatic charge on glass or transparent plastic on the front of the running cage. This is eliminated with an ungrounded wire screen between the glass or plastic and the rat.) Elimination of movement artifact in slow waves from the microelectrode was the most difficult problem.

Chapter VI

A TECHNIQUE FOR RECORDING SINGLE NEURONS FROM UNRESTRAINED ANIMALS

R. M. HARPER and D. J. McGINTY

THIS PAPER DESCRIBES a unit recording technique that was developed to study brain regions concerned with complex behaviors. Until recently the examination of neural firing patterns has been the province of specialized neurophysiologists who have been interested primarily in neurons of the sensory and motor systems in which the input and output relations of cells could be easily specified. The application of single cell techniques to the study of brain areas that are of great interest to behavioral scientists has been hindered by the difficulty in recording from conventional microelectrodes in behaving animals and by the expertise required for the manufacture and use of such microelectrodes. We are presenting here a technique for single cell recording which is suitable for the study of brain behavior problems and which can be used by behavioral scientists who lack specialized training.

Areas such as the hypothalamus, reticular formation, and other limbic structures of the brain have attracted the attention of brain scientists because of the functions they perform in the control of temperature regulation, feeding, sleep, sexual, and affective behavior. These regions are concerned with the integration of information from a wide variety of inputs and appear to select behavioral activities as a result of these inputs. The dis-

We wish to thank John O'Keefe, Tom Babb, Mary Fairbanks, David Kelly, and William Elferink for assistance during the development of this technique. This research was supported by USPHS Grant MH 10083 and by the U.S. Veterans Administration. Computational assistance was furnished by the Data Processing Laboratory of the Brain Research Institute, UCLA, which is supported by USPHS Grant NS-02501.

covery of the neuronal coding of these control functions provides a captivating challenge to the neuroscientist. However, the initial steps in a meaningful study of complex integrative mechanisms in behaving animals is difficult. We frequently must rely on lesion or stimulation experiments or slow wave recording studies to guide our investigations of these sites, in spite of the fact that lesioning and stimulation affect many different types of neurons simultaneously, and slow wave recording techniques sample electrical activity which is influenced by thousands of neurons. In many cases we do not know the specific anatomical connections of the sites under study.

Thus, our initial problem is to identify homogeneous groups of neurons, to determine the significant influences on these neurons from sensory systems or internal states, and to find correlations between specific neuronal activities and discrete behaviors. In addition, we must perform a variety of control procedures to rule out spurious correlations. For example, we may discover a class of neurons exhibiting accelerated firing during feeding behavior. These neurons should be studied also during comparable motor behaviors, postures, arousal levels, oropharyngeal sensations and autonomic states to determine the specificity of the accelerated spiking during feeding.

The technique described here provides three features to meet these requirements. First, it is imperative that the experimental subject be allowed to move freely without the influence of anesthetics, paralyzing agents, or restraints that both prevent the study of many behaviors and alter the discharge patterns of neurons that are concerned with such behaviors. Second, since we must study each neuron under a variety of experimental conditions, stable recordings must be maintained for at least several hours. Third, the technique must avoid specialized procedures that would overtax the resources of behavioral scientists.

One of the problems resulting from the need to record from freely moving animals over long periods is movement of the brain, since it is subjected to physiological pulsations and mechanical shock (4). With a stiff electrode, brain movement results in changes in the amplitude or wave shape of the recorded neuron. Another inherent difficulty in recording single neurons is the problem of obtaining noise free records from very low level signals composed of a broad range of frequencies (.2-10K Hz), especially since the signals are obtained from relatively high impedance electrodes attached to cables swinging with the moving animal.

For the past few years, we have been developing a technique for recording from single neurons that effectively solves many of the problems of chronic unit recording. We have been using bundles of 3-14 flexible insulated fine wires which were cut off bluntly at the tip and lowered to brain sites. These bundles were either firmly fixed in place by dental cement or are attached to a movable microdrive. The brain was effectively sealed except for the sliding surfaces of concentric hypodermic tubing in the case of the movable electrodes, and hence brain movements were minimized. At the same time the wires were flexible and moved with the brain when required. The wires were of lower impedance (100-150K ohm) than conventional microelectrodes. Consequently, extremely high input impedance amplifiers were not ordinarily used, and noise problems were subsequently reduced.

Several investigators have reported previously that single neurons can be recorded from relatively unrestrained animals with similar simple methods. Strumwasser (37) demonstrated that single neurons could readily be recorded from unrestrained squirrels using flexible wires of relatively gross diameter (80 μ). These neurons could be held for very long periods of time. Since then the fine wire procedure has been used for recording neurons with success in humans (22), rats (28, 33), and cats (27). In the procedure of Olds (28), individual fine wires are implanted surgically into brain sites. During implantation the recordings are monitored on an oscilloscope. When a single neuron is seen on the trace, the wire is cemented into place. Units often appear on the electrode after the animal has recovered from surgery. O'Keefe and Bouma (27) have used bundles of fine wires which are lowered to brain sites after the wires are adhered together with polyethylene glycol (Carbowax, Union Carbide), a soluable substance which melts at body temperature. Alternatively, the wires were lowered inside a hypodermic needle and cut off by the needle tip after reaching the desired brain area. Our technique evolved from the developments made by each of these predecessors.

Preparation of Electrodes

The specific procedures of electrode preparation and implantation vary, depending on the specific aims of the experiment. If extremely long term recordings are required, then permanent fixation of the electrodes to the skull, rather than attaching the bundles to a microdrive, may be desirable. On the other hand, if it is necessary to record from a large number of neurons by means of a penetration through a cell group, then use of the microdrive is appropriate.

We have used fine wires with a variety of metallic compositions in our studies, including stainless steel, nichrome with and without iron, and platinum in various alloys (platinum-iridium, platinum rhodium-rithenium). All of these materials seem to work successfully, and none appear to damage tissue grossly. If at least one wire in the bundle contains a little iron, it can be deposited with a small DC current (20 μ amp per 15 sec), so that a ferrocyanide stain can be produced to aid in histological examinations (3, 15). Preinsulated (heavy formvar) nichrome wire (Stablohm 675 stress relieved) can be obtained in small lots in any diameter from California Fine Wire.*

Preinsulated wires, cut to convenient lengths, are prepared for soldering by burning off insulation for about one eighth inch (with a small flame). Residue should be removed with a solvent or by scraping. The fine wires are then soldered to a standard connector and tied with small strings to form a bundle. The solder joints of the connector are sealed with dental cement to cover any uninsulated wire leads above solder points and to provide strength. These wires are cut off bluntly with a pair of sharp scissors or a razor to the desired length. Prior to implantation the wires are dipped either in polyethylene glycol, a sucrose solution, or saline so that they adhere to each other. The stiffened bundle

---

* California Fine Wire, P.O. Box 446, Grover City, California 93433.

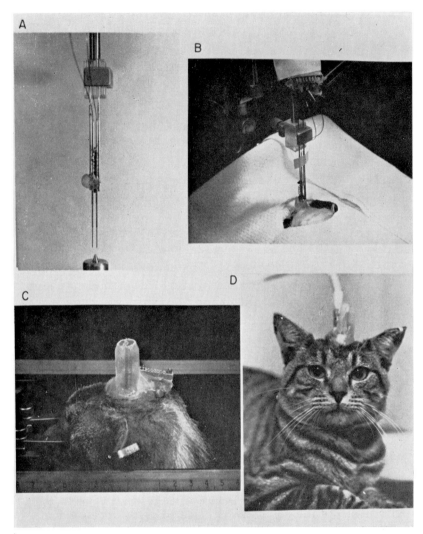

Figure 6.1. *A.* A double cannula microdrive, held in an electrode carrier by two side cannulae, is ready for calibration in the stereotaxic device. *B.* The microdrive is cemented in place after being lowered to the brain site. The microwire bundles have been placed within the inner cannulae. *C.* A plastic cylinder (a discarded hypodermic syringe cover) is placed over the protruding microdrive and caulk-encased microwire bundles for protection. *D.* Following recovery from surgery, the cable is attached to the freely moving cat. Adjustments to the microdrive are made through the open cylinder end.

may be calibrated for stereotaxic implantation like macroelectrodes.

Surgical Technique

Standard surgical procedures and stereotaxic techniques are utilized in this procedure (see Fig. 6.1). The animal is anesthetized, placed in a stereotaxic apparatus, and the skull bared. Holes are bored through the skull above the site and the dura underlying the burr hole cut. The bundle of wires or the microdrive is then lowered to a desired brain site stereotaxically. In the absence of a microdrive, a short length of stainless steel tubing (22-26 G) can be implanted to guide the bundle to increase stereotaxic accuracy. The microdrive or stainless steel tubing should end 5-10 mm above the recording site. The microwires are floating in the brain in the distance between the microdrive or guide and the recording site, providing the desired flexibility.

Microdrive

The microdrive which we use embodies a number of useful features including simple and inexpensive construction, compact size and low weight for chronic attachment. It can be constructed with a hand grinding tool (Dremel Moto-Tool), soldering iron,

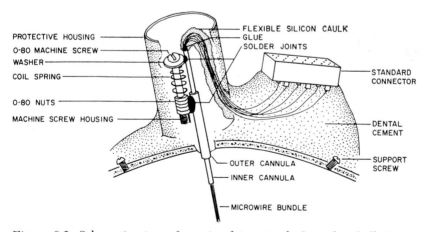

Figure 6.2. Schematic view of a microdrive attached to the skull. Rotation of the machine screw moves the sliding inner cannula, containing the microwire bundle, within the fixed outer cannula. For additional details, see text.

and stereotaxic holder with roughly twenty-five cents worth of materials.

This microdrive, which is seen schematically in Figure 6.2, consists of a movable *inner cannula* to which the fine wires are attached. This inner cannula can be lowered through a rigidly affixed *outer cannula* by means of a parallel machine screw. The mechanical connection is provided by a washer under the head of the machine screw, soldered to the inner cannula. A stiff compression coil spring pushes the washer against the screw head and maintains tension in the system to increase rigidity. The machine screw is threaded into a stack of matching nuts which are locked tightly together to increase rigidity further. The nuts are soldered to the outer guide cannula. Since the screw extends below the nuts in its lowest position, a protective guide projects below the nuts to prevent dental cement or other materials from obstructing the screw's path. The inner and outer cannulae should fit tightly to minimize the permanent opening to the brain. Tubing sizes can be selected according to the size of the microwires and number of wires in a bundle. A combination of 24 gauge and 20 gauge tubing is suitable for bundles of six 50 μ wires. The microdrive is constructed of stainless steel parts and may be sterilized.[†] This microdrive also may be used with macroelectrodes or for chemical stimulation of the brain.

During surgery the microdrive *inner cannula* may be stereotaxically implanted to a point above a brain site under investigation and the outer cannula cemented in position. The microelectrode bundle is then lowered *through* the inner cannula to a stereotaxically determined depth and the bundle glued to the inner cannula. Subsequent lowering of the inner cannula will also lower the microelectrode bundle.

After having been glued to the inner cannula, the microelectrode bundle is gently arched into position and covered with a flexible caulk (Silicon Seal, GE) for protection. The flexible caulk allows the bundle to bend further as the microdrive is lowered. Finally, a plastic cylinder, open at both ends, is cemented in place around the microdrive and bundle for protection.

A more complicated version of the microdrive is shown in

[†] Stainless steel tubing, machine screws, washers, and nuts may be obtained from Small Parts Inc., 6901 N.E. Third Ave., Miami, Florida 33138.

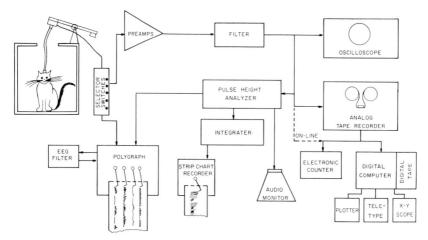

Figure 6.3. A flow diagram of the equipment used for recording, displaying, storing and analyzing data in typical unit recording experiments.

Figure 6.1. Two parallel cannulae are attached to the machine screw to allow simultaneous recording from closely adjacent sites. Two additional pieces of steel tubing are soldered on either side of the two outer cannulae to provide convenient attachment to the stereotaxic holder. Finally, in this case, the microwires are placed within the outer cannula before implantation, precut and stereotaxically calibrated, and then temporarily raised within the inner cannula for protection during surgery and implantation.

Chronic Recording Procedure and Equipment

The animals are typically run through an experimental paradigm in a sound attenuated chamber. The animal is connected by means of a 20 pin Amphenol connector with a low noise Microdot cable to a Lehigh Valley twenty track swivel connector suspended from a counterbalanced arm. The electrical activity from the various electrodes is passed through high impedance preamplifiers, typically Grass P15[‡] or equivalent preamplifiers. We have also used such medium impedance amplifiers as the Grass 7P5 (5 megohm input impedance polygraph amplifiers). Figure 6.3 shows the recording, data analysis, and data storage equipment.

---

‡ Grass Instrument Co., Quincy, Massachusetts.

Normally, EEG, EMG and EOG activity are recorded along with the activity of single cells. This activity is led to polygraph amplifiers and written on paper. The amplified activity of the single neurons is subjected to very narrow band pass filtering at 60 and 120 Hz with an electronic filter,[§] and to high pass filtering through a variable resistance-capacitance network to reduce the contribution to the signal from the line frequency and EEG.

We have found this filtering system preferable to sharp electronic filtering of all frequencies below 250 Hz and above 10 K Hz. With the electronic systems we have tried, the heavy filtering required to rid the signal of 60 Hz affects slow components of the spike wave form. Such filtering usually leads to differentiation of the spike or other distortation of the wave form which adds to the difficulty in separating the spike from noise and nearby spikes and recognition of wave form characteristics.

The amplified and filtered spike train is displayed on an oscilloscope and is taped on a multichannel tape recorder. We normally tape in the direct mode. However, when very low noise is required (*i.e.*, in separating two or more neurons on one electrode), FM recording may be used at a very high tape speed for the required band width.

The amplified and filtered spike signal is led to a window discriminator[§] with upper and lower thresholds for spike heights. One output of this discriminator is a lengthened pulse ($\sim$ 10 msec), which is led to the polygraph causing a pen deflection whenever a spike occurs. This technique cannot be used for precise analysis, especially when studying fast firing or bursting neurons, but it is useful for a quick look at the spike discharge pattern simultaneously with the EEG and EMG activity. Another output of the discriminator is a 50 μ sec pulse which is displayed on a dual beam oscilloscope simultaneously with the spike wave forms to insure adequate spike height discrimination.

The 50 μ sec output pulse is led also to an integrating device[§] which counts the number of discharges in a defined time period as a record on a cumulative recorder (Fig. 6.4). This provides an indication of changes in the rate of firing over time.

[§] Window discriminators, integraters and 60 and 120 Hz notch filters are available from Neurofeedback Instruments, 10535 Cedros Ave., Mission Hills, California 91340.

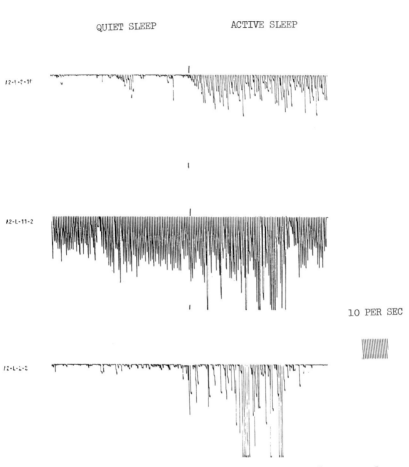

Figure 6.4. The integrater output is displayed by a strip chart recorder to produce a cumulative record of spike discharges. The integrater is reset at regular intervals (five seconds in this case) so that the length of each excursion indicates the number of spikes in the interval. The record is calibrated with a pulse train of known frequency. This type of record is useful for examining changes in the pattern of unit firing over long time periods. This figure shows increases in unit firing rate from quiet sleep on the left to active sleep (REM sleep) on the right. The increase is tonic in the top sample, but occurs only in bursts (phasically) in the center and bottom samples.

The wave form also is passed to an audio amplifier connected to a loud speaker. This is an important part of the instrumentation since, by listening to the pattern of firing, important aspects of the activity can be ascertained immediately. Moreover, the audio output aids in the recognition of artifacts since the wave shapes of neurons produce distinctive sounds.

Results

The usefulness of the fine wire technique would be severely limited if the quality of the recordings from single neurons was poor. It would seem that such large wires should yield very poor signal to noise characteristics relative to conventional microelectrodes with 1-5 μ tips. However, we have had extraordinarily good results with these wires. Figure 6.5 shows one example of a record taken from a Purkinje cell in the cerebellum. Both the simple and complex wave form (arrow) are visible (38). The second record is a red nucleus cell taken during quiet waking periods. Both are representative records, and they are comparable to results obtained with small tipped microelectrodes. Occasionally, two or more neurons do appear on one electrode. Sometimes these neurons can be separated by threshold gating techniques; on other occasions they must be discarded. Additional examples of neurons recorded with this technique are found in Chapters IX and XV of this volume. These brief samples with signal-to-noise ratios

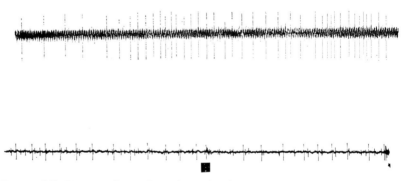

Figure 6.5. Traces of a red nucleus (top) neuron and a cerebellar Purkinje cell (bottom) recorded with 62.5 μ nichrome electrodes. The simple and complex (arrow) waveforms of the Purkinje cell are visible.

of 3/1-5/1 are typical of our better recordings, but S/N of 15/1 have been observed.

An additional benefit obtained by using the flexible wires is the excellent stability of the recordings. To demonstrate the stability of the records over an experimental session, we have monitored a neuron from a completely unrestrained cat through two sleep-wakefulness cycles that included two active sleep periods, several active movement sessions, and some feeding behavior. The recording of this neuron was digitized at 36KHz. Any wave form which crossed a selected voltage (after a forty-five second delay from the previous wave form) was stored on digital tape and plotted on an incremental plotter. Figure 6.6 illustrates the wave form for each discharge of the neuron (after each forty-five second delay) for the entire three hour record. It can be seen that the traces are remarkably stable from beginning to end and that, except for four artifacts from cable movements that triggered the sweep in the middle of the session (columns 4 and 8), the wave forms are very similar.

This figure illustrates three points. First, the wave forms can be very stable. Second, a single neuron, rather than two or more neurons of the same height, was recorded since different neurons would have slightly different shapes even if they had the same height. Third, even following movement indicated by cable noise, the wave forms were not altered. Of the two hundred forty wave forms sampled in this record, only four (less than 2 percent) appear to be different.

The great majority of several hundred neurons which we have studied have been stable throughout recording sessions of three to six hours. On occasion we have recorded neurons which, by a variety of criteria, appeared to be stable over a period of four days or more. We are presently studying the wave forms of such stable neurons to insure that these are indeed identical neurons.

Statistical Treatment of Spike Data

The taped spike records, together with the taped EEG and commentary on the animal's behavior, may be analyzed by a variety of procedures. For quick examination of the edited data, rates

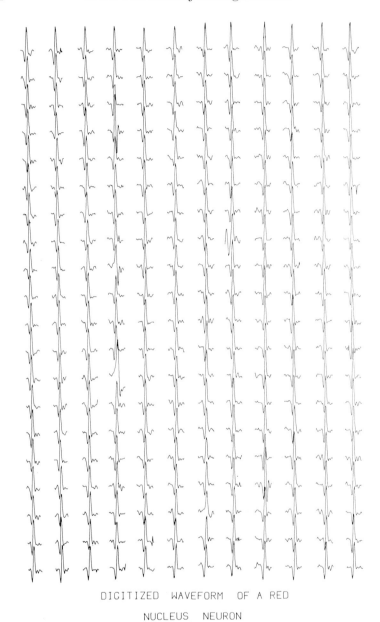

DIGITIZED WAVEFORM OF A RED

NUCLEUS NEURON

Figure 6.6. A continuous sample of waveforms of a red nucleus neuron during a three hour recording which included two sleep cycles and feeding, walking, and grooming behaviors. The computer display program ac-are calculated by an electronic counter. Selected samples of the data may be displayed by the integration device with its cumulative record and/or photographed with a kymograph camera. Most data, however, require some statistical processing of the spike train. For this we use a general purpose laboratory computer.

Our particular laboratory computer (Digital Equipment Corp., PDP-12)[||] is equipped with a display oscilloscope, digital magnetic tape, an analog to digital converter, digital sense lines, an incremental plotter, and a teletype. All of these accessories are useful for analysis of cell discharges.

The times of occurrences of the cell discharges should be stored on some mass storage device of the computer so that they can be subjected to a variety of analyses. Otherwise, for each analysis, one must go through the tedious process of digitizing the record and removing any source of artifact.

Our programs for acquiring and storing event times for spike discharges on the computer are designed to insure that only the activity for one neuron is being saved. We prefer to store times of occurrences of spike events rather than intervals between spikes. Although it is initially easier to store only intervals on a short word length computer, this procedure makes it more difficult to start analysis at any point on the spike train record. Furthermore, an artifact is easier to remove from a time of occurrence record than from an interval record.

We have used a variety of techniques to insure that the neurons we are recording are single neurons. One procedure was outlined in the results section. A record is digitized at a very high rate and the wave forms are frozen on the display scope for inspection, saved on the mass storage device (digital magnetic tape),

---

[||] PDP and FOCAL are registered trademarks of Digital Equipment Corp., Maynard, Massachussetts.

---

cepts each waveform exceeding a predetermined threshold after a forty-five second delay following the preceding sample. The columns of samples are continuous left to right. Note that the waveforms are similar at the beginning and end of the recording session. This unique waveform was selected to demonstrate the stability of recordings obtained with our microwire technique.

and plotted on an incremental plotter. With existing computer programs, the times of occurrence of the spikes can be stored at any discharge rate, but wave forms for each neuron can be saved only if the cell is relatively slow firing. However, we are developing procedures for storing the entire wave form, together with

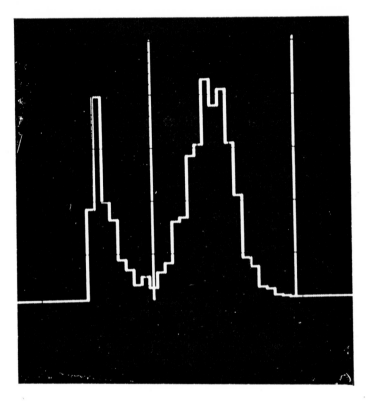

Figure 6.7. An amplitude histogram of the peak heights of all neuronal discharges above a minimum threshold during a specific time period. The frequency of occurrence of each spike height is displayed on an oscilloscope. The investigator can specify with the adjustable cursors (vertical lines) the upper and lower amplitude limits of spikes to be selected. The event times are saved on digital tape. In instances where two or more clearly discriminable amplitude distributions are observed, after selection of the first amplitude band, the display can be recalled for selection of a second amplitude band. This display was generated with the STAP-12 program of Wyss and Handwerker (41).

the time of occurrence for even rapidly firing neurons. In this way an entire record for a behavioral session could be scanned either visually or by a pattern recognition procedure to sort the spikes into neurons of one class or another.

Another way to sort spikes from records is by means of an amplitude histogram (Fig. 6.7). In this procedure the height of a spike is recorded together with its time of occurrence and a histogram of the number of spikes with respect to a specified amplitude is constructed. The times of occurrence of the spikes that appear between two criterion amplitudes can then be sorted by the computer. A number of programs have been developed for such amplitude sorting (8, 41). A sophisticated real time sorting routine which samples the amplitude at two points on the wave shape has also been developed (36).

Once the event times of discharge are stored on a mass storage device such as digital tape, they can be subjected to a wide variety of statistical analyses. We can, for example, examine instantaneous rate discharges at any point on the record as well as the overall rate for the complete record. Since our animals go through sequences of behaviors, the capability to look at short segments of the record is highly desirable. We can also examine the variations in rate or the distribution of intervals over the entire record or any segment of the period.

If the intervals or times of occurrences of spike discharges are stored on digital tape, they can then be accessed by high level easy-to-use languages such as FOCAL and FORTRAN. For example, Figure 6.8 is a scattergram of 256 intervals plotted in a linear and log form. This display was written by a two line FOCAL program; the intervals can be rearranged in a variety of ways to make it easier to recognize the spike firing pattern.

Since one of the chief advantages of using the fine wire bundle technique is that cells from interacting structures can be studied simultaneously, we use various statistical procedures to examine the interaction between two brain areas. We are interested, for example, in studying the interaction of orbital cortex and brain stem neurons or serotonergic neurons in the raphe and the cells to which these neurons project in the forebrain.

One very powerful spike train package which includes an am-

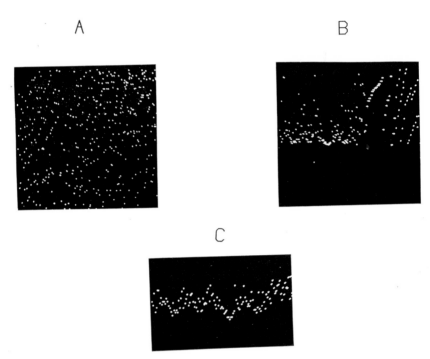

Figure 6.8. This figure demonstrates the ease of displaying interval discharges with a high level language on a small computer. The scattergrams display: A. The intervals of successive spikes plotted in a linear mode from a red nucleus neuron discharging during SWS. B. Intervals plotted in a linear fashion from a hippocampal neuron firing in a regular bursting pattern with EEG theta activity. C. The same intervals as B, plotted in a logarithmic scale. These display routines were written with a two line FOCAL program.

plitude histogram program, together with a wide variety of acquisition and analysis programs for single or multiple records, is a set or programs called STAP-12 (spike train analysis package). These programs were developed by Wyss and Handwerker (41). The event times of spike trains are stored on digital tape as labelled files and can be accessed by a wide variety of spike analyzer programs including interval histograms, frequency histograms, auto and cross correlation, and cross interval statistics. The labelled files can also be accessed by high level computer languages such as FOCAL and FORTRAN.

DISCUSSION

This technique has been used successfully in the amygdala (19, Chapter XVI of this volume), medial, lateral, and anterior hypothalamus, midbrain tegmentum and ventral tegmental area (18), hippocampus (13), VPL and anterior thalamus, red nucleus (Chapter IX, midbrain dorsal raphe nucleus (Chapter XV), and septum (14).

Success in resolving single neurons with the fine wire electrode procedure varies and probably depends on the size of neurons in the brain site and the density with which neurons are packed. In a recent study (14) which employed bundles of fourteen immovable wires of 62.5 μ diameter implanted in various diencephalic sites, a success ratio of one neuron for every eight wires was obtained. If the electrodes are connected to a microdrive, then a much larger number of neurons can be recorded (.5 to 2/wire).

We believe that the unit activity we are sampling does not differ from the recordings obtained with conventional microelectrodes. Very similar discharge patterns have been observed when conventional small tipped microelectrodes and fine wire microelectrodes have been employed in the same brain sites. For example, very slow neurons are seen in the amygdala (7, 19), thalamic relay neurons appear to have similar bimodal interval distributions during sleep (14, 26, 35), and raphe neurons appear to exhibit the same slow rhythmic pattern of firing (1, 2, Chapter XV). Our technique also meets the standards suggested by Evarts (9) for the recording of single neurons from intact animals: (1) The initial sign of the action potential is negative, indicating that the electrode tip is not impinging on the cell body; (2) the temporal pattern of the neural activity remains stable with small movements of the electrode (10-30 μ); and (3) the neurons can be separated as individual units. In addition, we offer two criteria that the firing pattern of neurons is not affected by the large tipped electrodes.

First, when we record neurons for long time periods, similar discharge patterns during similar behaviors are observed. That is, the recordings are stable, while injured neurons would be expected to deteriorate. Second, we do not see stereotyped dis-

charge patterns across different brain structures, but rather see
a variety of patterns depending on the brain site. For example, we
see slow regular neurons in the raphe with a unimodal distribution of intervals, medium rate neurons in the thalamus with a
bimodal interval distribution, and fast firing neurons in the cerebellum with a unimodal distribution. Injured neurons might be
expected to exhibit characteristic *injury* discharges.

These large tipped microelectrodes probably are selectively
biased toward larger neurons (39). We have used 25 μ, 50 μ, and
62.5 μ wires in our studies. Although we have not adequately
tested all of these electrode diameters on neurons of uniform
size to determine their efficacy in separating neurons from each
other and from surrounding noise, our impression is that smaller
wires are more efficient in obtaining single neurons. The difficulty in mechanical handling and soldering very small diameter
wire increases very rapidly with decreasing size, however, and
wires smaller than 25 μ do not readily penetrate the brain without deflecting. We have not explored the possibility of electro-
lytically etching the tips of the larger (40-60 μ) wires and exploit-
ing both a small tip diameter and the physical properties of larger
wires, but this remains a distinct possibility (22).

There appear to be some brain areas where the fine wire electrode technique is less successful. These areas include the cerebral
cortex and other subcortical sites like the lateral hypothalamus.
In the case of the dorsal cortex, the lack of a flexible section of
wire above the recording site appears to prevent stable recordings. The study of ventral cortex, approached through the brain,
has not been attempted. In the case of the lateral hypothalamus
the cells may be too small or the mixture of cells and fibers may
impede the approach to neurons by microwires. Whatever the
reasons, this technique cannot be universally recommended for
all brain sites. However, in those areas where it does work, it
works extremely well.

A number of additional problems have not yet been examined.
We have followed recordings from some subcortical neurons during microdrive movements of up to 300 μ. Fields of 100 μ have
been measured for cortical neurons (25). The difference may be
due to the type of neuron, the sensitivity of our relatively low im-

pedance electrodes, or uneven movement of our microwire within the brain leading to an overestimation of movement. Also needed is a systematic study of neuron size sampling (39). Although we obtain stable recordings, a histological study of the tissue damage created by the electrodes may indicate some limitations on the procedure, such as the undesirability of repeated penetrations.

Noise from cable movement artifacts in this system is minimized by the use of low noise cable. It may be necessary, however, for the study of very violent behaviors, such as that which may occur during sexual or aggressive activity, to mount small input amplifiers directly on the animal's head. These amplifiers normally should have high input impedance, low output impedance, and perhaps some gain. Just a reduction of impedance from the source electrodes is usually sufficient to make recording much easier. A number of miniaturized amplifiers using field effect transistors have been described (6, 29) and amplifiers mounted on a single transistor case are now available commercially (Transidyne, Haer).#

Some investigators, wishing to rid themselves of the restraints and the noise imposed by cables, have employed a telemetry system (5, 23, Chapter III). This appears to be the ultimate manner of recording for the investigator interested in unit concomitants of behavior. A limitation of the telemetry procedure is the number of channels of data that can be accommodated without cross talk between channels and without exceeding a reasonable bulk to be carried by the animal. In sleep research we normally record EMG, eye movement, and EEG activity of several macroelectrodes in addition to several channels of unit data. However, it should be possible to build a miniaturized FM multiplexer system for the low frequency data and to send this data over one FM channel with demodulation at the receiver into the separate data records. With the band width afforded by the McElligott transmitter (23), one such channel could probably handle six to ten slow wave records, leaving the remaining channels for unit data.

Transidyne General Corp., 462 S. Wagner Road, Ann Arbor, Michigan 48103; Frederick Haer & Co., P.O. Box 2138, Ann Arbor, Michigan 48106.

An FM/AM multiplexing system has already been developed for EEG telemetry (42).

A number of investigators have designed ingenious procedures for driving etched tip, stiff microelectrodes to brain sites. The procedures for lowering the microelectrodes through brain sites have incorporated both mechanical (17, 20, 40) and hydraulic microdrives (10, 16, 21, 30, 34). These microdrives have involved a degree of mechanical sophistication since they incorporate highly finished chambers and precision drilling. The procedure described here avoids this requirement. One advantage of the hydraulic microdrives is that electrodes can be advanced through the brain without disturbing the animal. However, since we normally record over several hours, through a complete behavioral sequence, we seldom need to move the electrode during testing.

The long term stability provided by this procedure has not been exploited. It should be possible to study the time course of activity in individual neurons produced by such changes as interruption of specific input pathways, experience or learning, long term biochemical changes, or development of seizures.

One of the chief advantages of using bundles of these fine wires is that large numbers of neurons can be recorded within the very limited area of the tips of the bundle (.25-.5 mm). We have on occasion recorded from eight neurons simultaneously in one brain site. Interactions can be studied between neurons within each site and between neurons recorded from bundles implanted in different sites. Using three implanted bundles we have seen as many as twenty neurons at one time on different electrodes from a single cat. If two or more neurons recorded from one electrode can be separated by threshold gates, then the total number of cells that can be recorded soon becomes very large indeed. This ability to examine interactions between brain areas will be of enormous use in studying how different brain areas affect each other. Moreover, we are now capable of examining the output of many neurons and relating this output to behavioral patterns. However, in order to utilize and interpret this information, statistical procedures for handling the discharge patterns of many neurons and interactions between groups of neurons must be developed.

Spike train statistics for handling the interactions of large groups of neurons are only at an early stage of development. There are a variety of single (24, 31) and multi-train statistics such as the cross correlation and cross interval histograms (11, 32). There are also scatter displays such as the joint peristimulus time histogram (12) for examining the interactions of two or more spike trains, and frequency histograms for looking at the total neuronal output of a group of spikes (41). We are moving in the direction of developing analytic procedures for handling large numbers of simultaneously recorded neurons.

SUMMARY

This chapter describes a single cell recording procedure for use in behaving animals which incorporates the use of bundles of flexible fine wires and a simple microdrive. This procedure provides three principal advantages: (1) stable recordings lasting hours or days; (2) simultaneous recordings of several neurons; and (3) simplicity of application. Long term recordings may be achieved even in actively moving animals. The quality of the recordings in terms of signal-to-noise ratio matches those which are seen by extracellular small tipped conventional microelectrodes in chronic animals. This paper describes the electrode material, implantation technique, recording facilities, data analysis procedures and discusses strengths and weaknesses of the technique.

REFERENCES

1. Aghajanian, G. K., W. E. Foote, and M. H. Sheard. Lysergic acid diethydamide: Sensitive neuronal units in the midbrain raphe. *Science*, 161:706-708, 1968.

2. Aghajanian, G. K., A. W. Graham, and M. H. Sheard. Serotonin-containing neurons in brain. Depression of firing by monamine oxidase inhibitors. *Science*, 169:1100-1102, 1970.

3. Akert, K., and W. I. Welkes. Problems and methods of anatomical localization. In D. E. Sheer (Ed.) *Electrical Stimulation of the Brain*. University of Texas Press, Austin, 1961, pp. 251-260.

4. Amassian, V. E. Microelectrode studies of the cerebral cortex. In C. Pfeiffer and J. Smythies (Eds.) *International Review of Neurobiology*. Academic Press, New York, 1961, pp. 67-136.

5. Beechey, P., and D. W. Lincoln. A miniature FM transmitter for the radio-telemetry of unit activity. *J. Physiol.*, 203:5-6, 1969.

6. Brakel, S., T. Babb, J. Mahnke, and M. Verzeano. A compact amplifier for extracellular recording. *Physiol. Behav.* 6:731-733, 1971.

7. Creutzfeldt, O. D., F. R. Bell, and W. R. Adey. The activity of neurons in the amygdala of the cat following afferent stimulation. *Prog. Brain Res.*, 3:31-49, 1963.

8. Dill, V. C., P. C. Lockemann, and K. I. Naka. An attempt to analyze multiunit recordings. *Electroenceph. clin. Neurophysiol.*, 28:79-82, 1970.

9. Evarts, E. V. Methods for recording activity of individual neurons in moving animals. In R. F. Rushmer (Ed.) *Methods in Medical Research*, Vol. 11. Medical Year Book Publishers Inc., Chicago, 1966, pp. 241-250.

10. Evarts, E. V. A technique for recording activity of subcortical neurons in moving animals. *Electroenceph. clin. Neurophysiol.*, 24:83-86, 1968.

11. Gerstein, G. L. Functional association of neurons: Detection and interpretation. In F. O. Schmitt (Ed.) *The Neurosciences Second Study Program.* Rockefeller University Press, New York, 1970, pp. 648-661.

12. Gerstein, G. L., and D. H. Perkel. Simultaneously recorded trains of action potentials: analysis and functional interpretation. *Science,* 164: 828-830, 1969.

13. Harper, R. M. Activity of single neurons during sleep and altered states of consciousness. *Psychophysiol.*, 7:312, 1971 (abstract).

14. Harper, R. M. Behavioral and electrophysiological studies of sleep and animal hypnosis. Ph.D. Thesis, McMaster University, Canada, 1968.

15. Hess, W. R. *Beiträge zur physiologie des hirnstammes.* Leipzig, Thieme, 1932.

16. Hubel, D. H. Single unit activity in striate cortex of unrestrained cats. *J. Physiol.*, 147:226-238, 1959.

17. Humphrey, D. R. A chronically implantable multiple microelectrode system with independent control of electrode position. *Electroenceph. clin. Neurophysiol.*, 29:616-620, 1970.

18. Jacobs, B. J., R. M. Harper, and D. J. McGinty. Neuronal coding of motivational level during sleep. *Physiol. Behav.*, 5:1139-1143, 1970.

19. Jacobs, B. J., and D. J. McGinty. Amygdala unit activity during sleep and waking. *Exper. Neurol.*, 33:1-15, 1971.

20. John, E. R. and P. P. Morgades. A technique for the chronic implantation of multiple movable microelectrodes. *Electroenceph. clin. Neurophysiol.*, 27:205-208, 1969.

21. Katsuki, J., K. Murata, N. Suga, and T. Tokenaka. Electrical activity

of cortical auditory neurons of unanesthetized and unrestrained cats. *Proc. Jap. Acad.*, 35:571-574, 1959.

22. Marg, E., and J. E. Adams. Indwelling multiple microelectrodes in the brain. *Electroenceph. clin. Neurophysiol.*, 23:277-280, 1967.

23. McElligott, J. G., J. R. Zweizig, and R. T. Kado. A miniaturized telemetry device for the transmission of the electrical activity of single nerve cells in the brain. *Proc. of the National Telemetry Conference*, Washington, D.C., 207-210, April 1969.

24. Moore, G. P., D. H. Perkel, and J. P. Segundo. Statistical analysis and functional interpretation of neuronal spike data. *Ann. Rev. Physiol.* 28:493, 1966.

25. Mountcastle, V. B., P. W. Davies, and A. L. Berman. Response properties of neurons of cat's somatic sensory cortex to peripheral stimuli. *J. Neurophysiol.*, 20:374, 1957.

26. Mukhametov, L. M., G. Rizzolotti, and A. Seitun. An analysis of the spontaneous activity of lateral geniculate neurons and of optic tract fibers in free moving cats. *Arch. ital. Biol.*, 108:325-347, 1970.

27. O'Keefe, J., and H. Bouma. Complex sensory properties of certain amygdala units in the freely moving cat. *Exper. Neurol.*, 23:384-398, 1969.

28. Olds, J. Operant conditioning of single unit responses. *Proc. XXIII Int. Congr. Physiol. Sci.*, Tokyo, 372-380, 1965.

29. Oomura, Y., H. Ooyama, and K. Yoneda. Minaturized high input impedance preamplifier. *Physiol. Behav.*, 2:93-95, 1967.

30. Oomura, Y., H. Ooyama, F. Naka, and T. Yamamoto. Microelectrode positioners for chronic animals. *Physiol. Behav.*, 2:89-91, 1967.

31. Perkel, D. H., G. L. Gerstein, and G. P. Moore. Neuronal spike trains and stochastic point processes. I. The single spike train. *Biophysical Jr.*, 7:391-418, 1967.

32. Perkel, D. H., G. L. Gerstein, and G. P. Moore. Neuronal spike trains and stochastic point processes. II. Simultaneous spike trains. *Biophysical Jr.*, 7:419-440, 1967.

33. Phillips, M. I., and J. Olds. Unit activity: motivation dependent responses from midbrain neurons. *Science*, 165:1269-1271, 1969.

34. Ricci, G., B. Doane, and H. H. Jasper. Microelectrode studies of conditioning: technique and preliminary results. In *Premier Congrès International des Sciences Neurologiques*, Bruxelles, 1957 Réunions Plénières (Brussels: Editions "Acta Medica Belgica," 1957), pp. 401-415.

35. Sakukura, H. Spontaneous and evoked unitary activities of cat lateral geniculate neurons in sleep and wakefulness. *Jap. J. Physiol.*, 18: 23-42, 1968.

36. Simon, W. The real time sorting of neuro-electric action potentials in

multiple unit studies. *Electroenceph. clin. Neurophysiol.* 18:192-195, 1965.

37. Strumwasser, F. Long term recording from single neurons in brain of unrestrained mammals. *Science,* 127:469-470, 1958.

38. Thatch, W. T., Jr. Discharge of Purkinje and cerebellar nuclear neurons during rapidly alternating arm movements in the monkey. *J. Neurophysiol.,* 31:785-797, 1968.

39. Towe, A. L., and G. W. Harding. Extracellular microelectrode sampling bias. *Exper. Neurol.,* 29:366-381, 1970.

40. Wall, P. D., J. Freeman, and D. Major. Dorsal horn cells in spinal and freely moving rats. *Exper. Neurol.,* 19:519-529, 1967.

41. Wyss, U. R., and H. Handwerker. STAP-12: A library system for on-line assimilation and off-line analysis of event/time data. *Computer Programs in Biomedicine,* 1:209-218, 1971.

42. Zweizig, J. R., R. T. Kado, J. Hanley, and W. R. Adey. The design and use of an FM/AM radio telemetry system for multi-channel recording of biological data. *IEEE Trans. on Bio. Med. Engng.* *BME-14,* 4:230-238, 1967.

Chapter VII

IMPLANTABLE MONOLITHIC WAFER RECORDING ELECTRODES FOR NEUROPHYSIOLOGY

R. LLINÁS, C. NICHOLSON and K. JOHNSON

O NE OF THE KEY PROBLEMS in the understanding of the function of the nervous system is that neural information is not solely organized in a temporo-spatial pattern of nerve impulses in a single fiber but is disseminated by a parallel multichannel system.

In order to study the properties of "messages" transmitted through many channels in parallel, one solution is to monitor the information from as many of these parallel channels as possible. The usual electrophysiological techniques, although allowing almost perfect recording of a single channel, are incapable of handling extensive multichannel recording. For this reason, we are studying the possibility of developing a novel method of recording electrical activity from the brain. The method is based on the well known fact that transected nerves, especially in lower vertebrates, tend to grow back to their correct target centers after apposition of the distal and proximal stumps (see review by Jacobson, 1967).

Recent research by A. Marks (1971 and personal communication) at Johns Hopkins University and by R. Stein (personal communication) at the University of Alberta has demonstrated that nerves will grow through a gold tube or other barriers such as Gelfoam® (Upjohn). These observations led us to consider a recording electrode in the form of a thin film of an insulating material with a large number of small holes in it, each of which has a dis-

Preparation of this report was partially supported by U.S.P.H.S. research grant NS 09916 from the National Institute of Neurological Diseases and Stroke.

crete conductive surround (*e.g.,* gold) that may be connected to an individual amplifier. This film is interposed in the path of a bundle of growing fibers so that they will traverse the holes as they grow toward their neural targets. The fibers will then be accessible for recording, since each nerve impulse generates an all-or-none action current across the nerve membrane which can be picked up by the conductive surround of the holes in the form of a potential difference between a gold nerve interface and an indifferent electrode (see below).

GENERAL CONCEPT OF WAFER ELECTRODES

In the simplest form, a wafer electrode for single extra-axonal recording would consist of a glass or ceramic substrate 1 to 2 mm in diameter, as shown in Figure 7.1. Deposited on the sub-

SIMPLE ELECTRODE

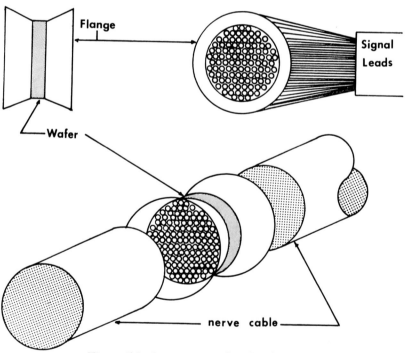

Figure 7.1. Construction of wafer electrode.

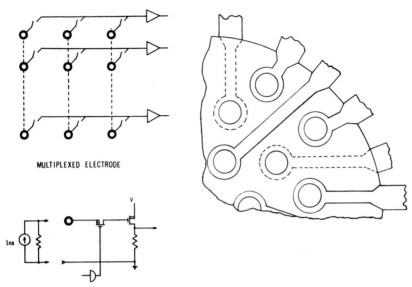

Figure 7.2. Connection of sensing rings.

strate is a gold film from which circles 50-60 μ in diameter have been etched. Through the center of each circle a 25 μ hole is drilled by pulsed laser, leaving a gold ring. A lead from each ring runs to the edge of the substrate and terminates on the supporting flange. These connecting leads are covered with an insulating material, leaving only the gold rings around each hole exposed. A terminating cable wired to the supporting flange is used to sense the presence of a signal on each gold ring.

The entire wafer is inserted between the ends of a severed and expanded nerve. As the process of regeneration takes place, the nerve ends will attempt to grow back to their target cells and, in doing so, will pass through the holes in the wafer and make contact with the gold rings. When the animal responds to some external stimulation, different nerve fiber paths will be activated, and if one of the fibers passes through a hole in the wafer and conducts action potentials, the signal is sensed by a gold ring.

This approach, although simple, has several inherent problems. The first limitation is in the number of leads that can physically be terminated on the wafer. Secondly, the size of the cable leading from the brain to the external amplifier is limited and, finally, noise levels and cross talk increase with the number of wires. A better approach is to multiplex the leads from a large number of sensing rings down to a practical number (10-30) on the wafer, as shown in Figure 7.2. This involves masking multiplex gates, amplifiers and a counter circuit onto the wafer via monolithic techniques.

The number of sensing rings and/or multiplexed leads is not critical. Multiplexing of the leads can be accomplished in groups of ten to thirty because a low sampling rate of only 100 kHz is required. Likewise, the number of sensing rings is a flexible quantity since one cannot hope to sample all fibers in a bundle. For example, a typical sensory nerve bundle (1 mm in diameter) may have twenty thousand individual fibers ranging in size from 0.2 to 5.0 μ in diameter. Assuming a wafer of two hundred holes was available, an average of two to five fibers would grow through each hole; the other fibers around the electrode. An *as required* electronic system can be built around the wafer to convert the biological data into suitable form for analysis.

MONOLITHIC WAFER

As shown in Figure 7.2 (lower left), an equivalent model of the biological signal source can be represented by a current source of 1 nano-amp into a 1 megohm resistor. This signal source appears as a pulse of current crossing the membrane of the nerve fiber and sensed by the gold ring. The gold ring is connected to a MOSFET multiplex gate and MOSFET source follower. A functional schematic of the complete circuit is shown in Figure 7.3. By fabricating the gold rings alternately on each side of the wafer and bonding to the MOSFET multiplex gates, a possible physical arrangement might appear as shown in Figure 7.4. From a practical standpoint, placing the rings alternately on each side effectively doubles the recording surface area. Assuming this layout is practical, the number of rings that could be placed on a wafer is a function of the MOSFET device size. For the properties shown, gold rings 50 μ square, with 75 μ centers, would represent about one hundred thirty holes per circular millimeter area. The following paragraphs attempt to outline a fabrication which appears practical. However, since the actual details

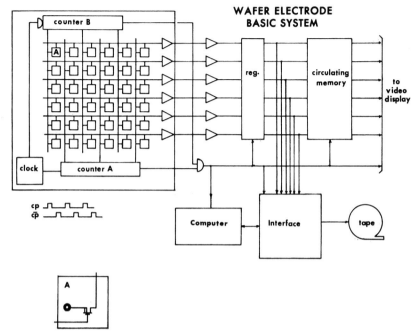

Figure 7.3. Diagram of multiplex electrode system.

TOP VIEW - NOT ENCAPSULATED

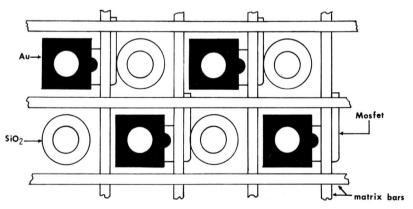

Figure 7.4. Detail of integrated MOSFET sensing ring array; top view.

CROSS SECTION - ENCAPSULATED

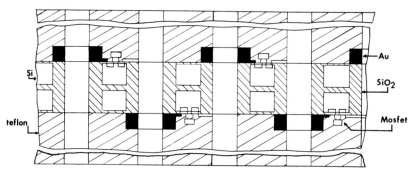

Fig. 7.5. Detail of integrated MOSFET sensing ring array; side view showing double sandwich construction.

of the monolithic manufacturing process are not available outside the manufacturing firms this procedure serves mainly as a description of the problem.

As shown in Figure 7.5, a cross sectional area of the complete unit appears as a sandwich of two silicon wafers placed back to back and insulated by a thick layer of silicon dioxide. Initially, 50-75 μ holes are drilled in the sandwiched wafer. Since contact between the nerve fiber and the silicon substrate would effectively short circuit the signal, the holes must be refilled with a silicon dioxide insulator. Next, the wafer is covered on both sides with gold and etched, leaving the square pads shown in Figure 7.5. Conventional techniques can then be employed to make the MOSFET devices and interconnecting matrix leads. Last, a layer of dielectric substance with suitable inert biological properties (*e.g.*, Teflon) is used to encapsulate the entire device and 25 μ holes are drilled through all five layers. The total thickness of the wafer is critical. It must be thick enough to have mechanical stability, but not so thick that the nerve fibers cannot find their way through the holes. A practical thickness appears to be 0.5 mm and will depend, in part, upon the type of pulsed laser available for hole drilling.

CONCLUSION

It is evident that the development of a monolithic wafer recording electrode, although technically difficult, is within the state of the art for modern electronic technology. Due to the specialized nature of the wafer electrode, its development is beyond the economic capabilities of research groups in most universities. However, its ultimate usefulness in brain research, artificial protheses and possible brain computer hybridization could make the development of an electrode such as that outlined here a worthwhile project.

REFERENCES

Jacobson, M.: Starting points for research in the ontogeny of behavior. In *Major Problems in Developmental Biology*, ed. M. Locke, pp. 339-383. Academic Press, New York, 1967.

Marks, A. F.: Acceptance of implanted plastic structures by the brain of the mature rat. *Anatom. Rec.* 169:375a, 1971.

PART TWO

UNIT ACTIVITY STUDIES

UNIT ANALYSIS OF THE EFFECTS OF MOTIVATING STIMULI IN THE AWAKE ANIMAL: PAIN AND SELF STIMULATION

K. L. CASEY and J. J. KEENE

THE TECHNIQUE OF UNIT analysis in the awake animal is especially suited for the study of neural mechanisms related to pain and other motivational stimuli. The study of other sensory systems such as vision, audition, and the discriminative somesthetic senses, is facilitated by the ability to manipulate discrete physical parameters of the stimulus and subsequently relate the neural responses to the discriminative capacity of the behaving organism subjected to the same stimuli. Noxious stimuli, however, do not have well defined physical parameters and may elicit responses in neural populations mediating somatic or autonomic reflexes which may be independent of the more complex aversive behavior of the whole organism. In the awake animal, however, an operational definition may be employed: a painful or noxious somatic stimulus is one which the organism will work to escape and avoid. In studying the neural mechanisms of pain, therefore, it is especially important to ultimately relate the activity of a neural population to the aversive behavior of the organism. The same rationale applies to the study of other systems mediating nonaversive or approach behaviors.

In this report, we will briefly summarize the approach which has been and is currently being used in this laboratory in studying pain and other neural systems of motivational significance.

THE PAIN SYSTEM

Peripheral Fibers

Experimental and clinical observations in man have shown that finely myelinated (A-delta) and unmyelinated (C) afferent fiber activity is necessary for pain sensation (10, 25). These observations have been supported by single fiber recordings in cat and monkey: both A-delta and C fiber populations include afferents responding only to thermal or mechanical stimuli which are presumably noxious to the awake animal (2, 20). The exploration of central nervous system (CNS) structures forming part of the pain system can, therefore, be reasonably guided by the responses of central cells to A-delta and/or C fiber input.

Central Pathways: Guiding Observations

It is well established that lesions of the anterolateral quadrant of the spinal cord interfere with normal pain sensation (26). Spinal cord cells responding primarily to presumably noxious stimuli and to A-delta or C fiber input have been identified (9, 22), but the course of their ascending projections and their role in reflex or sensory mechanisms remains to be clarified. Ideally, it would be desirable to relate the activity of spinal neurons to measures of aversive behavior in the awake animal. Although spinal unit recording has been accomplished in the awake rat (27), the associated technical problems have not encouraged its general use.

The study of supraspinal structures, however, can be guided by the ascending projections of the anterolateral cord (16) and by the cellular responses to noxious stimuli or to A-delta or C fiber input. Spino-thalamic projections of the anterolateral cord, for example, terminate not only in the ventrobasal thalamus (VB), but also in the intralaminar and posterior (PO) group of thalamic nuclei (16). In the anesthetized cat, some PO neurons respond only to presumably noxious stimuli (21) and, in man, electrolytic lesions in medial and intralaminar thalamus interfere with normal appreciation of pain (15). Unit activity has been recorded from the PO and medial-intralaminar thalamus of awake squirrel monkeys seated in a restraining chair during the application of noxious stimuli defined on the basis of consistent withdrawal of the stimulated body part (8). Under those conditions, it could be shown that units which appeared to respond only to noxious stimuli during sleep or light anesthesia responded to light tactile stimuli when the animal was awake. No units were found to respond exclusively to noxious stimuli, but twenty-eight units, recorded principally from the medial-intralaminar and posterolateral thalamus, responded to noxious stimuli with discharges which were consistently and distinctly more rapid and prolonged than the responses to innocuous stimuli. Control recordings during active and passive movement showed that the increased responses could not be attributed to the withdrawal movement itself (8).

The above observations suggested the importance and feasibility of using the awake preparation in the unit analysis of pain mechanisms. Since anatomical (16), physiological (1), and behavioral data (11, 18) indicated that the medullary reticular formation in the region of the nucleus gigantocellularis (NGC) might form part of the central pain sensory system, unanesthetized decerebrate and cerebellectomized cats could be used to examine the responses of NGC units to natural and electrical somatic stimuli (6). In this preparation, anodal polarization of a cutaneous nerve was used to deliver isolated A-delta and C fiber inputs (4). The results showed that sixty-three of the ninety-six units responding to somatic stimuli were affected primarily or exclusively by A-delta fibers and by presumably noxious stimuli (6). The anatomical evidence that NGC receives somatic input via the anterolateral cord was also confirmed. These findings provided the basis for unit analysis of NGC activity in the awake cat (5, 7).

Bulboreticular Unit Recording in the Awake Cat

Technical Aspects

The essential features of the method have been presented elsewhere (5, 7). The cats were trained in a two way barrier-crossing escape task, using electrical stimulation of the superficial radial nerve via an implanted silastic cuff electrode as the aversive stimulus. NGC unit activity was recorded by advancing a stainless steel microelectrode through a permanently mounted rubber sealed mercury pool which contacted the uninsulated part of the electrode shaft as the tip entered the medulla. The electrode was fastened within a hollow nylon screw which could

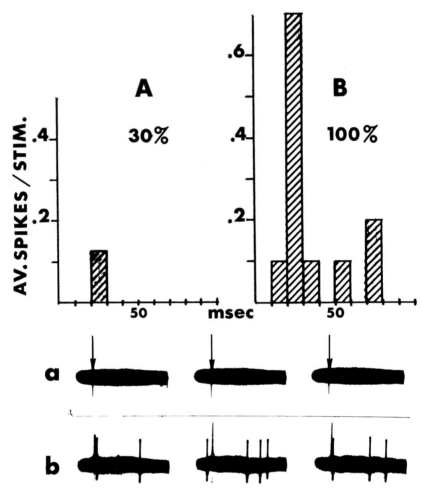

Figure 8.1. NGC unit response to cutaneous nerve stimulation in the awake cat. A: Poststimulus histogram constructed from thirty stimulus trials using 30 percent of the current which elicited escape during observation of this unit. Initial three sweeps of unit response shown in (a). B: Same as (A) except stimulating current elicited escape on the twenty-fifth trial (100 percent escape current); unit response shown in (b).

be left in place, permitting subsequent stimulation at the recording sites. Electrolytic lesions were used to identify electrode position at histology.

Results

In agreement with the results of the acute experiments, a population of NGC units were found to respond either exclusively
or primarily to mechanical stimuli which caused withdrawal and
vocalization. Of fifty-three cells systematically tested with nerve
stimulation, thirty-nine showed increasing poststimulus responses as the stimulus current was raised to levels eliciting escape
(Figs. 8.1 and 8.2). Figure 8.3 summarizes the results of the nerve
stimulation experiments, showing that the poststimulus response
of the pooled population increases with stimulus intensity and
reaches the maximum observed for each cell when escape current
is attained. Figure 8.4 shows that interstimulus activity also increases as the animal orients toward the barrier and prepares to

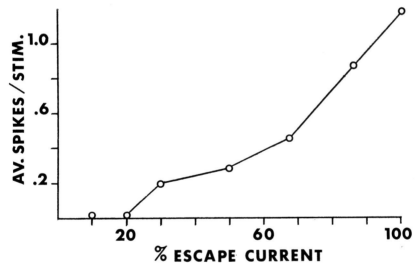

Figure 8.2. Graph of stimulus response function of NGC unit shown in
Figure 1. Stimulus strength expressed as percent of current required to
elicit escape. Response function averaged from the sum of unit discharges
appearing within one hundred msec following a total of thirty stimuli at
each current strength.

escape. Statistical measures indicate that the time locked response to the nerve stimulus also increases near escape levels; control observations fail to reveal any relation between a specific motor act and unit discharge (5). In addition, stimulation applied through the microelectrode was shown to be an effective escape stimulus, the sites with lowest thresholds for eliciting escape (25 μA, 0.2 msec. duration pulses at 100/sec) overlapping with the location of escape related unit activity (3). NGC stimulation could be

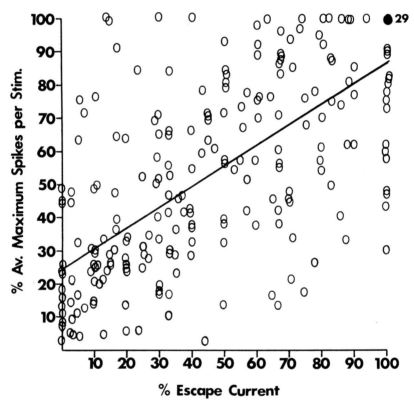

Figure 8.3. Pooled stimulus response relation of thirty-nine NGC units each with excitatory responses tested at several stimulus strengths (percent escape current). The response measure is expressed as a percentage of the maximum response observed for each unit. Note that twenty-nine points overlap at the upper right 100 percent intersection. Analysis of variance shows the regression is significant ($P < 10^{-10}$); $r = 0.69$.

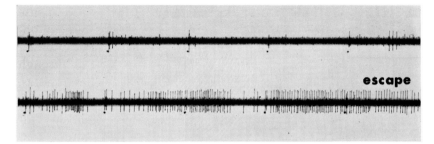

Figure 8.4. NGC unit activity during nerve stimulation in awake cat. Upper record shows low level of unit response and interstimulus discharge during one per second stimulation (dots below records) below escape current levels. Lower record, at escape current levels, shows consistent unit driving and increased interstimulus discharge for at least four seconds before escape was executed.

used as the unconditioned stimulus in avoidance training, shaping operant behavior, and usually elicited escape on the initial NGC stimulus trials (3). The results thus confirmed previous observations that NGC stimulation elicited escape in the rat (13).

These experiments in the cat have encouraged us to use NGC stimulation as an aversive stimulus in further studies of CNS mechanisms related to pain and their interaction with other neural systems of motivational significance.

THE SELF-STIMULATION SYSTEM

NGC neurons (24) and a major system of collaterals from the medial forebrain bundle (MFB) in the lateral hypothalamus (17) both project into medial thalamus (MT). Intracranial stimulation of NGC and MFB elicits escape (3, 13) and self stimulation (19) respectively. The projections from these structures to the MT region may play a role in the production of escape and self stimulation behavior.

NGC and MFB Effects on MT Units in the Acute Rat

Data obtained from rats demonstrate a direct effect of NGC and MFB stimulation on MT units (12). In the anesthetized rat, NGC stimulation at sites responding to peripheral noxious stimuli has elicited, at latencies as low as 5.0 msec, excitation of thir-

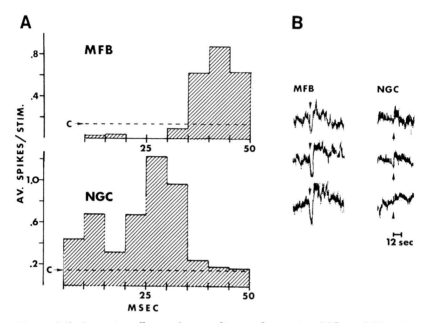

Figure 8.5. Opposite effects of rewarding and aversive ICS on MT units. MFB and NGC stimulation (.5 msec pulses, 500 μ A) elicited (1) self-stimulation and escape behavior, respectively, and (2) opposite post-stimulus patterns of excitation and inhibition (A) as well as (3) opposite changes in discharge rate lasting several seconds (B) in MT units. A: Post-stimulus histograms for one of several similar units in posterior dorsal medial thalamus. During the period that MFB inhibits the unit with reference to control rate (C), NGC excites it. During the following period in which MFB excites the unit, NGC has no effect. B: Polygraph records of integrated marker pulses triggered by a parafascicularis unit showing discharge rate over time. Trains (60 Hz, .2 sec) of MFB stimulation (arrows), identical to those for which the animal selfstimulated, consistently inhibited the spikes for five seconds. Similar trains of NGC stimulation (arrows) consistently increased the spike rate for at least five seconds.

ty-five of sixty-nine units in MT regions including parafascicularis and the dorsal medial and intralaminar nuclei. In anesthetized and cerveau isole rats, unit recording in MT regions including the anterior, dorsal medial, ventral medial, reunients, and para-fascicularis nuclei, reveals that seventy-two of ninety-two units respond to MFB stimulation with latencies as low as 1.2 msec. MFB stimulation has been observed to produce three kinds of responses in the dorsal medial nucleus of thalamus: (1) slow wave recruiting with repetitive stimulation at 8 Hz, (2) excitation in the first forty to fifty msec. after the stimulus, followed by inhibition lasting up to one hundred msec and (3) decreased excitation with higher frequency (20 to 100 Hz) stimulation. These three effects usually occur together and may be uniquely associated with MFB stimulation since stimulation in medial hypothalamus or cerebral peduncle does not produce all three of these responses.

In the anesthetized and cerveau isole rat, it has also been found that stimulation of areas eliciting escape (NGC or the reticular formation lateral to the posterior commissure) and self stimulation (MFB) both affect thirty-five of the fifty-one units driven by one of these inputs to the dorsal medial and intralaminar nuclei of thalamus (Figs. 8.5 and 8.6). One half of the cells responding to both reticular and MFB stimulation show similar responses. These effects include poststimulus patterns of excitation and inhibition as well as increases or decreases in discharge

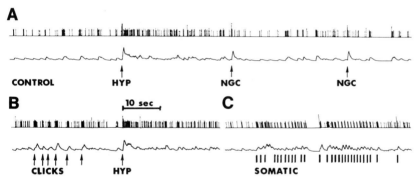

Figure 8.6. Convergence of sensory and motivational systems on a unit in the region of the anterior dorsal and anterior ventral nuclei of thalamus. A-C: sections of a continuous polygraph record of pulses (upper) and their integration (lower) marking discharge of the unit. HYP: Trains (60 Hz, .2 sec, 350 μ A) of far lateral hypothalamic stimulation produced excitation of the unit for more than ten seconds; the rat bar pressed for these trains. NGC: Similar trains of dorsal medial NGC stimulation, suprathreshold for eliciting escape behavior, suppressed unit discharge for more than ten seconds. Auditory stimuli (clicks) and light brushing of the hair (somatic) also consistently produced bursts of spikes.

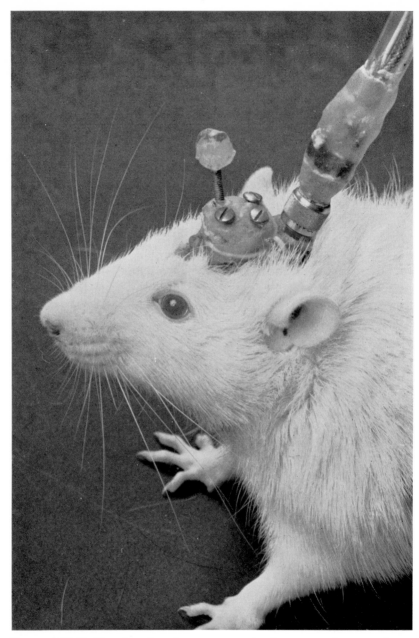

Figure 8.7. Skull pedestal and connections for brain stimulation and mi-croelectrode recording in the awake rat. The screw projecting from the

rate with higher frequencies of supra-threshold stimulation. The remaining half of the units show opposite responses to reticular and MFB stimulation.

Unit Recordings in the Awake Rat

These unit responses are currently being explored by correlating the behavioral effects of NGC and MFB stimulation with the activity of MT units. MT units are being recorded in awake, unrestrained rats with movable microelectrodes and stimulating electrodes in NGC and MFB. A modification of the system for chronic unit recording with a moveable microelectrode developed by Ranck (23) is shown in Figure 8.7. This modification allows four different paths of electrode excursion in the brain.

Units recorded thus far in the awake rat show responses (Fig. 8.5A) to NGC stimulation similar to that seen in acute experiments. In Figure 5B, a brief NGC stimulus train elicits a prolonged increase in discharge rate of a parafascicularis unit. In contrast, an anterior MT unit responded with a prolonged decrease in spike rate to a similar NGC stimulus train (Fig. 8.6). As shown in Figure 8.8 (A and B), NGC stimulation with increasing currents increased the escape rate and also increased the discharge rate of this unit to a maximum of approximately seventy spikes per second. Data obtained thus far from awake rats also indicates that the threshold intensity of MFB stimulation required to elicit MT unit responses is comparable to that required to elicit self stimulation.

NGC-MFB interaction is shown in Figure 8.5A where NGC and MFB stimulation produces opposite poststimulus patterns of unit discharge. Brief trains of MFB and NGC stimulation also elicits opposite changes in spike rate lasting several seconds (Figs. 8.5B and 8.6). The majority of MT neurons receive

---

anterior part of the pedestal drives a tungsten microelectrode; the three short flat head screws temporarily protect the openings of three additional trajectories into the thalamus. MFB and NGC bipolar stimulating electrodes are covered by the pedestal. Stimulating and recording leads are fastened to a receptacle which is mounted posteriorly and is shown connected to the coaxial cable containing field effect transistors mounted in dental acrylic.

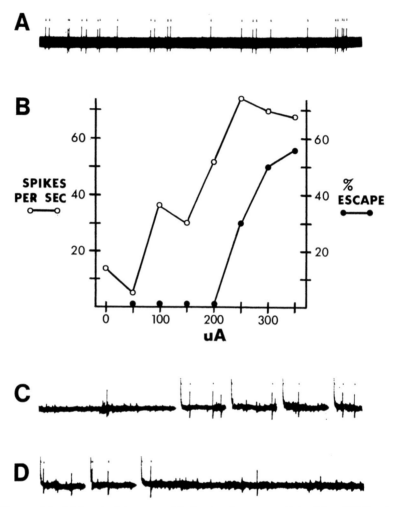

Figure 8.8. MT unit driving and behavioral escape elicited by NGC stimulation. A: Spontaneous activity of a unit in the ventral medial (VM) nucleus of thalamus. Pulses shown above the spikes are generated by a level
detector and are used to measure spike rates and generate poststimulus
histograms. B: NGC stimulation above 250 μ A (20 Hz, .5 msec pulses)
elicits escape (percentage escape = percent of test time rat has turned
stimulus off) and fixed latency unit driving above sixty spikes per second.
C and D: VM thalamic unit in the same animal. At the onset of 350 μ A
NGC stimulation (C), the spike rate increases and (D) decreases after
the last pulse.

sensory input (14). The experiments thus far also indicate that many MT units receive input from NGC and MFB. The extent of the overlap of these two populations remains to be determined. Figure 8.6, for example, shows an anterior MT unit affected by stimulation of different sensory modalities as well as NGC and lateral hypothalamic inputs of opposing motivational valence. A number of studies utilizing lesion, stimulation, and recording techniques have implicated MT in the interrelated phenomena of learning and motivation. Further study of the interaction of sensory and motivational systems on single MT neurons may lead to increased understanding of the role MT structures might play in these phenomena.

SUMMARY

Unit recording in the awake animal is an especially valuable technique for investigating central neural mechanisms which may subserve pain and other motivational systems. Such experiments are often best guided by the results of more conventional studies in acutely prepared animals and by the effects of brain stimulation in the awake preparation. The results of experiments based on this approach have shown that unit activity in bulboreticular and medial thalamic areas may be related to the motivational effects of noxious stimuli. Experiments now in progress indicate that central systems mediating self stimulation and escape behavior interact in medial thalamic structures.

REFERENCES

1. Bowsher, D., A. Mallart, D. Petit and D. Albe-Fessard. A bulbar relay to the centre median. *J. Neurophysiol.* 31:288-300, 1968.
2. Burgess, P. R. and E. R. Perl. Myelinated afferent fibres responding specifically to noxious stimulation of the skin. *J. Physiol.* 190:541-562, 1967.
3. Casey, K. L. Escape elicited by bulboreticular stimulation in the cat. *Intern. J. Neurosci.* 2:29-34, 1971.
4. Casey, K. L. and M. Blick. Observations on anodal polarization of cutaneous nerve. *Brain Res.* 13:155-167, 1969.
5. Casey, K. L. Responses of bulboreticular units to somatic stimuli eliciting escape behavior in the cat. *Intern. J. Neurosci.* 2:15-28, 1971.
6. Casey, K. L. Somatic stimuli, spinal pathways and size of cutaneous

fibers influencing unit activity in the medial medullary reticular formation. *Exp. Neurol.* 25:35-56, 1969.

7. Casey, K. L. Somatosensory responses of bulboreticular units in awake cat: relation to escape-producing stimuli. *Science* 173:77-80, 1971.

8. Casey, K. L. Unit analysis of nociceptive mechanisms in the thalamus of the awake squirrel monkey. *J. Neurophysiol.* 29:727-750, 1966.

9. Christensen, B. N. and E. R. Perl. Spinal neurons excited specifically by noxious or thermal stimuli: Marginal zone of the dorsal horn. *J. Neurophysiol.* 33:293-307, 1970.

10. Collins, W. F., F. E. Nulsen and C. T. Randt. Relation of peripheral nerve fiber size and sensation in man. *Arch. Neurol. Psychiat.* 3: 381-385, 1960.

11. Halpern, B. P. and J. D. Halverson. Elevated escape latencies after hindbrain lesions. *Physiologist* 10:193, 1967.

12. Keene, J. J. Unpublished observations.

13. Keene, J. J. and K. L. Casey. Excitatory connection from lateral hypothalamic self-stimulation sites to escape sites in medullary reticular formation. *Exp. Neurol.* 28:155-166, 1970.

14. Krupp, P. and M. Monnier. The unspecific intralaminary modulating system of the thalamus. In: C. C. Pfeiffer and J. R. Smythies (Eds.). *International Rev. Neurobiol.,* Vol. 9, Academic Press, New York, 1966, pp. 45-94.

15. Mark, V. H., F. R. Ervin and P. I. Yakovlev. Stereotactic thalamotomy. *Arch. Neurol.* (Chicago) 8:528-538, 1963.

16. Mehler, W. R., M. E. Feferman and W. J. H. Nauta. Ascending axon degeneration following anterolateral cordotomy. An experimental study in the monkey. *Brain* 83:718-750, 1960.

17. Millhouse, O. E. A Golgi study of the descending medial forebrain bundle. *Brain Res.* 15:341-363, 1969.

18. Mitchell, C. L. and W. W. Kaelber. Effect of medial thalamic lesions on responses elicited by tooth pulp stimulation. *Am. J. Physiol.* 210:263-269, 1966.

19. Olds, M. E. and J. Olds. Approach avoidance analysis of rat diencephalon. *J. Comp. Neurol.* 120:259-295, 1969.

20. Perl, E. R. Myelinated afferent fibers innervating the primate skin and their response to noxious stimuli. *J. Physiol.* 197:593-615, 1968.

21. Poggio, G. F. and V. B. Mountcastle. A study of the functional contributions of the lemniscal and spinothalamic systems to somatic sensibility. Central nervous mechanisms in pain. *Johns Hopk. Hosp. Bull.* 106:266-316, 1960.

22. Pomeranz, B., P. D. Wall and W. V. Weber. Cord cells responding to fine afferents from viscera, muscle and skin. *J. Physiol.* 199:511-532, 1968.

23. Ranck, J. B., Jr. (Chapter V—this volume.)
24. Scheibel, M. E. and A. B. Scheibel. Anatomical basis of attention mechanisms in vertebrate brains. In: G. C. Quarton, T. Melnechuk and F. O. Schmitt (Eds.) *The Neurosciences.* Rockefeller Univ. Press, New York, 1967, pp. 577-601.
25. Swanson, A. G., G. C. Buchan and E. C. Alvord. Anatomic changes in congenital insensitivity to pain. *Arch. Neurol.* (Chicago) 12:12-18, 1965.
26. Sweet, W. H. Pain, In: J. Field, H. W. Magoun and V. E. Hall (Eds.) *Handbook of Physiology,* Vol. I, American Physiol. Soc., Washington, 1959.
27. Wall, P. D., J. H. Freeman, and D. Major. Dorsal horn cells in spinal and freely moving rats. *Exp. Neurol.* 19:519-529, 1967.

Chapter IX

RELATIONSHIP OF NEURONAL ACTIVITY TO EEG WAVES DURING SLEEP AND WAKEFULNESS

R. M. HARPER

A VARIETY OF BEHAVIORS are associated with distinctive EEG patterns which occur during wakefulness. For example, specific patterns of EEG activity in the hippocampus are associated with movement and with sitting (11, 16, 34, 37, 38). There are also waves in the posterior cortex associated with reinforcement (9, 27) and others in the anterior cortical region which are accompanied by a group of specific behaviors involving somatic immobility, reduced neck tone and decreased heart rate (8, 32, 40). Sleep states are also characterized by unique EEG patterns. Quiet sleep consists of several behavioral stages with each stage accompanied by specific patterns of EEG waves. Active or rapid eye movement (REM) sleep is distinguished by desynchronization of certain cortical areas and highly regular 4-7 Hz theta activity in the hippocampus (19).

For the past few years we have been studying the spontaneous discharge patterns of single neurons in forebrain structures and attempting to relate these patterns of firing to specific behaviors. Since we are interested in describing unit concomitants of behavior, it is necessary to determine those aspects of behavior which influence neuronal firing. These behaviors are composed

A large number of these studies were carried out at McMaster University over the period 1964-1968 in the laboratory of Dr. Woodburn Heron and were supported by the Canadian National Research Council Grant No. AP0053. Additional studies in this chapter were supported by USPHS Grant MH-10083 and the Veterans Administration. Computational assistance was furnished by the Data Processing Laboratory of the Brain Research Institute, UCLA, which is supported by USPHS Grant NS-02501.

I would like to thank Rebecca Harper, Mary Fairbanks and Doctors M. Chase, D. McGinty and M. B. Sterman for their assistance in this project.

of a number of different subset activities and are associated with a number of physiological signs, among which are EEG pattern changes.

It is the aim of this chapter to demonstrate that the spontaneous firing of many neurons in a variety of structures is closely related to EEG activity. These units appear to be correlated with discrete behaviors that are associated with specific EEG patterns. It also will be demonstrated that, with various pharmacological and naturally occurring manipulations, certain EEG patterns can be dissociated from the behavior that is normally associated with such activity. In this regard many neurons were found to be related to the EEG patterns rather than to the behavioral activity.

The following studies then will (a) examine unit activity in various brain structures during periods of atropine dissociation, that is, when EEG activity normally associated with quiet sleep is seen during the alert state; (b) describe the discharge pattern of neurons during the presence of various frequencies of hippocampal EEG activity associated with specific behaviors; and (c) examine unit activity during the presence of conditioned 12-14 Hz rhythms over the sensorimotor cortex.

These studies are offered both as a descriptive evaluation of the spontaneous activity of neurons under the above conditions and to indicate the kinds of control procedures needed to measure neuronal discharge patterns during various behaviors.

Neuronal Activity During Atropine Dissociation

Of the behavioral states which are accompanied by specific EEG patterns, quiet sleep is perhaps the best known due to the prominence of the slow wave EEG activity. This state is characterized by a variety of indices such as reduced neck muscle tone, closed eyes, slowed heart rate, as well as changes in body posture (lying down). Very large waves (1.0-2.5 Hz) and 12-14 Hz spindle activity develop over many parts of the brain during quiet sleep. One can, however, induce slow waves and spindles in an alert animal with large doses of an anticholinergic drug, atropine (25, 39). Such a drugged animal can exhibit slow waves similar to those seen during sleep while clearly awake and alert.

Since atropine induces slow waves and spindles in an alert animal, this condition has been termed a *dissociated state, i.e.,* the behavioral state and EEG state are dissociated from the normal condition where alert behavior is characterized by a desynchronized cortical EEG. Neurons in thalamic and cortical structures begin to discharge in distinctive burst-pause patterns in slow wave sleep, as contrasted to the more regular firing patterns seen during the alert state. (See Chapter XI.) The question arises whether the neuronal discharges are related to the specific state of the animal, sleep or alert, or whether they are related to the slow waves. We tested these alternative possibilities by recording from single neurons during atropine dissociated, sleep, and alert states in rabbits.

Method

Seven rabbits were surgically prepared with fine wire microelectrodes (62.5 μ, see Chapter XI) placed stereotaxically in the hippocampus, midline and anterior thalamus, and pontine and midbrain reticular formation. Eye movement and neck muscle electrodes also were inserted according to standard procedures (see Chapter XI). After recovery from the surgical procedures (at least two weeks), the rabbits were allowed to sleep through two consecutive sleep-wake cycles. They then were injected intravenously with large doses of atropine sulfate (5 mg/kg). The slow electrical activity recorded from the cortex and the depth microelectrodes (EEG), together with single cell activity, were monitored for two hours after the injection. Three minute samples of EEG and single unit activity were taken while the animals were alert and still; these records were compared with three minute records taken while the animals were in slow wave sleep and while alert and still, but not under the influence of drugs. The unit records were subjected to an analysis of mean rate, variance, and distribution of intervals. These analyses were carried out with a computer of average transients in a histogram mode and on a PDP-12 computer using programs written by Wyss and Handwerker (41).

Slow wave electrical activity was recorded through the microelectrode tips together with the activity of single units; the activity between .2 Hz and 30 Hz was subjected to power spectral analysis. A description of the slow electrical changes during the various conditions studied here has been reported elsewhere (16). Twenty-eight cells were recorded from the animals. The greatest number of cells were recorded from thalamic, tegmental and pontine reticular, and hippocampal sites. A few cells were recorded from sensorimotor cortex, septum and central grey.

RESULTS

Large doses of atropine produced slow waves and spindles in the alert animal (Figs. 9.1, 9.2, 9.3). These waves were remarkably similar to those obtained from slow wave sleep records if the ani-

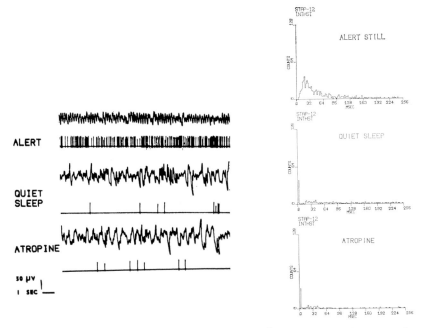

Figure 9.1. (Left) Activity of an anterior thalamic neuron (n. ventralis anterior) during periods when the animal was sitting alert and still, in quiet sleep, and while alert, under the influence of atropine. This neuron was characterized by a striking decrease in the rate of discharge during slow wave development, regardless of whether the slow waves were caused by the onset of sleep or atropine administration.

(Right) First order interval histograms of the unit activity under the same three conditions. The atropine and slow wave sleep histograms are very similar, and both of these histograms are different from the distribution of intervals in the alert state.

mal remained still. If the animal moved, however, the slow waves would disappear and reappear after the movement had been completed.

The activity of single units during slow wave sleep in a variety of thalamic, hippocampal or reticular sites was very similar to the atropine condition. Changes in rate and the burst pause pattern were clearly seen on the polygraph pen deflection records.

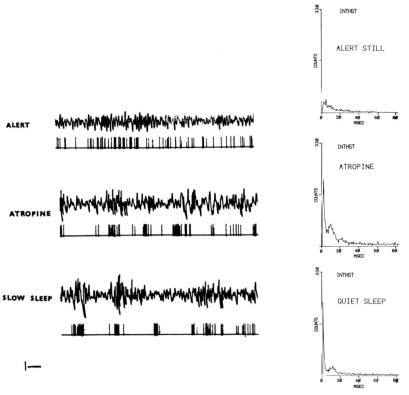

Figure 9.2. (Left) EEG and single unit records of a neuron in the medial thalamus (n. paracentralis) during three states. During the atropine condition the neurons fired in patterns of long pauses and bursts, similar to that seen in quiet sleep.

(Right) First order interval histograms for this neuron under the three conditions. The histograms for the atropine and slow wave sleep states differed only slightly, while the histogram for the alert condition was very different calibration 50 µv, 1 sec.

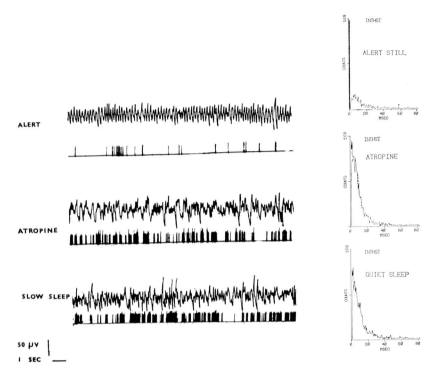

Figure 9.3. Records and first order interval histograms of units recorded from a hippocampal cell during three states. This neuron increased in rate during slow wave sleep. It also fired in long bursts at very high rates. The interval histograms for the corresponding states on the right demonstrated the similarity of the firing patterns under the sleep and atropine states, and the difference between these two states and the alert condition.

Differences in pattern were confirmed in the rate and interval distribution measures. The neuronal activity of an anterior thalamic neuron during three conditions, quiet sleep, atropine dissociation, and alert, still conditions is shown in Figure 9.1. This cell slowed from a rate of fifteen per second during the alert state to a discharge rate of less than one per second during quiet sleep. The rate of firing during the atropine condition was virtually identical (t-test, $P < .7$) to the rates during quiet sleep. The interval histograms for the spike discharges under the three conditions are shown also in Figure 9.1. The histogram shapes are very similar during the quiet sleep and atropine condition; these two histograms are dissimilar to the distribution of intervals seen in the alert still condition.

Cells which fired in a similar fashion under quiet sleep and atropine did not uniformly slow down in passing from the alert to the quiet sleep or atropine condition. Another cell which altered its discharge pattern from the alert state to the quiet sleep and the atropine condition with little change in rate is shown in Figure 9.2. The discharge rate during these two slow wave conditions was similar to that of the alert state, but the pattern of firing was very different. This neuron was located in the thalamic midline complex (n. paracentralis).

Figure 9.3 shows a record of a hippocampal cell which fired at low rates during the alert, still condition (4/sec) and increased its discharge rate markedly during the slow wave conditions, either quiet sleep (30/sec) or atropine dissociation (24/sec). The discharge rates and the burst pause patterns were very much alike under these latter two conditions as indicated by the interval histograms. The distribution of intervals for the alert condition, however, was very different.

The direction of the rate change in passing from the alert to quiet sleep condition was not a good predictor of the degree to which a cell would discharge in a similar fashion during the atropine condition as during quiet sleep.

Seventeen of the twenty-eight neurons examined under the atropine condition had patterns of discharge which were similar to the slow wave sleep state, and different from those seen in the normal alert state. Of the remaining neurons, six cells fired in the same pattern across all three conditions and five assumed spontaneous rates and patterns which were distinctive for each of the three states, *i.e.*, the cells fired differently under the atropine state from either the alert or quiet sleep condition, while the remaining neurons fired as if the animal were normally alert and not under the influence of atropine.

Seven of ten hippocampal cells, all four tegmental reticular neurons, five of seven thalamic neurons and one of three septal neurons fired in the same fashion during the atropine state as during quiet sleep.

These studies indicate that certain neurons will fire in similar patterns when similar background conditions of EEG prevail rather than when the behavioral state of the animal changes. The findings also demonstrate that changes in unit activity from one state to the next may be a reflection of one or more unique components of that total state. For example, the change in unit firing from the alert state to quiet sleep may be due to a related change in a specific component of physiology, such as slow wave development.

Neuronal Activity During Hippocampal Theta

The electrical activity of the hippocampus is characterized by a variety of EEG frequencies, but especially prominent are synchronous 4-7 Hz waves known as hippocampal slow activity (RSA) or theta waves. This synchronous pattern predominates the hippocampal electrical activity when an animal is moving about (16, 34, 37, 38) or in active sleep (16, 19). It is so reliably associated with active sleep that it has become one of the distinctive classification signs of that state.

During the course of a sleep study it became apparent to us that a large number of neurons in the forebrain were very sensitive to the occurrence of this hippocampal rhythm, and were sensitive even to variations in the frequency of the rhythm.

The following study describes neuronal activity during behavioral patterns that are associated with theta activity. These experiments attempted to examine the degree of relationship between neuronal discharge and theta activity, and to determine the extent to which changes in unit firing activity in sleep-wakefulness patterns are accounted for by state related changes in synchronous hippocampal rhythms.

Method

Ten rabbits were prepared with microelectrodes placed in the hippocampus, anterior and medial thalamus, and midbrain reticular formation. Electrodes for recording eye movement and neck EMG were also present. Seven of the ten rabbits were later used for the atropine study just described. EEG recordings were obtained from each rabbit during two sleep-wakefulness cycles, *i.e.*, quiet sleep followed by active sleep. Additional records were obtained when the animals were sitting alert and still, and while they were moving about. Slow electrical activity occurring at the microelectrode tips was taped together with the activity of single neurons.

Results

Theta activity (4-7 Hz) was very prominent in the rabbit brain, not only in the hippocampus but also in a number of forebrain and reticular structures. In fact, only scattered areas of the rabbit brain exhibited EEG records free of the theta rhythm. The frequency changes in hippocampal theta have been described elsewhere (16) and will only be outlined here. Hippocampal theta was present in the rabbit when the animal was alert and still, but its frequency (5.5-6.5 Hz) was lower than if the animal moved. Theta activity was also present in the EEG of slow wave sleep, although its presence was masked by larger slow waves and spindles. It can be detected easily, however, by power spectral techniques, and its frequency during quiet sleep was similar to that seen when the animal was alert and still. During active sleep other waves on the hippocampal EEG disappeared and theta became very prominent. Its frequency increased in REM sleep and increased even further during the phasic twitches of that state, to a frequency as high or higher than that seen during movement.

There were a number of frequency changes noted in hippo-

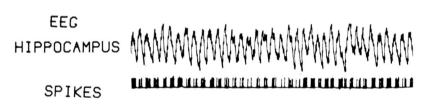

Figure 9.4. A dorsal hippocampal neuron which fired in short bursts synchronous with waves of theta. This sample of EEG was taken during REM sleep. Calibration 50 μv, one second.

campal theta during the transition from wakefulness to the various stages of sleep. If cell firing is directly related to the frequency of theta waves, then any change in discharge pattern as the animal goes through the various behavioral states may be related to the theta activity changes.

An examination of fifty neurons in various diencephalic and reticular structures revealed that the discharge pattern of nineteen cells was related in some way to the theta waves. Sixteen neurons, divided approximately equally among the pontine and tegmental reticular formation, hippocampus, thalamus and cortex, fired in a bursting fashion in which the frequency of bursts was related to the frequency of theta. Figure 9.4 is an example of such a neuron located in the dorsal hippocampus of a rabbit. This figure illustrates the regularity of theta activity during active sleep and demonstrates the close relationship of burst discharges of the neuron to the theta waves.

Some of these neurons continue to fire in bursts with theta waves during all behavioral states including quiet sleep. Autocorrelations from one such neuron are presented in Figure 9.5. It can be seen by the autocorrelograms that the intervals between bursts of these neurons are shorter in active sleep and when the animal is moving. Theta is faster (7-8/sec) in these conditions than when the animals are alert or in quiet sleep (5-6/sec). The autocorrelation of units during quiet sleep indicated that neurons fire in bursts with intervals between the bursts corresponding to those seen while the animals were not moving, but alert. During both these conditions theta is slower in frequency (5-6 Hz).

Active sleep and waking movement conditions are both characterized by high frequency theta, *i.e.*, theta with shorter wave lengths. These neurons fired with shorter interburst intervals in these two different states. During quiet sleep and alert still conditions, the frequency of theta decreases; the interburst interval of neurons increases, reflecting the increased length of the waves. It appears that the cell discharge patterns were correlated with the theta waves rather than with the particular behavioral state.

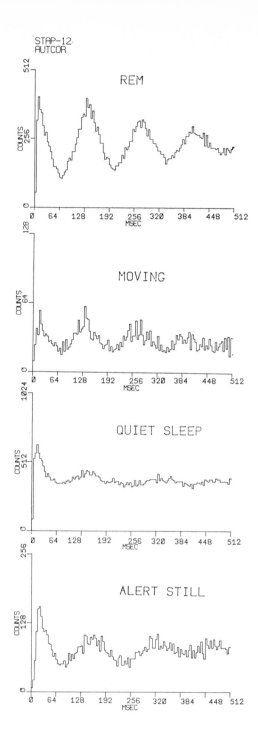

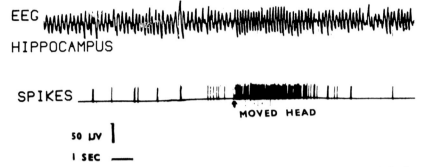

Figure 9.6. This is a dentate neuron which fired in a long burst with high-er frequencies of theta, such as the theta which occurred during a head movement. The neuron fired in this manner during any behavior which caused higher frequencies of theta, including REM sleep and whole body movements.

Three hippocampal neurons were found which did not fire in phase with theta waves, but rather fired in a long sustained burst as fast theta appeared during a particular movement of the animal. Figure 9.6 shows a cell of this kind. This cell was fairly silent during the alert state but discharged in a sustained burst during a head movement. This neuron fired also in long sustained bursts during the rapid theta of active sleep.

The finding that neurons will fire in bursts in which the inter-val between bursts bears a direct relationship to the frequency of theta apparently is not confined to neurons in the rabbit brain; in a preliminary study in acute cats, we have found units in the basal forebrain (preoptic) area which burst in conjunction with hippocampal theta (Fig. 9.7). These units have longer burst in-tervals than observed in the rabbit, reflecting the fact that theta activity in the cat is correspondingly slower (3.5-5.5 Hz).

These studies suggest that some neurons in hippocampal, re-ticular, thalamic, and cortical structures will fire in bursts in which the interburst interval is related to the wave length of

---

Figure 9.5. Autocorrelograms of a hippocampal neuron which fired in synchrony with theta waves throughout all behavioral states. During the REM and movement states the intervals between bursts were shorter than during quiet sleep and alert still states.

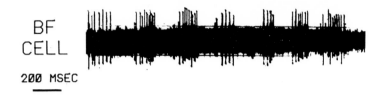

BF
CELL

200 MSEC

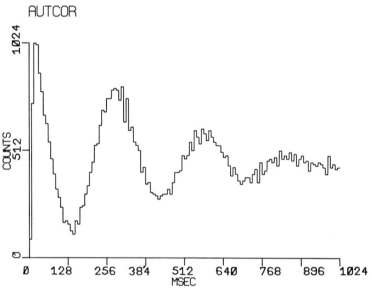

AUTCOR

Figure 9.7. A neuron in the basal forebrain of a cat which discharged very synchronously with hippocampal theta. The autocorrelation of the unit below indicates burst intervals of 280 msec. The frequency of theta in the cat is lower than in the rabbit (3.5-5.5 Hz vs 5-8 Hz).

theta activity. In addition, certain hippocampal cells appear to fire in long bursts in conjunction with high frequency theta. Theta activity can occur in different behavioral states, and may determine the type of discharge pattern that is seen in these neurons during that state.

Neuronal Activity During Conditioned 12-14 Hz Sensorimotor Rhythm (SMR)

The electrical activity of the sensorimotor cortex during periods of quiet immobility in the cat is characterized by trains of high amplitude 12-14 Hz activity (27, 32). This activity can be brought under operant control by a conditioning paradigm in which reward is contingent upon the generation of the sensori-motor rhythm that normally occurs during periods of immobil-ity (40).

A variety of visceral and somatic changes take place during the presence of this rhythm; heart rate slows, neck muscle tone de-creases, and respiration becomes much more regulated and tied to the onset and termination of the rhythm (8). The generation of this rhythm is thus accompanied by a variety of visceral and somatic changes. We have examined the activity of single neurons in various parts of the brain, particularly the thalamic relay nuclei and the red nucleus during the generation of the rhythm.

Methods

Cats were implanted with the usual array of electrodes plus two leads over the sensorimotor area of the brain. The surgical pro-cedure is described in detail elsewhere (17). After recovery from surgery, they were placed in a chamber and conditioned in a free operant paradigm to generate 12-14 Hz EEG activity. When the duration and amplitude of the cortical rhythm met certain cri-teria, the animals automatically were presented with .2 cc of milk from an automatic dispenser. The cats were readily trained to produce the rhythm of up to ten seconds in duration. Follow-ing a session of at least sixty reinforcements of four second epochs of SMR, the cats were allowed to sleep through two con-secutive sleep cycles (quiet sleep followed by active sleep).

Our description of neural discharge patterns during these SMR studies rely on film strips and polygraph outputs since the statistical description of the activity of neurons during such training of waves is difficult because of limited time (3-10 sec) during which cats produce the rhythm. A sufficient number of spikes for an interval histogram does not occur in this short peri-od. We are, however, developing procedures for averaging across short term histograms, and these data will be presented else-where.

Results

During the SMR, neurons in the thalamic relay nuclei began to discharge in short high frequency bursts of two to seven spikes with long pauses between the bursts. An example of such a neuron is shown on the top half of Figure 9.8. The presence of the rhythm on the EEG is indicated by the relay deflection and by the increase in 12-14 Hz output of the filter. The VPL cell fires in a regular fashion before the onset of the rhythm. As the 12-14 Hz activity increases, the neuron begins to pause in its discharge pattern and then to fire in very high frequency bursts followed by more long pauses. The burst-pause discharge pattern was not related just to sitting still since the cat was sitting still prior to the generation of the rhythm. The single unit activ-

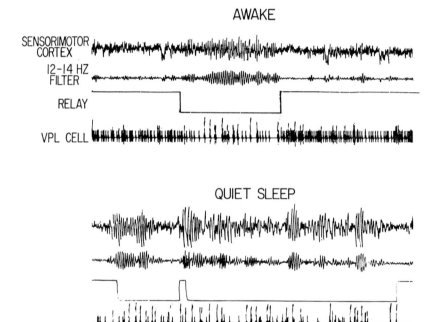

Figure 9.8. An epoch of conditioned sensorimotor rhythm (top) and quiet sleep (bottom). The relay deflection and the increase in amplitude of the filter output help to delineate the period of SMR. The neuron from the VPL nucleus of the thalamus began to fire in a pattern characterized by pauses and short, high frequency bursts. The bursts of activity are indicated by the lengthened pen deflections which cannot follow the high frequency of the spike discharge. During quiet sleep the neuron showed very similar activity to that seen during the conditioned epoch.

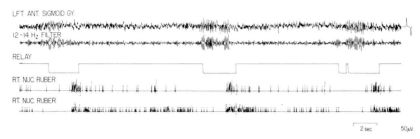

Figure 9.9. Records from two red nucleus neurons recorded simultaneously during three epochs of conditioned SMR. Both neurons slowed during the rhythm.

ity seen during the SMR was remarkably similar to that seen during slow wave sleep (bottom trace of Fig. 9.8).

Another characteristic change in firing pattern was seen in cells of the red nucleus. These neurons slowed during the production of this rhythm. An example of two such neurons is shown in Figure 9.9.

These neurons fired at fairly regular rates, then slowed during the presence of the SMR. They resumed firing at the offset of the train. At the cessation of the rhythm a large transient increase in the rate of discharge typically occurred.

Discussion

Specific classes of behavior are characterized by unique trains of EEG activity in certain areas of the brain. We have found that these unique EEG patterns are frequently accompanied by specific modes of unit discharge. In some cases, illustrated here with neurons that discharged in bursts with the theta rhythm, the patterns of discharge are related to a particular aspect of the wave form or slope of the EEG trace. In other cases, such as in atropine dissociation and with some of the hippocampal neurons during theta, the spontaneous discharge pattern of the neuron changes to a different pattern during time periods when trains of a particular EEG frequency occur. These patterns, however, are not necessarily related to a specific phase of the wave form.

There has been some controversy whether unit activity bears

any relationship to EEG waves. Li and Jasper (20) argue against such a relationship, pointing out that during hypoxia and anesthesia slow waves continue to occur, even when spikes disappear. Moreover, they found deep cortical neurons which had little relation to surface slow waves. Buchwald et al. (7) were able to find relationships between unit activity and waves only during certain circumstances; in general, the two kinds of neural activity were found to be independent.

There is growing evidence, however, that the probability of spike discharge is very much related to the slow potentials recorded from the microelectrode tip. Much of the evidence for a high degree of correlation between spike discharges and slower waves has been demonstrated by evoked activity studies. Fox and O'Brien (13) have shown that averaged evoked potentials of slow waves and post stimulus histograms of single units in the visual cortex have a high degree of similarity. A similar correlation has been seen in conditioning studies involving multiple units (18). Verzeano et al. (36) have demonstrated that if multiunit post stimulus histograms are compared to evoked potential responses in the lateral geniculate, the histogram peaks are highly correlated with the negative peaks of the first derivative of the slow potential. Thompson (33), using multiunit records, has shown that small units tend to fire at periods of maximum negative slope of the gross potential, while larger units tend to occur at or just beyond the peak of the negativity.

The very large waves typically seen in such evoked potential studies probably bias the results toward the correlation of spikes and waves. However, there is evidence that spontaneous waves are related to spike firing on the condition that the amplitude of the waves is large. For example, spikes appear to be related to slow activity if large amplitude spindles are present (7); convulsoid waves appear to be associated with bursts of spikes at particular points on the waves (10).

Even when the amplitude of the EEG waves is not abnormally large, a relationship between unit activity and slow waves seems to exist. Fox and Norman (12) have developed a measure of congruence based on amplitude of the slow wave and probability of cell discharge. Both the rate of discharge of cortical spikes

(14, 26) and the probability of onset of a burst of spikes (30) are related to the degree of negativity (surface positivity) at the microelectrode tip. Our findings in the present studies, then, should not be unexpected in light of the number of reported relations between spikes and slow waves.

Theta Activity

We have found that the frequency of theta waves reflects the ongoing behavior of the animal. We have also found that single neurons in a wide variety of brain areas fire in relation to the theta rhythm and that the firing patterns are altered by changes in the frequency of theta.

A number of investigators have reported that hippocampal and septal cells fire in bursts with the hippocampal theta rhythm in restrained animals (15, 21, 24). Fujita and Sato (15) have shown that bursts of spikes accompany the depolarization phase of intracellular membrane potentials of hippocampal pyramidal neurons. These membrane potentials are synchronous with the theta rhythm, and the hyperpolarization and depolarization of these potentials correspond to the positive and negative phases of the EEG theta rhythm. Macadar et al. (21) have found cells in the septum and hippocampus of rats which are highly correlated with the theta rhythm.

We have extended these observations to show correlations between unit activity and theta as the theta frequency varies with the behavior of the animal. Thus, changes in unit discharge in different behavioral states are associated with theta frequency. This correlation between unit discharge and theta frequency may dominate over any other state related changes. We also have found theta related neurons in a variety of locations—medial and anterior thalamus, limbic cortex and reticular structures—all structures which lie outside the septum and hippocampus.

The reason why so many neurons in such diverse areas are so sensitive to the theta rhythm is puzzling. Initially, we thought that these findings were specific to the rabbit because the theta rhythm is such a dominant and large rhythm in many brain areas of that animal. However, we are finding theta related neurons, such as the neuron shown in Figure 9.7, in the cat.

One may wonder what behavioral function is encoded with these cells which fire in bursts with the burst repetition rate of the theta frequency. Their principle mode of response, it appears, is to change in their burst repetition rate with various behaviors. Such an undifferentiated response would lead one to think that these neurons in these widely scattered areas are concerned with only broad regulatory mechanisms, since finely differentiated behaviors would almost certainly involve much more differentiated activity from such a wide number of neurons. From the data furnished by Vanderwolf (34) and others (11, 16, 37, 38), it may be surmised that the regulatory role is one of initiating *start* or *stop* behaviors, since theta amplitude and frequency seem to be so finely attuned to changes in movement.

Atropine

Quiet sleep is characterized by slow waves and unique patterns of unit discharge in thalamic and cortical areas. When slow waves were generated in an alert animal by means of atropine administration, then the majority of neurons examined appeared to fire as if the animal were asleep. The cell discharge during atropine dissociation did not appear to be related to a certain aspect of the EEG wave. Instead, the neurons fired in a particular pattern when slower waves were generated; these patterns were similar to those seen during quiet sleep.

The change in discharge pattern during atropine dissociation could be caused by mechanisms other than those related to slow wave generation such as peripheral effects of the anticholinergic agent. However, this explanation does not appear likely since, if the animal moved while under the influence of atropine, the slow waves disappeared and the cells returned to normal discharge patterns. It thus appears that whatever factors are causing the cortex to synchronize in the absence of movement are also affecting the patterning of cell discharge. This effect may be exerted indirectly by excitation of the neurons through the slow potentials, or it may be caused directly through other mechanisms.

The atropine dissociation effect has attracted the attention of investigators of memory and learning functions since it has been suggested that an animal can exhibit differential memory to a task which is presented to it either in the normal state or under a dissociating drug (22, 23). One of the possible interpretations of the action of dissociating drugs in memory is that the drugs act to change neuronal background activity. Sensory input in a learning task is imposed upon a background of spontaneous neural activity and is encoded together with that background activity. A state change such as a change from the atropine alert state to the normal alert state brings about different spontaneous activity in the neurons, and similar stimuli can be paired with totally incompatible responses to the responses learned under a different state.

Sensorimotor Rhythm (SMR)

During epochs of conditioned SMR, neurons in thalamic relay nuclei altered their discharge pattern from a relatively random mode to a pattern characterized by long pauses and short high frequency bursts. At the same time, neurons in the red nucleus slowed and occasionally ceased firing.

The SMR has been localized by macroelectrode techniques to the somatosensory system (17); cortical recordings of SMR are maximal from the somatosensory area. This area receives input from thalamic relay cells (6, 29). The VPL nucleus, from which most of the recordings in this study were taken, is a primary somatosensory relay nucleus (28). There is increasing evidence that cortical synchronization is governed by thalamic neurons (1, 2, 35). One possible mechanism for generation of synchronous cortical waves involves generation of long lasting inhibitory post synaptic potentials (IPSPS) by thalamic relay nuclei. High frequency discharge bursts of these relay neurons could be caused by rebound of excitation from these prolonged IPSPS (3, 4, 5). The burst of cell firing could recycle the process, setting up synchronous waves or spindles. The burst-pause pattern seen in these thalamic neurons during the generation of synchronous SMR spindles might well be a reflection of such a mechanism.

The slowing of the red nucleus cells indicates that the motor system is also intimately involved in the generation of this rhythm.

Both patterns of neural activity seen during the generation of the SMR were in the direction of changes seen during sleep. Although sleep spindles tend to be recorded maximally over motor areas rather than the somatosensory areas where SMR is found (17), the two kinds of spindles are similar in frequency. Moreover, conditioning of SMR in waking animals facilitates the production of spindles in quiet sleep (31). The conditioning of SMR may represent a conditioning of synchronization in the waking state of neural elements that normally synchronize during sleep.

Experimental Controls

These experiments show that, in the course of the study of unit correlates of any behavior, it is necessary to specify to what aspect of behavior the units are sensitive. For example, quiet sleep may be accompanied by changes in spike discharge rates by a factor of fifteen or more from the alert state; REM sleep may have even higher changes in rate from waking states. However, quiet sleep is accompanied by a variety of changes, among which is slow wave development. Unit discharges, as we have seen, may be related to the slow wave development rather than behavioral sleep. Changes seen in REM sleep may reappear during motor behaviors of waking animals.

We have also shown that in subcortical structures EEG waves can change across behaviors or be very similar in two quite different behaviors. Theta rhythms are very similar in REM sleep and in awake moving conditions; the frequency of theta is lower and very similar in quiet sleep and alert still states. We have demonstrated that some neurons fire in close relation to aspects of that rhythm. As the state of the animal changes, the neuronal discharge patterns may change; but the alteration may be reflecting frequency shifts in EEG waves.

Consequently, in describing unit changes across behavioral states, it is necessary to find to what particular aspect of brain physiology the cells are sensitive. We now have the ability to relate spike activity to aspects of EEG waves, and even to generate certain aspects of states on demand by pharmacological or conditioning procedures. These tools allow us to dissect components of behavior to which neurons are responsive.

SUMMARY

This chapter discussed studies concerned with evaluation of the activity of single neurons in various brain structures during the presence of spontaneous and conditioned EEG waves.

A majority of neurons sampled in thalamic, hippocampal and reticular structures of the rabbit discharged in the same fashion during slow wave EEG activity produced either by quiet sleep or by atropine administration to alert animals.

A large number of neurons in hippocampal, anterior thalamic and reticular structures discharged with specific stereotyped patterns during the presence of theta rhythm. Three types of discharge patterns were observed. Some cells would fire in bursts with the intervals between bursts approximating wave lengths of theta; others would discharge in such bursts with theta activity only during some states, while other neurons fired only in long sustained periods of discharge with a particular frequency of theta.

Neurons in specific thalamic nuclei and in the red nucleus altered their pattern of discharge during the presence of conditioned sensorimotor rhythm. These changes were frequently in the direction seen in quiet sleep.

These studies suggest that the firing pattern of a high proportion of neurons in the forebrain are related to EEG activity. They also suggest that certain neurophysiological components of states can be dissected with behavioral or pharmacological techniques, and that the neural substrates of these components can be examined in detail.

REFERENCES

1. Andersen, P. and S. A. Andersson. *Physiological Basis of the Alpha Rhythm.* Appleton-Century-Crofts, New York, 1968.
2. Andersen, P., S. A. Andersson, and T. Lomo. Some factors involved in the thalamic control of spontaneous barbiturate spindles. *J. Physiol.,* 192:257-281, 1967.
3. Andersen, P. and J. C. Eccles. Inhibitory phasing of neuronal discharge. *Nature,* 196:645-647, 1962.
4. Andersen, P., J. C. Eccles, and T. A. Sears. The ventro-basal complex of the thalamus: Types of cells, their responses and their functional organization. *J. Physiol.,* 174:375-399, 1964.

5. Andersen, P. and T. A. Sears. The role of inhibition in the phasing of spontaneous thalamo-cortical discharge. *J. Physiol.*, 173:459-480, 1964.

6. Andersson, S. A., S. Landgren, and D. Wolsk. The thalamic relay and cortical projection of group I muscle afferents from the forelimb of the cat. *J. Physiol.*, 183:576-591, 1966.

7. Buchwald, J. S., E. S. Halas, and Sharon Schramm. Relationships of neuronal spike populations and EEG activity in chronic cats. *Electroenceph. clin. Neurophysiol.*, 21:227-238, 1966.

8. Chase, M. H. and R. M. Harper. Somatomotor and visceromotor correlates of operantly conditioned 12-14 c/sec sensorimotor cortical activity. *Electroenceph. clin. Neurophysiol.*, 31:85-92, 1971.

9. Clemente, C., M. B. Sterman, and W. Wyrwicka. Post-reinforcement EEG synchronization during alimentary behavior. *Electroenceph. clin. Neurophysiol.*, 16:355-365, 1964.

10. Creutzfeldt, O. D., J. Watanabe, and H. D. Lux. Relations between EEG phenomena and potentials of single cortical cells. II. Spontaneous and convulsoid activity. *Electroenceph. clin. Neurophysiol.*, 20:19-37, 1966.

11. Dalton, A. J. Discriminative conditioning of hippocampal electrical activity in curarized dogs. *Commun. Behav. Biol., Part A*, 3:283-287, 1969.

12. Fox, S. S. and R. J. Norman. Functional congruence: an index of neural homogenity and a new measure of brain activity. *Science*, 159: 1257-1259, 1968.

13. Fox, S. S. and J. H. O'Brien. Duplication of evoked potential waveform by curve of probability of firing of a single cell. *Science*, 147: 888-890, 1965.

14. Fromm, G. H. and H. W. Bond. Slow changes in the electrocorticogram and the activity of cortical neurons. *Electroenceph. clin. Neurophysiol.*, 17:520-523, 1964.

15. Fujita, Y., and T. Sato. Intracellular records from hippocampal pyramidal cells in rabbit during theta rhythm activity. *J. Neurophysiol.*, 27:1011-1025, 1964.

16. Harper, R. M. Frequency changes in hippocampal electrical activity during movement and tonic immobility. *Physiol. Behav.*, 7:55-88, 1971.

17. Howe, R. C. and M. B. Sterman. Cortical-subcortical correlates of suppressed motor behavior during sleep and waking in the cat. *Electroenceph. clin. Neurophysiol.*, 32:681-695, 1972.

18. John, E. R. and P. P. Morgades. The pattern and anatomical distribution of evoked potentials and multiple unit activity elicited by conditioned stimuli in trained cats. *Commun. Behav. Biol., Part A*, 3: 181-207, 1969.

19. Jouvet, M. Neurophysiology of the states of sleep. *Physiol. Rev.* 47: 117-177, 1967.
20. Li, C.-L., H. Mclennan, and H. H. Jasper. Brain waves and unit discharge in cerebral cortex. *Science*, 116:656-657, 1952.
21. Macadar, O., J. A. Roig, J. M. Monti, and R. Budelli. The functional relationship between septal and hippocampal unit activity and hippocampal theta rhythms. *Physiol. Behav.*, 5:1443-1450, 1970.
22. Overton, D. A. State dependent learning produced by depressant and atropine-like drugs. *Psychopharmacologia*, 10:6-31, 1966.
23. Overton, D. A. State dependent or "dissociated" learning produced with pentobarbital. *J. Comp. Physiol. Psychol.*, 57:3-12, 1964.
24. Petsche, H. and C. Stumpf. Hippocampal arousal and seizure activity in rabbits: toposcopical and microelectrode aspects. *In Physiologie de l'Hippocampe*. Colloques Internationales CNRS No. 107, pp. 121-134, 1962.
25. Podvoll, E. M. and S. J. Goodman. Averaged neural electrical activity and arousal. *Science*, 155:223-225, 1967.
26. Robertson, A. D. J. Correlation between unit activity and slow potential changes in the unanesthetized cerebral cortex of the cat. *Nature*, 5012:757-758, 1965.
27. Roth, S., M. B. Sterman, and C. D. Clemente. Comparison of EEG correlates of reinforcement, internal inhibition and sleep. *Electroenceph. clin. Neurophysiol.*, 23:509-520, 1967.
28. Rose, J. E. and Mountcastle, V. B. The thalamic tactile region in the rabbit and cat. *J. Comp. Neurol.*, 97:441-490, 1952.
29. Rosen, I. Excitation of group I activated thalamocortical relay neurones in the cat. *J. Physiol.*, 205:237-255, 1969.
30. Smith, G. K. Slow potential correlates of cortical neurone excitability. *Proc. Can. Fed. Biol. Soc.*, 9:48-49, 1966.
31. Sterman, M. B., R. C. Howe, and L. R. Macdonald. Facilitation of spindle-burst sleep by conditioning of electroencephalographic activity while awake. *Science*, 167:1146-1148, 1970.
32. Sterman, M. B. and W. Wyrwicka. EEG correlates of sleep: evidence for separate forebrain substrates. *Brain Res.*, 6:143-163, 1967.
33. Thompson, R. F., L. A. Bettinger, H. Birch, and P. M. Groves. Comparison of evoked gross and unit responses in association cortex of waking cat. *Electroenceph. clin. Neurophysiol.*, 27:146-151, 1969.
34. Vanderwolf, C. H. Hippocampal electrical activity and voluntary movement in the rat. *Electroenceph. clin. Neurophysiol.*, 26:407-418, 1969.
35. Verzeano, M. and I. Calma. Unit activity in spindle-bursts. *J. Neurophysiol.*, 17:417-428, 1954.
36. Verzeano, M., R. C. Dill, E. Vallecalle, P. Groves, and J. Thomas.

Evoked responses and neural activity in the lateral geniculate. *Experientia* (Basel), 24:696-698, 1968.

37. Whishaw, I. Q. and C. H. Vanderwolf. Hippocampal correlates of movement. *Proc. Can. Fed. Biol. Soc.*, 13:48, 1970.

38. Whishaw, I. Q. and C. H. Vanderwolf. Hippocampal EEG and behavior: effects of variation in body temperature and relation of EEG to vibrissal movement, swimming and shivering. *Physiol. Behav.*, 6:391-397, 1971.

39. Wilker, A. Pharmacologic dissociation of behavior and EEG "sleep patterns" in dogs: morphine, N-allylnor-morphine and atropine. *Proc. Soc. Exptl. Biol. Med.*, 79:261-265, 1952.

40. Wyrwicka, W. and M. B. Sterman. Instrumental conditioning of sensorimotor cortex EEG spindles in the waking cat. *Physiol. Behav.*, 3:703-707, 1968.

41. Wyss, U. R. and H. Handwerker. STAP-12: A library system for on-line assimilation and off-line analysis of event/time data. *Computer Programs in Biomedicine*, 1:209-218, 1971.

Chapter X

ACTIVITY OF MIDBRAIN RETICULAR FORMATION UNITS DURING CONDITIONED FREEZING

P. J. BEST, L. E. MAYS and C. E. OLMSTEAD

THE IMPORTANCE OF the midbrain reticular formation (MRF) in behavioral arousal was first demonstrated by the discovery that stimulation of the MRF caused desynchronization of the electrocorticogram, accompanied by waking and alertness (Moruzzi and Magoun, 1949). It was also found that lesions in the midbrain tegmentum abolished activated desynchronized cortical activity (Lindsley, Bowden and Magoun, 1949) resulting in lethargic, somnolent or comatose animals (Lindsley, Shriner, Knowles and Magoun, 1950). The view that a unitary ascending reticular activating system is simultaneously responsible for maintenance of desynchronized activated cortex, the waking state and behavioral arousal has had to be modified for a number of reasons. Not the least of these is the discovery by Dement and Kleitman (1957) that during sleep, cortical slow waves (S sleep) periodically give way to activated desynchronized patterns (D sleep). During these periods of D sleep most MRF neurons show higher rates of firing than during any other time (Huttonlocher, 1961; Mink, Best and Olds, 1967).

Nevertheless, the MRF is still considered to play an active role in behavioral arousal (see Jouvet, 1969). A number of recording studies have found increases in neural activity in MRF and related structures during awake aroused conditions. Bulboreticular cells in cats show selective sensitivity to aversive footshock (Casey, 1971), and cells in midbrain central gray of cats

This study was supported by USPHS grant MH 16478. The authors are grateful to M. Best and A. Mickley for help in all stages of this investigation.

are activated during aggressive behavior (Adams, 1968). In rats, MRF activity is augmented during operant responding for food (Best and Olds, 1968; Olds, Mink and Best, 1969). Tonal stimuli which signal food presentation have been found to cause sustained increase in MRF activity in rats (Hirano, Best and Olds, 1970; Phillips and Olds, 1969). The study of Phillips and Olds showed that tone signalling food caused a greater augmentation in MRF activity, in hungry animals, than tones signalling water presentation. But when the rats were made thirsty, the tone signalling water caused a greater augmentation of MRF unit activity. The authors concluded that the units were responding to the signal appropriate to the animal's motivational state.

The present study attempts to extend our understanding of conditioned changes in MRF response by presenting tones followed by footshock. The paradigm has been called conditioned freezing (CF) because after a few conditioning trials the tone acquires sufficient motivating properties to suppress ongoing operant behavior (Estes and Skinner, 1941; also see various chapters in Brush, 1971). From Phillips and Olds' conclusion, and the classical view of the MRF, one might predict that tones signalling footshock might cause an increase in activity since the tone acquires intense motivating properties. Another possible interpretation of the Phillips and Olds study is that the MRF units were responding to the relative valence of the tones; responding at higher rates to the more positively reinforced signal. One would then predict that tones signalling aversive footshock would lead to a decrease in MRF activity. The current study was designed to investigate the responses of MRF units to aversive footshock, to tones signalling aversive footshock, and to compare results with the changes in MRF activity that accompany D sleep.

METHODS

Twenty male Sprague-Dawley derived albino rats, weighing 250-300 gms were each implanted with five to eight indwelling microelectrodes following the procedure of Olds, Mink and Best (1969). The microelectrodes were prepared from factory insulated sixty-two micron nichrome wire stock (Johnson Matthey), which were soldered to Amphenol *reliatac* male pin connectors and further insulated with Epoxy-lite. The recording surface was the cut cross section of the tip. An indifferent electrode was similarly constructed from 250 micron nichrome wire but was left uninsulated.

The subjects were anesthetised with Sodium Pentobarbital (40 mg/kg) and mounted in a stereotaxic instrument. Six to nine holes ($\frac{1}{32}$" diam.) were drilled in the exposed cranium for electrode placement, and six holes ($\frac{3}{64}$" diam.) were drilled to receive self tapping anchoring screws (0-80 stainless steel). After the screws were in place, the ground electrode was lowered into the forebrain and fastened to the skull.

Each recording electrode was aimed under stereotaxic guidance at the desired area. The electrode was moved under electrophysiological guidance into the region of recordable neural activity, which was monitored via a Grass P15 preamplifier and integrated circuit amplifier. The neural activity was displayed on oscilloscopic and auditory monitors. Stable unit activity of greater than 100 μvolt amplitude and a signal-to-noise ratio of at least 3:1 were the primary criteria used in accepting or rejecting a cell within a desired area. If the activity persisted for three to five minutes, the electrode was secured to the skull with cranioplastic cement. The electrodes were then brought together in an Amphenol 9-pin *Tiny Tim* connector and secured with cranioplastic. A $\frac{3}{8}$" long (4-40) hex nut was included in the final assembly to provide for the later connection to the recording apparatus. Following the completion of the surgical procedure subjects were returned to their home cage.

The recording chamber contained a 35 cm diameter plexiglass cylinder. An array of nine shielded noise-free *microdot* cables was led from the electrode assembly on the animal's head to a Lehigh Valley brush commutator mounted on an overhead counter balanced arm. An additional unshielded *noisy* wire was loosely draped around the *microdot* cables and attached open-ended to the assembly on the animal's head. High impedance, solid state preamplifiers were mounted via phonojacks on the commutator assembly. The preamplified impulses were led to solid state amplifiers (-3db @ 750 Hz and 2000 Hz).

The animals were placed in the experimental chamber from

two to five days following surgery. All electrodes were tested according to amplitude, signal-to-noise ratio (minimum 3:1), and the absence of EMG and EKG artifact. The amplified impulses from the four or five most satisfactory electrodes were passed through special purpose electronic circuitry which discriminated unit signals from background activity on the basis of amplitude and wave form. The discriminator circuits give a digital pulse when specific amplitude and falltime criteria are met.

Following the setting of the discriminator circuits for each electrode, photographic records were made of the analog signal and discriminator settings. The animal was then given a period of twelve or more hours of habituation to the experimental chamber.

Four second samples of single cell activity were taken at various intervals during each recording session. The outputs from the unit discriminators were recorded on punched paper tape along with marks signifying stimulus presentations and/or behavioral states. The punched paper tapes were read off line by a Burroughs 5500 general purpose computer. A Grass 6-channel polygraph was used to record cortical and hippocampal EEG and the signal from the noisy movement wire continuously during all phases of the experiment.

On the first day of recording, all animals were observed during naturally occurring states of sleep and waking. The state of the animal was classified on the basis of experimenter observation and EEG activity. Data were taken during at least two sleep sessions. Paradoxical sleep was defined by the presence of synchronized theta in the hippocampal EEG and low voltage fast activity in neocortex.

Following the second sleep session, cellular activity was recorded during presentations of a 5400 kHz, 75 db, 2.5 sec duration tone in the absence of footshock. The tone was presented about thirty times on a random schedule with three to ten minutes between presentations, in one or two habituation sessions. On the following day another habituation session was run and then followed by the first CF session. During each CF session the tone was presented about thirty times at a slower rate (eight to fifteen minutes between tones) and each presentation was immediately followed by footshock (.6 ma .1 sec pulsed D.C. 120 Hz). One or two CF sessions were run on each of the next three to five days yielding between four and eight sessions per animal.

During stimulus presentation periods, four second samples were taken prior to, during and following the tone, as well as at various periods between tone presentations. Upon completion of training, the animals were sacrificed and perfused in formalin. Frozen sections were taken and Nissl stained to verify electrode placement.

RESULTS

The response of most units during both habituation and CF was a sharp increase in activity at tone onset followed by a reduction in activity. (This brief orienting response has been noted by Hirano, Best & Olds, 1970.) Table 10.1 shows the median percent change in activity with respect to pretone levels as well as the number of cells that showed a reliable increase or decrease in rate of firing from the pre-tone baseline. The cells labelled *medial* were located immediately lateral or ventral to central gray. The cells labelled *lateral* were typically found 1-2 mm lateral to the midline. Figure 10.1 shows the four typical response types found during CF.

The presentation rate during habituation was slow enough such that no habituation or sensitization was observed except for

TABLE 10.1

MEDIAN PERCENT CHANGE IN RATE OF FIRING OF MEDIAL AND LATERAL MRF UNITS AND NUMBER OF UNITS THAT SHOWED INCREASE (+), DECREASE (−), AND NO CHANGE (0) WITH RESPECT TO PRE-TONE LEVEL, DURING FIRST ½ SEC (ONSET) AND LAST 1 SEC (LATE) OF TONE PRESENTATION

		Habituation Onset	Late	*Conditioning* Onset	Late
Median percent change		+10	0	+100	− 5
Medial	+	4	3	7	4
(N = 10)	0	6	6	2	3
	−	0	1	1	3
Median percent change		+10	0	+220	−10
Lateral	+	7	6	13	6
(N = 17)	0	9	9	2	6
	−	1	2	2	5

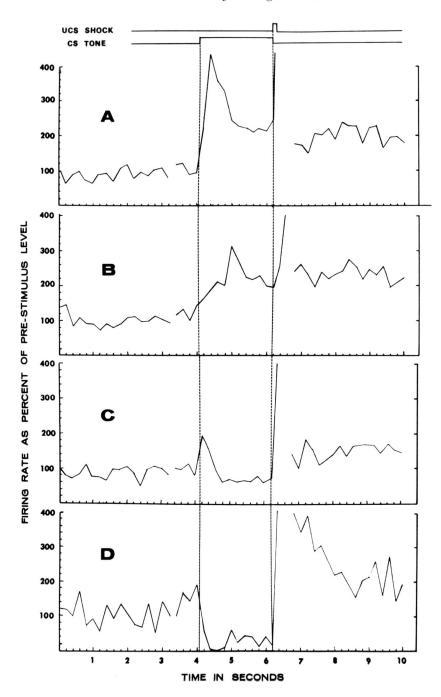

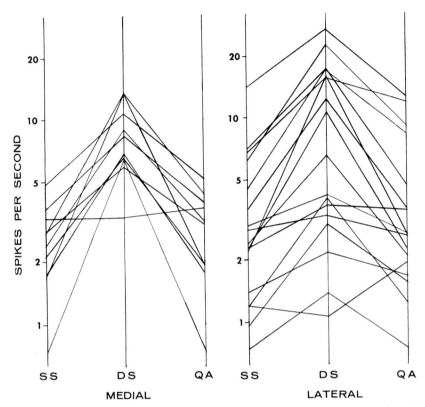

Figure 10.2. Absolute rate of firing per second of all medial and lateral MRF cells during S sleep (SS), D sleep (DS) and Quiet Awake (QA) same animal.

a reduction in the exaggerated response typically found during the first one or two tone presentations, which were frequently accompanied by gross movement artifact. The data from habituation therefore indicate unconditioned responses to the tone. Of the twelve cells that showed either augmented or diminished activity during habituation, ten showed the same response dur-

Figure 10.1. Rate of firing of typical MRF neurons during CF procedure. The rates are summed over thirty tone presentations and expressed as percent of mean pretone rate. Unit A and C are two lateral cells from the periods. Rates are plotted on a logarithmic scale.

ing CF. Although no independent operant behavior was used in the procedure, a definite freezing response was observed in all animals after three to five tone-shock pairings.

The right segment of Figure 10.1 shows the enhanced activity typically seen following footshock. Note that the fast rise in activity within one-half second of footshock is due to shock movement artifact. Twenty-three of the twenty-seven cells showed a prolonged enhanced activity. In five cells this enhanced activity was still reliably above the pretone baseline fifteen minutes after footshock. However, the postshock rate exceeded that found in D sleep in only three of the twenty-three cells.

The rates of firing of all the cells during S sleep, D sleep and quiet awake are shown in Figure 10.2.

DISCUSSION

These data differ from the results of studies measuring MRF activity in appetitive situations. Studies using tone-signalled food delivery (Hirano, Best & Olds, 1970; Phillips and Olds, 1969) or operant-contingent food delivery (Olds, Mink and Best, 1969), found that every MRF unit showed a sustained increase in activity as food delivery became imminent. The results indicate that some MRF units may be responsive to the acquired valence of the tone, *i.e.,* augmented during positive signals and diminished during negative signals, while other neurons in the same location, or a similar location in the same animal, are sensitive to the level of arousal produced by the tone. Phillips (1971) has come to a similar conclusion from analyzing the response of MRF to two tones, one signalling food, the other inescapable footshock. He found general augmentation to the food stimulus, but a preponderance of reduced late responses to tones signalling footshock.

These results indicate that the rate of activity of midbrain reticular neurons may be a reliable index of arousal or motivation level in the awake animal under conditions where appetitive drives are manipulated. However, it is not a reliable index under conditions in which noxious stimuli are presented, nor is it a reliable index of the relative level of arousal between different states of consciousness, such as waking, D sleep or S sleep.

It is very likely that different inputs operate on MRF neurons during paradoxical sleep than during painful stimulation. Hobson (1971) has shown that neurons in the gigantocellular tegmental field of the pons in cats show a greater augmentation in activity during D sleep than has been reported anywhere else in the brain. He suggests that these neurons play an active role in the production of rate changes elsewhere in the brain during D sleep. Casey (1971) has shown that cells in nucleus gigantocellularis of the bulboreticular formation in cats are selectively sensitive to footshock intense enough to cause escape responses.

Perhaps the MRF units are driven by the bulbar units during aversive stimulation in the waking animal, by pontine cells during D sleep and by still other neurons during conditioned tone presentations. Furthermore, it is likely that different MRF units have different arrays of these inputs.

SUMMARY

Rate of activity in twenty-seven single cells in reticular formation (MRF) was measured during conditioned freezing to a tone CS (2½ sec., 5.4 kHz, 75 db, US was .6 ma footshock) and during other sleep and waking conditions. During tone presentation eight units showed decreased activity, ten increased and nine were unchanged. Following the footshock, twenty-three units showed prolonged augmented activity, but only three showed rates exceeding those found in rapid eye movement sleep. It was concluded that increases in behavioral arousal are not necessarily accompanied by increases in MRF activity.

REFERENCES

Adams, D. B. Cells related to fighting behavior recorded from midbrain central gray neuropil of cat. *Science*, 1968, 159, 894-896.

Best, P. and Olds, J. Change in neural activity during *ad libitum* eating and sleeping in albino rats. *Proc. of Amer. Psychol. Assoc.*, 1968, 283-284.

Brush, F. R. (Ed.) *Aversive Conditioning and Learning*, Academic, New York, 1971.

Casey, K. L. Somatosensory responses of bulboreticular units in awake cat: relation to escape producing stimuli. *Science*, 1971, 173, 77-80.

Dement, W. and Kleitman, N. Cyclic variation in EEG during sleep and their relations to eye movements, bodily motility, and dreaming. *EEG Clin. Neurophysiol.*, 1957, 9, 673-690.

Estes, W. K. and Skinner, B. F. Some quantitative properties of anxiety, *J. Exper. Psychol.*, 1941, 29, 390-400.

Hirano, T., Best, P. and Olds, J. Changes in activity of subcortical units during auditory discrimination learning and extinction. *EEG Clin. Neurophysiol.*, 1970, 28, 127-135.

Hobson, J. A. Neural activity of pontine brain stem during sleep and waking. *Proc. of First Annual Meeting, Society for Neuroscience*, 1971, 152.

Huttonlocher, P. Evoked and spontaneous activity in single units of medial brain stem during natural sleep and waking. *J. Neurophysiol.*, 1961, 24, 451-468.

Jouvet, M. Biogenic amines and the states of sleep. *Science*, 163, 1969, 32-41.

Lindsley, D. B., Bowden, J. and Magoun, H. W. Effect upon EEG of acute injury to the brain stem activating system. *EEG Clin. Neurophysiol.*, 1949, 1, 475-486.

Lindsley, D. B., Schreiner, L. H., Knowles, W. B. and Magoun, H. W. Behavioral and EEG changes following chronic brainstem lesions in the cat. *EEG Clin. Neurophysiol.*, 1950, 2, 483-498.

Mink, W., Best, P. and Olds, J. Neurons in paradoxical sleep and motivated behavior. *Science*, 1967, 158, 1335-1337.

Moruzzi, B. and H. W. Magoun. Brainstem reticular formation and activation of the EEG. *EEG Clin. Neurophysiol.*, 1949, 1, 455-473.

Olds, J., Mink, W. and Best, P. Single unit patterns during anticipatory behavior. *EEG Clin. Neurophysiol.*, 1969, 26, 144-158.

Phillips, M. I. Unit activity study of positive and negative conditioning in chronic rats. *Proc. Amer. Psychol. Assoc.*, Vol. 6, part 2, 1971, 796-797.

Phillips, M. I. and Olds, J. Unit activity: Motivation-dependent responses from midbrain neurons. *Science*, 1969, 165, 1269-1271.

Chapter XI

BRAIN SINGLE UNIT ACTIVITY DURING SLEEP-WAKEFULNESS— A REVIEW

B. L. JACOBS, D. J. McGINTY and R. M. HARPER

THE STUDY OF the activity of single neurons during sleep has been a major theme in the growing literature on unit recordings in behaving animals. In this chapter we will review and assess these studies, both to assist investigators unfamiliar with the specific concepts in sleep research and to outline some of the major issues in this area. Sleep has been a popular subject of unit recording studies in part because it furnished a conveniently stable and quiescent condition for investigation. In addition, we believe that sleep research can serve as an important conceptual focus for basic brain research.

Sleep provides a naturally occurring experiment for the examination of significant general questions concerning the neuronal bases of brain function: do neurons fatigue and require periods of inactivity; how do complex neural systems achieve the restoration which, we believe, underlies the need to sleep; what underlies the process of sensory gating which appears to protect sleep from interruption; what is the nature of interactions within nerve nets in the absence of sensory signals; and what is the basis of unconsciousness itself? These are complex questions whose solutions are still distant, but we believe that they may be profitably explored within the context of the phenomenon of sleep.

Definitions

Sleep in adult mammals consists of two distinct phases which show regular alternation within a continuous sleep epoch. In the

This research was supported by USPHS Grant MH 10083 and by the U.S. Veterans Administration. Computational assistance was furnished by the Data Processing Laboratory of the Brain Research Institute, UCLA, which is supported by USPHS Grant NS-02501.

first of these, slow wave sleep (SWS), the electroencephalogram (EEG) is dominated by high voltage slow waves and 12-14 Hz waves called sleep spindles. In man, slow wave sleep is subdivided into stages II, III and IV according to the frequency of occurrence of spindles and slow delta waves (47). Respiration and heart rate become slower and more regular than in wakefulness, and there is a complete absence of phasic muscle activity with tonic muscle tonus being slightly reduced below the level in quiet waking.

The second state, which occupies 12-25 percent of total sleep time in most mammals, is termed rapid eye movement (REM) sleep and is distinguished by both tonic and phasic properties (27). The tonic properties include low voltage fast activity in the EEG similar to that of wakefulness and a powerful tonic inhibition of motoneuron activity (45). Phasic properties include an increase in the variability of respiration and heart rate, the appearance of rapid eye movements, twitches of distal muscles, and closely associated monophasic waves in the pons, lateral geniculate body and visual cortex. Hippocampal theta rhythm also appears during REM sleep and is prominent in rodents. These properties are characteristic of the sleep of a wide variety of adult mammals including rodents, carnivores, and primates.

This description emphasizes the differences between SWS and REM. That *both* states are marked by the absence of voluntary motor activity, sensory gating, and subjective continuity of sleep is often overlooked. There is controversy as to the relationship between the two phases of sleep, especially whether they represent two distinct behavioral events or a sleep continuum with certain noncritical differences (26). A useful point of view is that sleep, like the nutritional process, may represent a sequence of behavioral and physiological events. The nutritional process includes: accumulation of a hunger drive, search for, and selection of a food supply, ingestion, digestion, post-prandial depression, and metabolism. Similarly, sleep may include a sequence of seemingly different processes which are directed toward the satisfaction of the same physiological need. However, the alternative that the two phases of sleep serve at least two distinct functions cannot be rejected.

The Sleep Center Problem

Certain brain structures appear to play a central role in initiating and/or maintaining sleep or causing certain of the manifestations of the sleep state. Brain sites at several levels of the neuraxis, including the medullary (31) and pontine reticular formation (2), locus coeruleus (25), brainstem raphe system (28), and basal forebrain (35, 49) have been proposed as sleep *centers*. This list is not meant to exclude other brain sites, a number of which will almost certainly be added as our knowledge of sleep expands, nor does it mean that these structures will eventually be found to be exclusively concerned with aspects of sleep behavior. Rather, it represents contemporary theories of the sites that are important in sleep.

If the neural control of sleep is organized like other basic adaptive behaviors such as aggression and copulation, then it is likely that neural mechanisms subserving different levels of adaptation are involved in sleep. Reflexive, regulatory, and anticipatory mechanisms would be organized at different levels of the neuraxis. Consequently, the finding of such alternative *centers* is expected. The exact contribution of each level remains to be established. Unit studies of *centers* at each level may contribute to the understanding of this hierarchical organization if we search for correlations between unit activity and specific elements of the process of sleep initiation and maintenance. This approach has not yet been applied to unit studies and sleep.

With the exception of the raphe neurons discussed in Chapter XV of this volume, there are no unit studies which describe the activity of the proposed sleep *centers* in relation to sleep. Therefore, this review will not be concerned with neural mechanisms controlling sleep; instead, we will look for clues as to the nature of the state of sleep, that is, how the brain changes during sleep and how these changes may account for the properties of sleep.

Literature Review

This section will contain a review of selected unit studies of the brain during sleep and waking. In order to simplify matters, we will discuss only single unit studies on intact, non-anesthetized, non-flaxedilized animals.*

The classical sensory and motor cortices, the thalamus and hypothalamus, and the midbrain reticular formation have been the principal targets of unit studies during sleep, while elements of the association cortex, extrapyramidal motor system, limbic system, and the pons and medulla of the brain stem remain virtually unexplored. The cat has been the experimental subject in most of these studies.

Discharge Rates

The majority of neurons in most brain loci exhibit higher discharge rates in REM than in quiet waking (W), and higher rates during W as compared to SWS. Thus, in most sites SWS appears to be a period of reduced activity. However, these neurons do not cease firing during SWS, but maintain appreciable rates. Further, as is discussed more fully below, very slow firing neurons often fire faster in SWS than in W. In addition, most studies report that a minority of neurons in each site exhibit faster discharge rates during SWS than W. This minority could represent smaller neurons which are underrepresented in samples from heterogeneous sites (50). There also are some brain sites where the majority of neurons exhibit increased firing during SWS compared to W and REM (4, 22, 24, 43). It may be noteworthy that, in four of five of these exceptions to the rule of decreased firing rate in SWS, the recordings were from limbic structures: amygdala (24), hippocampus (36), and from a closely related structure, the medial hypothalamus (23, 43). These results may be characteristic of structures whose function is to control or suppress behavior. The amygdala (7, 16), hippocampus (34), and medial hypothalamus (37) are often characterized as inhibitory structures.

The dramatic augmentation of unit activity throughout the brain during REM is an important finding. In most sites, units exhibit similar activity during W and REM. This observation sup-

---

* For a comprehensive annotated bibliography on the subject of sleep and unit activity, the reader is referred to *Neuronal Activity in Sleep* by Hobson and McCarley, available from the UCLA Brain Information Service.

ports the concept that the brain becomes aroused during REM while behavioral expression is blocked by inhibition of motoneurons. The somewhat higher rates in REM as compared to W may result from the common use of samples from quiet waking rather than active waking or periods of stimulation. The similarity of unit activity during W and REM makes the discovery of exceptions to this rule of special interest, because they are correlated with sleep behavior rather than arousal of the brain.

Several recent studies have reported that the increase in discharge rate during REM, as compared with SWS, is totally accounted for by the bursts which appear in association with the phasic activities of REM, such as eye movements or muscle twitches (20, 21, 29, 51). This has not been found in a number of other studies which report that units discharge at higher rates in REM even in the absence of phasic activity (4, 20, 23). This distinction between tonic and phasic changes during REM may prove indicative of tonic and phasic functions. It should also be pointed out that several studies report no increase in discharge rate in association with phasic activity (4, 33, 40) and in some cases a decrease has been found (24, Chapter XV of this volume).

It is interesting to note that discharge rates during all states tend to be higher in the thalamus (38, 39, 48) and in brain stem structures such as the midbrain reticular formation (23, 29), vestibular nuclei (4), and the cerebellum (20, 32, 33), as compared to cortical areas (10, 12, 14, 21), the hypothalamus (15, 23, 43) and the limbic system (24, 40). Mean discharge rates in the former structures are typically twenty-five to fifty spikes/sec in REM and ten to thirty spikes/sec in SWS, while the mean rates in the latter structures are typically less than fifteen spikes/sec in REM and less than ten spikes/sec in SWS. There are important exceptions to this particular generalization such as the slow firing brain stem raphe neurons discussed in Chapter XV of this volume, but future studies may suggest some meaningful principles relating discharge rate to organization or function.

A number of investigators have attempted to deduce morphological and functional characteristics of neurons from both discharge rates during quiet waking and the changes in rates as the animal goes through several sleep states. Evarts (13) has provided us with data from monkey pyramidal tract neurons which indicate that cells which are slow firing during W tend to: have large cell bodies, be phasically active, and increase in discharge rate during SWS, while those that are faster firing during W discharge slower during SWS, and tend to be smaller cells. The relationship between level of spontaneous activity during W and the direction of rate change in going into SWS also holds for cells in visual and association cortex (9, 14, 21), reticular formation (22) and amygdala (24, Chapter XVI). These findings do not mean that all large cells in the brain have low firing rates during W and speed up during SWS, or that all small cells tend to increase their rates of firing as they pass from quiet waking to SWS. For example, Mano (32) showed that cerebellar Purkinje cells (rather large neurons) that had mean discharge rates covering a range of five/sec to sixty-five/sec undergo negligible rate changes from W to SWS.

To examine the generalization that fast cells slow down in the transition from W to SWS one must study a group of neurons from a homogeneous population and realize that defining absolute rates for neurons across the entire brain as fast or slow is not meaningful in making the "speed up, slow down" generalization. Moreover, the study of a structure such as the cortex without identifying a homogeneous group of neurons as a basis of classification may be inappropriate.

These results bear on the problem of the encoding of information by fast firing and slow firing cells. One often finds cells that are virtually silent during W, but this is rarely seen during SWS (8, 22, 24). Closely related to this is the finding that slow firing cells have been found to discharge at high rates in response to phasic motor activity or sensory input (13, 24, 29). Evarts (8, 11) has suggested that a decrease in discharge rate of slow firing cells during W may be a manifestation of an increase in the signal to noise ratio of the nervous system. Conversely, the regression toward a mean during SWS (fast cells—slow down, slow cells—speed up) reflects a decreased signal to noise ratio within the brain. According to this approach, changes in rate of firing during sleep are reflections of altered information transmission rather than of restoration or fatigue of the neuron.

Discharge Patterns

The most pervasive changes in unit activity during sleep are in firing patterns. Most neurons exhibit a burst-pause pattern during SWS. This pattern is characterized by bursts of two to twenty spikes at rates of up to several hundred spikes/sec followed by a relative or complete decrease in discharge rate lasting from several hundred msec up to several seconds. It appears that the tendency to show this burst-pause pattern is much stronger in the forebrain, especially the thalamus and cortex, than in the brain stem. The thalamus has, in fact, been theorized to be the generator of this pattern (1), but the issue remains open. Unit activity during W is often described as *regular*. As stated above, during REM, units tend to burst in association with phasic activities; the only exceptions to this rule are cells in the amygdala (24), hippocampus (40), cerebellum (33), raphe nucleus (see Chapter XV) and lateral vestibular nucleus (4). In the absence of phasic activity, cells are typically described as having a *regular* pattern of discharge like that during quiet waking. Exceptions are reported in studies of cells in the pyramidal tract (12), midbrain reticular formation (22), superior colliculus (22), and thalamus (3, 48).

In pyramidal tract neurons (12) and in neurons of the ventroposterolateral nucleus of the thalamus (3), the pattern of activity during REM, an exaggerated burst-pause pattern, is described as being more similar to that seen during SWS than W. This type of finding is significant because it is an example of a phenomenon shared by SWS and REM.

Interactions Between Cells

Two recent papers by Noda (41, 42) provide data on an interesting aspect of unit activity across sleep-wakefulness. In studies of the cat association cortex and hippocampus, he reported that neighboring cells (those which could be recorded simultaneously from a single microelectrode) tended to show less of a relationship, *i.e.*, minimal cross-correlations, during REM as compared to SWS. During arousal the cross-correlation was even lower than that seen in REM. These findings suggest that, when the brain is aroused, neighboring cells show little relationship, and this relationship among cells greatly increases when the brain is at rest. As stated above, a large part of the brain shows a burst-pause pattern during SWS. This has been interpreted as being indicative of neuronal systems which are functionally unavailable for the processing of neural information (46). The high cross correlation observed between cells during SWS is consistent with this notion. It is as though the cells within a group were being driven in a synchronous, automatic fashion, and were unable to conduct any functional throughput. It would indeed be interesting to gather data similar to Noda's from a variety of other structures.

Brazier (5) has demonstrated by means of EEG coherence techniques that the degree of correlation of EEG activity in specific frequency bands between hippocampal and amygdala structures is decreased in the transition from wakefulness to slow wave sleep. If one could examine the neural activity at the single cell level between these structures, then it should be possible to see in what manner the coherence breaks down. It appears from the Noda studies that the degree of relationship may increase between cells *within* a structure. There is a possibility, then, based on EEG evidence, that relationships of cells between certain structures such as the hippocampus and amygdala may decrease during slow wave sleep. This reciprocal change in within-structure and between-structure interactions may be an important property of sleep.

Experimental Controls

Although most brain sites exhibit striking changes in activity during sleep, many of these changes may represent passive consequences of sleep or correlates of secondary aspects of behavior during sleep. A trivial example would be unit activity changes that are correlated only with lying postures or absence of movement. Since these postures may occur in the waking animal, unit activity should be studied in comparable situations during sleep and wakefulness. Indeed, we must consider the variety of autonomic and peripheral changes that take place during sleep. A sleeping animal is usually lying down with many consequent changes in proprioceptive, visual, and tactile stimuli; he usually chooses a place of rest where he is subjected to lesser intensities of external stimuli; because he is still, there is usually reduced cardiac and respiratory output and neuronal motor outflow to certain muscle groups is altered. Moreover, brain structures concerned with such acts as the initiation of movement are altered in function (18). Control of most of these variables is easily achieved since animals exhibit brief spontaneous EEG arousals during SWS with minimal somatic and autonomic changes. Nevertheless, most investigators have failed to report specifically on these experimental controls.

Unit Activity and EEG Synchronization

SWS is closely associated with EEG synchronization; however, there are some special instances in which we can dissociate the EEG and behavioral aspects of sleep. For example, atropine given in sufficient dosage to an alert animal will synchronize the EEG and produce slow waves and spindles while the animal is awake (17, 52). It was found that during atropine dissociation a great proportion of the neurons in diencephalic structures exhibited a firing pattern like that in SWS (17, Chapter XV). Thus, these units were related to EEG patterns rather than to the particular behavioral state of the animal.

Specific aspects of the sleeping EEG such as the 12-14 Hz spindle activity appearing over the sigmoid gyrus can be conditioned in an alert animal (6, 53). During conditioning of this rhythm some units from VPL and red nucleus change their discharge pattern to that seen during sleep (19). These changes may result from the EEG synchronization or the accompanying changes in visceral and somatic functions associated with EEG conditioning or both.

Some neurons appear to fire in a direct relationship to particular aspects of an EEG wave. For example, neurons in the hippocampus, anterior thalamus and septum (17, 30, 44) are related to certain aspects of the wave shape of hippocampal theta. During sleep there are a variety of EEG changes, including an increase in the amplitude and frequency of theta during REM sleep (18). The spontaneous activity of those neurons should be considered in the light of their relationship to this very specific EEG frequency. The relationship of unit activity to EEG patterns is discussed fully in Chapter IX of this volume.

Natural sleep itself provides examples of dissociation of EEG ac-

tivity and behavior. REM sleep is characterized by a desynchronized EEG typical of wakefulness. Indeed, REM sleep has been
known by the term paradoxical sleep since, paradoxically, the
EEG was desynchronized during a period of obvious sleeping.
Many neurons exhibit similar patterns during REM and wakefulness. The activity of these neurons appears to be correlated
with a state of brain arousal rather than behavior.

SUMMARY

Studies of spontaneous unit activity during sleep and wakefulness have neglected proposed sleep centers. However, the review
of investigations of a variety of cortical and subcortical sites suggests some tentative characteristics of the sleeping brain and provides some insights into basic properties of brain function.

During SWS most brain sites exhibit reduced firing compared
to W, but neurons do not become silent. Slow firing neurons often
increase in rate from W to SWS. Neurons in some limbic sites, as
well as a minority of neurons elsewhere, also exhibit increased
firing in SWS. A burst-pause pattern of firing pervades much of
the brain during SWS.

During REM, most neurons exhibit high rates of firing, comparable to or higher than active waking. Bursts of firing, particularly in relation to phasic events, characterize this state. The majority of neurons in the amygdala (Chapter XVI), dorsal raphe
nucleus (Chapter XV), as well as a minority of neurons elsewhere, exhibit slowing in REM.

The experimental dissociation of EEG synchronization and
sleep reveals that the firing of a large number of neurons is correlated with EEG patterns rather than sleep behavior.

REFERENCES

1. Andersen, P. and S. A. Anderson. *Physiological Basis of the Alpha Rhythm.* Appleton-Century-Crofts, New York, 1968.
2. Batini, C., G. Moruzzi, M. Palestini, G. F. Rossi, and A. Zanchetti. Effects of complete pontine transections on the sleep-wakefulness rhythm, the midpontine pretrigeminal preparation. *Arch. ital. Biol.* 97:1-12, 1959.
3. Benoit, O. Spontaneous repetitive discharge of thalamic units during sleep in cats. *Psychophysiology* 7:310-311, 1970 (abstract).

4. Bizzi, E., O. Pompeiano, and I. Somogyi. Spontaneous activity of single vestibular neurons of unrestrained cats during sleep and wakefulness. *Arch. ital. Biol.* 102:308-330, 1964.

5. Brazier, M. A. B. Studies of the EEG activity of limbic structures in man. *Electroenceph. Clin. Neurophysiol.* 25:309-318, 1968.

6. Chase, M. H. and R. M. Harper. Somatomotor and visceromotor correlates of operantly conditioned 12-14 c/sec sensorimotor cortical activity. *Electroenceph. Clin. Neurophysiol.* 31:85-92, 1971.

7. Egger, M. D. and J. P. Flynn. Effects of electrical stimulation of the amygdala on hypothalamically elicited attack behavior in cats. *J. Neurophysiol.* 26:705-720, 1963.

8. Evarts, E. V. Effects of sleep and waking on spontaneous and evoked discharge of single units in visual cortex. *Fed. Proc.* 19:828-837, 1960.

9. Evarts, E. V. Effects of sleep and waking on activity of single units in the unrestrained cat. In G. E. W. Wolstenholme and C. M. O'Connor (Eds.) *The Nature of Sleep.* Little, Brown, Boston, 1960, pp. 171-187.

10. Evarts, E. V. Activity of neurons in visual cortex of the cat during sleep with low voltage fast EEG activity. *J. Neurophysiol.* 25:812-816, 1962.

11. Evarts, E. V. Photically evoked responses in visual cortex units during sleep and waking. *J. Neurophysiol.* 26:229-248, 1963.

12. Evarts, E. V. Temporal patterns of discharge of pyramidal tract neurons during sleep and waking in the monkey. *J. Neurophysiol.* 27:152-171, 1964.

13. Evarts, E. V. Relation of discharge frequency to conduction velocity in pyramidal tract neurons. *J. Neurophysiol.* 28:216-228, 1965.

14. Evarts, E. V., E. Bental, B. Bihari, and P. R. Huttenlocher. Spontaneous discharge of single neurons during sleep and waking. *Science,* 135:726-728, 1962.

15. Findlay, A. L. R. and J. N. Hayward. Spontaneous activity of single neurons in the hypothalamus of rabbits during sleep and waking. *J. Physiol.* (London) 201:237-258, 1969.

16. Fonberg, E. and J. M. R. Delgado. Avoidance and alimentary reactions during amygdala stimulation. *J. Neurophysiol.* 24:651-664, 1961.

17. Harper, R. M. Activity of single neurons during sleep and altered states of consciousness. *Psychophysiology* 7:312, 1971.

18. Harper, R. M. Frequency changes in hippocampal electrical activity during movement and tonic immobility. *Physiol. Behav.* 7:55-58, 1971.

19. Harper, R. M. Relationship of neuronal activity to EEG waves during sleep and wakefulness. Paper presented to First International

Congress of the Association for the Psychophysiological Study of Sleep, Bruges, 1971.

20. Hobson, J. A. and R. W. McCarley. Spontaneous unit activity of cat cerebellar Purkinje cells in sleep and waking. *Psychophysiol.* 7:311, 1970.

21. Hobson, J. A. and R. W. McCarley. Cortical unit activity in sleep and waking. *Electroencephalog. Clin. Neurophysiol.* 30:97-112, 1971.

22. Huttenlocher, P. R. Evoked and spontaneous activity in single units of medial brain stem during natural sleep and waking. *J. Neurophysiol.* 24:451-468, 1961.

23. Jacobs, B. L., R. M. Harper, and D. J. McGinty. Neural coding of motivational level during sleep. *Physiol. Behav.* 5:1139-1143, 1970.

24. Jacobs, B. L. and D. J. McGinty. Amygdala unit activity during sleep and waking. *Exper. Neurol.* 33:1-15, 1971.

25. Jouvet, M. Recherches sur les structures nerveuses et les mecanismes responsables des differentes phases du sommeil physiologique. *Arch. ital. Biol.* 100:125-206, 1962.

26. Jouvet, M. Etude de la dualite des etats de sommeil et des mechanismes de la phase paradoxical. In M. Jouvet (Ed.) *Aspects Anatomo-Fonctionnels de la Physiologie Du Sommeil,* Centre National de la Research Scientific, Paris, 1965, pp. 397-450.

27. Jouvet, M. Neurophysiology of the states of sleep. *Physiol. Rev.* 47: 117-177, 1967.

28. Jouvet, M. Biogenic amines and the states of sleep. *Science* 163:32-41, 1969.

29. Kasamatsu, T. Maintained and evoked unit activity in the mesencephalic reticular formation of the freely behaving cat. *Exper. Neurol.* 28:450-470, 1970.

30. Macadar, O., J. A. Roig, J. M. Monti, and R. Budelli. The functional relationship between septal and hippocampal unit activity and hippocampal theta rhythms. *Physiol. Behav.* 5:1443-1450, 1970.

31. Magnes, J., G. Moruzzi, and O. Pompeiano. Synchronization of the EEG produced by low-frequency electrical stimulation of the region of the solitary tract. *Arch. ital. Biol.* 99:33-67, 1961.

32. Mano, N. I. Changes of simple and complex spike activity of cerebellar Purkinje cells with sleep and waking. *Science* 170:1325-1327, 1970.

33. Marchesi, G. F. and P. Strata. Climbing fibers of cat cerebellum: modulation of activity during sleep. *Brain Res.* 17:145-148, 1970.

34. McCleary, R. A. Response-modulating functions of the limbic system: initiation and suppression. In E. Stellar and J. M. Sprague (Eds.) *Progress in Physiological Psychology,* Vol. I. Academic Press, New York, 1966, pp. 209-272.

35. McGinty, D. J. and M. B. Sterman. Sleep suppression after basal fore-brain lesions in the cat. *Science* 160:1253-1255, 1968.
36. Mink, W. D., P. J. Best, and J. Olds. Neurons in paradoxical sleep and motivated behavior. *Science* 158:1335-1337, 1967.
37. Morgane, P. J. The function of the limbic and rhinic forebrain-limbic midbrain systems and reticular formation in the regulation of food and water intake. *N.Y. Acad. Sci. Annals* 157:806-848, 1969.
38. Mukhametov, L. M., G. Rizzolatti, and A. Seitun. An analysis of the spontaneous activity of lateral geniculate neurons and of optic tract fibers in free moving cats. *Arch. ital. Biol.* 108:325-347, 1970.
39. Mukhametov, L. M., G. Rizzolatti, and V. Tradardi. Spontaneous activity of neurons of nucleus reticularis thalami in freely moving cats. *J. Physiol.* (London) 210:651-667, 1970.
40. Noda, H., S. Manohar, and W. R. Adey. Spontaneous activity of cat hippocampal neurons in sleep and wakefulness. *Exper. Neurol.* 24:217-231, 1969.
41. Noda, H., S. Manohar, and W. R. Adey. Correlated firing of hippo-campal neuron pairs in sleep and wakefulness. *Exper. Neurol.* 24: 232-247, 1969.
42. Noda, H. and W. R. Adey. Firing of neuron pairs in cat association cortex during sleep and wakefulness. *J. Neurophysiol.* 33:672-684, 1970.
43. Oomura, Y., H. Ooyama, F. Naka, T. Yamamoto, T. Ono, and N. Koba-yashi. Some stochastical patterns of single unit discharges in the cat hypothalamus under chronic conditions. *N.Y. Acad. Sci. Annals* 157: 666-689, 1969.
44. Petsche, H. and C. Stumpf. Hippocampal arousal and seizure activ-ity in rabbits: toposcopical and microelectrode aspect. *In Physio-logie del' Hippocampe Colloques Internationales,* CNRS, No. 107, pp. 121-134.
45. Pompeiano, O. The neurophysiological mechanisms of the postural and motor events during desynchronized sleep. In S. S. Kety, E. V. Evarts, and H. L. Williams (Eds.) *Sleep and Altered States of Consciousness.* Williams and Wilkins, Baltimore, 1967, pp. 351-423.
46. Purpura, D. P. Operations and processes in thalamic and synaptically related subsystems. In F. O. Schmitt (Ed.) *The Neurosciences: Second Study Program.* Rockefeller University Press, 1970, pp. 458-470.
47. Rechtschaffen, A. and A. Kales (Eds.) *A Manual of Standardized Terminology, Techniques and Scoring System for Sleep Stages of Human Subjects.* Public Health Service, U.S. Printing Office, 1968.
48. Sakakura, H. Spontaneous and evoked unitary activities of cat lateral

geniculate neurons in sleep and wakefulness. *Jap. J. Physiol.* 18: 23-42, 1968.

49. Sterman, M. B. and C. D. Clemente. Forebrain inhibitory mechanisms: sleep patterns induced by basal forebrain stimulation in the behaving cat. *Exper. Neurol.* 6:103-117, 1962.

50. Towe, A. L. and G. W. Harding. Extracellular microelectrode sampling bias. *Exper. Neurol.* 29:366-381, 1970.

51. Valleala, P. The temporal relation of unit discharge in visual cortex and activity of the extraocular muscles during sleep. *Arch. ital. Biol.* 105:1-14, 1967.

52. Wikler, A. Pharmacologic dissociation of behavior and EEG "sleep patterns" in dogs: morphine, N-allylnor-morphine and atropine. *Proc. Soc. Exptl. Biol. Med.* 79:261-265, 1952.

53. Wyrwicka, W. and M. B. Sterman. Instrumental conditioning of sensorimotor cortex EEG spindles in the waking cat. *Physiol. Behav.* 3:703-707, 1968.

Chapter XII

NATURAL FUNCTIONS OF CEREBELLAR CIRCUITS

W. T. THACH

THE CEREBELLUM IS particularly suited to single unit analysis. The cell types are segregated into layers or masses; their connecting fibers are also to some extent segregated. This design allows one to record with a microelectrode from identifiable cell types under different experimental conditions.

One may also electrically stimulate identifiable inputs to a cell and see how they affect the behavior of the cell. In the hands of Eccles, Ito and others, this experimental method has shown which synapses are excitatory and which inhibitory (4, 11-14, 28). Along with the anatomic methods of Nauta and Golgi stains and electron microscopy (*e.g.*, 6-9), this approach is drawing a remarkably complete diagram of the cerebellar circuitry (Fig. 12.1). The design appears fundamental throughout the cerebellum, one area differing from another chiefly in its input and output connections (Fig. 12.2). Yet the diagram renders the actual circuitry deceptively simple, for it omits entirely the crucial features of convergence and divergence as cells project to and receive from one another. Lacking this information (and surer knowledge of the membrane and synaptic properties), one is limited in trying to deduce from the circuit diagram its overall function, or even the circuit function of any one of its components.

One approach to the problem is to learn what one can by recording from single cells during conditions with which the circuit would seem (according to classic ablation experiments) to be mainly concerned: natural posture and movement. To this end, Evarts' techniques (15-17) have been used to record the discharge of single neurons in the cerebellum of rhesus macaques trained to maintain postures and perform movements with the arms. Under

179

these conditions, one can learn about the properties of the cerebellar output by recording from cerebellar nuclear cells which, along with some Purkinje cells, generate and distribute the cerebellar output. One can learn about the synthesis of that output by recording from Purkinje cells which, along with collaterals from mossy and climbing fibers, control the nuclear cell. It is more difficult to record directly from the climbing and mossy fibers themselves, but one can learn something about their behavior by recording from the Purkinje cell, since each input to the cerebellum appears to cause (or influence the occurrence) of a different kind of spike potential in the Purkinje cell (Fig. 12.3). The Purkinje cell generates two kinds of spike potential, a fact that has been proven by recording them not only extra- but also intracellularly

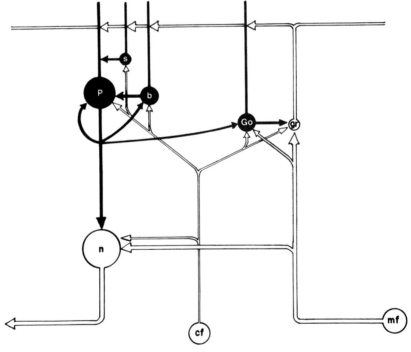

Figure 12.1. Simplified diagram of cerebellar circuitry. MF = mossy fiber; cf = climbing fiber; gr = granule cell; Go = Golgi cell; b = basket cell; s = stellate cell; P=Purkinje cell; n = nuclear cell. White cells are excitatory; black, inhibitory.

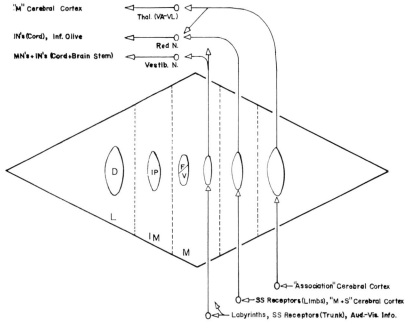

Figure 12.2. Simplified diagram of the mossy fiber input and output connections of different parts of the cerebellum. Cortical zones: L = lateral; IM = intermediate; M = medial. Deep nuclei: D = dentate; IP = interposed; F/V = fastigial and vestibular. Outputs: *M* = motor; VA-VL = ventrolateral and ventroanterior nuclei of the thalamus; IN = interneuron; MN = motor neuron; N = nucleus. Inputs: SS = somatosensory; M + S = motor and sensory. The *reticular formation* sends to and receives from all parts of the cerebellum.

from a Purkinje cell reliably identified by its antidromic response to an electric shock to its axon in the cerebellar nuclei (20). One spike potential is of short duration and simple contour (hence, *simple spike*), and occurs in anesthetized and awake animals at frequencies as high as 100/sec. Its occurrence may be increased by stimulating the axons of granule cells (13, 29), which suggests that it is caused by input from granule cells. The simple spike discharge is at intervals interrupted by a second kind of spike potential of longer duration and more complex contour (hence, *complex spike*), which occurs sporadically at a rate averaging around 1/sec (34). Its occurrence may be caused by stimulating

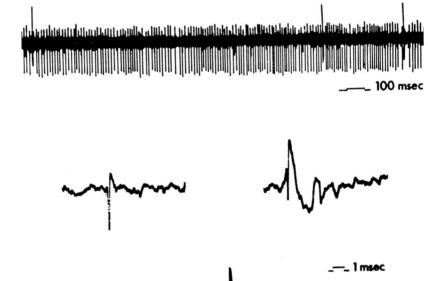

100 msec

1 msec

Figure 12.3. Maintained discharge of a Purkinje cell. Many units in or near the Purkinje layer generate spikes of two different shapes (*simple,* left; *complex,* right) that occur in a distinctive firing pattern (top). These discharge properties are similar to those that have been recorded intracellularly in antidromically identified Purkinje cells and serve not only to identify the Purkinje cell but also tell something about the activity of its two excitatory inputs. From *J. Neurophysiol.* 31:785-797, 1968.

the inferior olive (14) which, along with other evidence (cf. 18) suggests that it is the response of the Purkinje cell to a spike or a burst of spikes (3, 5) in a climbing fiber coming from the inferior olive (32). These spikes serve as indices of activity in the two excitatory inputs to the Purkinje cell—climbing fiber, and the mossy fiber-granule cell relay. In addition, the distinctive two-spiked pattern of discharge also suffices (along with histologic verification refs. 34, 35) to identify a Purkinje cell encountered with an extracellular microelectrode without other experimental manipulation. Nuclear cells may be identified when a negative cell-spike is recorded in the nuclei (with histologic verification); this identification is aided by the fact that in our hands the glass-coated platinum-iridium microelectrode (39), unlike the lacquer-coated tungsten microelectrode (23), passes long distances through white matter without recording from fibers. These apparent differences between the two types may be due to the former being rounded and the latter very sharp at the tip, which may determine whether the tip pushes aside or cuts through myelinated fibers. Whatever the cause, the differences in their ability to record from fibers make both electrodes useful.

Monkeys were trained to grasp a vertical rod and move it in a horizontal plane in return for a fruit juice reward. In one experiment (35) the movement was a self paced rapid alternating movement at the wrist (flexion-extension) or shoulder (pushing-pulling); in a second experiment (36, 37) prompt movement of the wrist (flexion or extension) from a maintained posture (extension or flexion) in response to a signal (light or buzzer). When the monkeys had learned the task, steel bolts were surgically placed in the skull. These were then attached during the training sessions to bars on the sides of a special primate chair, so as to restrain the head. After a monkey had learned to perform with the head held, a hole was cut in the skull over the cerebellum and a steel cylinder fixed to bone over the hole. On recovery from this operation, the monkey was placed in the chair with head fixed and allowed to perform the task as the microelectrode was advanced through dura, cerebrum, tentorium, and into the cerebellum.

What parts of the cerebellum are concerned with movement of the arms? Penetrations passed vertically through the *intermediate zone* (IM) cortex, whose Purkinje cells project chiefly to the interposed nucleus (27). The penetrations were then continued deeper into the interposed nucleus or the dentate (both being under the IM zone cortex), which receives from Purkinje cells more in the lateral zone cortex. Both zones—intermediate and lateral—might be supposed to be involved in arm movements. The intermediate zone receives *arm* information over mos-

sy fibers from two major sources: from receptors in the arm relayed by spinocerebellar tracts, and from motor and sensory cerebral cortex relayed by ponto-cerebellar paths (27). Its output
(generated by the interposed nucleus) is distributed principally
to the magnocellular part of the red nucleus, which is thought
(cf. 18) to project to spinal cord interneurons and to aid the
cortico-spinal tract in the control of movements of the limbs (and
not trunk). The lateral zone receives its major mossy fiber input
from frontal, temporal, parietal and occipital *association* areas
of the cerebral cortex after a synapse in the pontine nuclei; its
coding is not known. Nevertheless, the output of the lateral zone
(generated by the dentate nucleus) projects to VA-VL thalamus
which is the major driving input to motor cortex (cf. 18), and
would appear to contribute to arm movement via corticospinal,
corticorubrospinal, and corticoreticulospinal controls. Since these
different parts of the cerebellum might be expected to differ in
their relation to arm movements, a marking method (35) was developed for analyzing subsequent histological sections that accurately identified which part of the cerebellum each of the many
penetrations in a single monkey traversed.

What questions, using this technique, may one ask of neurons
in these parts of the cerebellum? The properties and possible uses
of cerebellar output may be studied by looking at its frequency of
discharge, coding and timing. One might have predicted that the
frequency of discharge of both nuclear and Purkinje cells even
in the absence of movement would be high (averaging around 40-
70/sec, respectively). Comparably high frequencies had previously been seen in anesthetized or decerebrate animals. During
movement, changes in discharge would occur over a wide range
(0-500/sec). Somewhat less predictable were the observations
made on the coding of discharge. During each of two maintained
postures (wrist flexion vs. extension), about 90 percent of nuclear
cells discharged at one frequency, suggesting that those cells did
not distinguish between the postures. But 10 percent of the cells
(Fig. 12.4) discharged as much as five times faster for one posture as the other, suggesting that these cells—and thus probably
the cerebellum generally—can distinguish between and contribute differentially to (and thus help select or maintain) two dif-

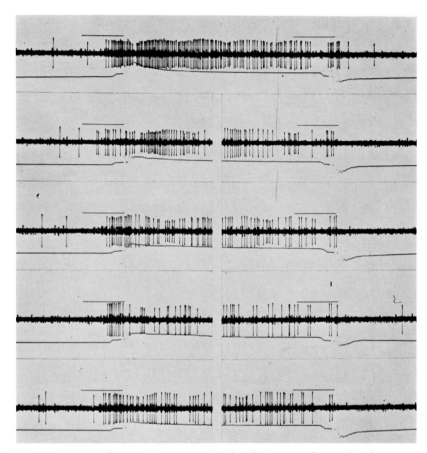

Figure 12.4. Discharge of a neuron in the dentate nucleus related to consecutive flexor (left) and extensor (right) movements of the ipsilateral
wrist. Top line = onset and duration (350 msec) of the light signal; middle line = discharge of the unit (positivity up); bottom line = force exerted
on the vertical rod (up is flexion; down is extension). Change in frequency
is better time locked to the movement than to the signal to move, precedes the movement (and even the first change in force), and is different
in pattern for movement in the two different directions. The maintained
frequency during maintained flexion (middle) was greater than that during maintained extension (ends). From *J. Neurophysiol.* 33:527-536, 1970.

ferent postures. During the stereotyped repeated movements (self-paced rapidly alternating or prompt signal-triggered) the pattern and frequency of discharge varied from cell to cell for a given movement and for a given cell for two different movements. The diversity of pattern suggests that many cells may contribute to any one movement, but that each cell must preferentially be linked to some particular aspect of the movement whose full occurrence is related to a maximum (or minimum) discharge frequency in that cell. What these particular aspects of movement are and what the precise cerebellum-movement relationship (or code) is has not been further determined. Least predictable were the observations on timing: while some neurons changed discharge frequency only after the movement had begun, others changed well before the movement—as early as 90 msec before any EMG change in trunk or limbs. This suggests that these *early* neurons could not have been caused to change by feedback from the movement; instead they may have themselves helped cause the movement, participating at an early stage in its initiation. On the other hand, changes in the *late* neurons could either have been related to and caused by feedback from the onset of movement, or related to and helping cause some later components of the movement—or both, one movement triggering another movement in a chain reflex. Of great interest was the finding that the *early* neurons were preferentially grouped in the dentate and the *late* neurons in the interposed nuclei (Fig. 12.5). One may consider these timing differences in light of the theories on cerebellar function of Herrick (21), Holmes (22), and Ito (24). According to Herrick's first mechanism, the late neurons in interpositus could well have been triggered from receptors in the limb by the onset of movement, and be used to help attain or maintain (regulate) a final position or prevent oscillation of the limb at the end of movement. According to Herrick's second mechanism, the earlier neurons in interpositus, changing at the time of or slightly before movement, could well have been initiated by the input to this area from the motor cortex—perhaps to be compared in the cerebellum with information from the peripheral receptors about the steady state posture existing before movement, and the output used to help the corticospinal tracts initiate and maintain movement appropriate to the pre-existing posture. The earliest cells were in the dentate, which receives its input principally from association cortex (and to a lesser extent from motor cortex—10), and sends to motor cortex after a synapse in VA-VL thalamus. According to Gordon Holmes, dentate upon receipt of information from the association area would synthesize the first motor command, that would be fed through thalamus where further specifications could be added on, and then used to initiate a change in motor cortex output. In this mechanism changes in dentate would precede and initiate changes in motor cortical output. According to Ito, motor cortex would initiate the first command for movement: a sample of the command would be fed to dentate where it would be compared with input from association cortex, which might represent steady state conditions in body and environment, properties of the stimulus, memory of past performance, etc. On the basis of the comparison, a judgement might be made as to whether the movement that had been ordered by the cerebral cortex were appropriate to these various contexts. If inappropriate, an *error* signal would be sent rapidly back to motor cortex to change the command. The change would occur after the initiation of the command, but before movement—and cerebellar output would occur after motor cortex output. In simple language these hypotheses may appear fanciful; yet any or all could be correct, and they are in large part testable simply by looking for differences in timing that may exist between different elements of the motor system as each enters into the genesis of a prompt movement. This does not imply that the sequence will be the same for all movements —it may, for example, be different for volitional movements and involuntary startle responses (31). But the observed differences between interpositus and dentate (Fig. 12.5) suggest that timing differences do exist, and, as Evarts suggested (16), that they may be measured in this way.

What may one say about the synthesis of cerebellar output? The output of Purkinje cells, which along with mossy fibers and climbing fibers control the nuclear cells, was in general *similar* to that of the nuclear cells to which it projects. In the absence of movement, there was a high average maintained frequency of

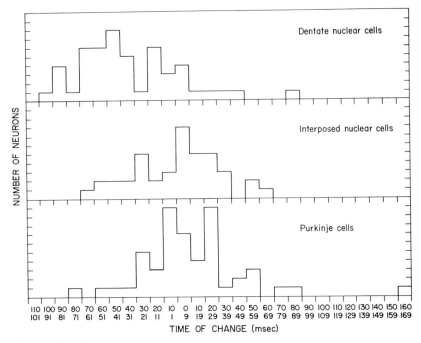

Figure 12.5. Distribution of the time of change of discharge frequency in relation to flexion or extension (whichever earlier) for all neurons in the dentate and interposed nuclei and Purkinje cells of the intermediate zone. Onset of movement = 0 msec. From *J. Neurophysiol.* 33:537-547, 1970.

discharge; during each of two maintained postures, 10 percent of Purkinje cells discharged higher for one posture than the other; during movement, there was wide variation in discharge pattern from cell to cell in relation to a given movement, and for one cell in relation to each of two movements; the time of change could be before or after the movement (Fig. 12.6). Given the similarity of properties of the Purkinje cells and the nuclear cells to which they project, the question arises: do the Purkinje cells cause these changes in the nuclear cell? Since the nuclear cell has ongoing discharge in the face of ongoing inhibitory discharge from the Purkinje cell, it must either have strong pacemaker activity or tonic excitatory drive from mossy fibers. Given the capacity for maintained discharge (whatever the cause), changes in Purkinje cell input would cause changes in nuclear cell output, and since the synapse is inhibitory, the changes would be opposite in sign. This question was examined by comparing the changes that occur in the intermediate zone Purkinje cells and in the interposed nuclear cells to which they project in relation to the signal-triggered prompt movement (37).

As expected, Purkinje cells changed discharge at about the same time as did the nuclear cells to which they project (Fig. 12.5). But contrary to expectations, the initial change in frequency for *both* populations was more commonly (76 percent of Purkinje cells and 76 percent of nuclear cells) an increase rather than a decrease. This suggests that the Purkinje cell and the nuclear cells to which it projects initially change frequency in the same direction. At rest, the Purkinje cell inhibition must tonically oppose the maintained firing of the nuclear cell; during movement, it must change in opposition to the change that also occurs in the nuclear cell. Thus, rather than *initiate* the change in the nuclear cells, the Purkinje cell must *modify through restraint* the already initiated output of the nuclear cell. This mechanism has received further experimental support in the observations of Mortimer (31). In his experiments, the discharge of intermediate zone Purkinje cells and interposed nuclear cells were recorded in monkeys before and during a *start* in response to a loud noise. He observed that for over 90 percent of the nuclear cells and 60 percent of the Purkinje cells the first change was an increase rather than a decrease in activity; and that the nuclear cells changed a few milliseconds *before* the Purkinje cells. These plus the above observations suggest that the first changes in nuclear cell activity must be initiated by prior changes in their mossy fiber inputs. It must be the mossy and not the climbing fiber inputs because 1) climbing fibers discharge at too low a frequency to account for the high frequency output of the nuclear cell, and 2) from Mortimer's data, climbing fiber activity (as indicated by the complex spike of the Purkinje cell) changes much later than the first changes in nuclear cell output and in the simple spike discharge of the Purkinje cell. If, in relation to movement, changes in mossy fiber activity cause most of the changes both in nuclear cell and Purkinje cell output, it seems likely also for the changes that

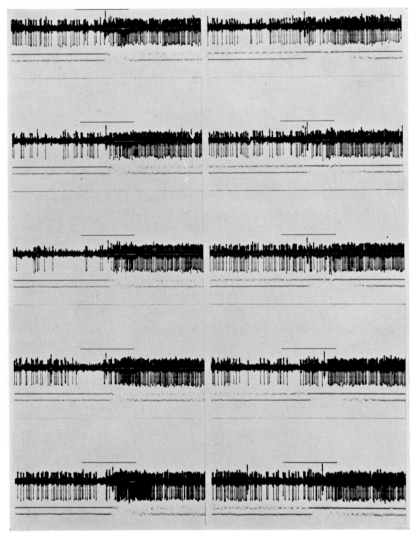

Figure 12.6. Discharge of a Purkinje cell related to consecutive flexor (left) and extensor (right) movements. First line = onset and duration (350 msec) of the light signal; second line = discharge of the unit; third line = EMG recorded from the ipsilateral surface of the forearm; fourth line = EMG from the extensor surface of the forearm. Both the complex (more positive) and simple (more negative) spikes occur in relation to the movement. From *J. Neurophysiol.* 33:537-547, 1970.

occur in relation to two different postures, and probably also that a maintained discharge frequency in the absence of movement drives the tonic firing of the nuclear cell. These predictions about mossy fiber activity during posture and movement can be tested by recording from their cells of origin during these conditions.

Given that the Purkinje cell is a *feedforward inhibitory frequency controller* superimposed on the straight through line, what might it be used for? Possibilities have been mentioned elsewhere (38): it may differentiate the input, giving an output with a transient at its leading edge perhaps to overcome the inertia of the body in initiating movements; or it might increase the specificity of the nuclear cell response to its input by a filtering process similar to lateral inhibition; or it might change the input-output properties of the straight through circuit by changing the degree of restraint from the Purkinje cell by a process akin to learning. It might perform all three of these functions, and a number of others.

The role of the climbing fiber, and of the inferior olive whence it largely comes, remain a mystery. Some of the clues are: 1) the climbing fiber is excitatory (14, 28); 2) it apparently contacts not only the Purkinje cell but also every other (stellate?) cellular element in the cerebellum (9); 3) it may change frequency of firing in relation to some kinds of movement (startle response and signal triggered prompt movement—31, 37) and not to others (self paced rapid alternating movement—35); 4) it may change before or after the movement (37), and 5) preferentially in relation to one movement (flexion) and not another (extension) (37); 6) its firing frequency even when increased in relation to movement is a low 0.5-2.0/sec (37); 7) when increased in frequency it may be associated with many different patterns of change in simple spike activity in the Purkinje cell, and the simple spike may change without the complex spike changing—hence, no unique relationship between the two (37); 8) simple spike change may precede complex spike change (31); 9) the small secondary wavelets which are often seen on the slow after-wave of the complex spike have been observed to come down the axon in about half the Purkinje cells and not to come down in another half (25); 10) the small secondary wavelets each appear to be caused by a spike within the variable burst of spikes that comes up the climbing fiber from the inferior olive (3, 5); 11) the number of small secondary wavelets in the complex spike does not correlate with the immediately prior firing frequency of the simple spike and thus seems independent of the state of excitability of the Purkinje cell (29). Moreover, the inferior olive would appear essential to *all* of cerebellar function (and not simply learning), since its ablation apparently results in a motor deficit indistinguishable from that following cerebellar ablation (31b). It is difficult to see what these properties add up to beyond rejecting some of the popular hypotheses on climbing fiber function and setting some narrow constraints on future proposals.

What direction will further studies take? One worthwhile question is that raised by Evarts (16) of the relative timing of changes in discharge of various components of the motor system. Is there a sequence of changes that betrays a causal chain? Does a change in cerebellar output precede and initiate or does it follow and modify the changes that also occur in the target neurons? Does the dentate nucleus (and lateral cerebellar cortex) cause the initial command from the motor cortex or only correct it after it has begun? A second question is the code of cerebellar unit discharge and its relation to movement and posture. Several approaches may be taken: one is similar to that of somesthetic and visual sensory physiologists who record from neurons at various stages in a linear array. The aim is to determine how the cells at successive stages specifically respond to a *best* natural peripheral stimulus and to deduce what functions are being developed in each of the various stages and by the entire linear array of stages. Some earlier attempts at this in anesthetized animals failed to drive many cells (34), but in decerebrate animals Purkinje cells (*e.g.*, 4b, 33) and nuclear cells (2) can respond sensitively to natural peripheral stimulation, and this approach is currently being used by several groups. A second approach, begun by Fetz (19), mirrors the first, and would consist of an attempt to characterize the behavior of single cells in parts of the motor system in relation to activity in output (rather than input or receptive) fields composed of specific muscle groups. Success would depend on being able to train animals either to perform a wide repertoire of stereotyped movements or to vary their behavior continuously at the will of the experimenter. Man, at the time of neurosurgery, would theoretically be a good candidate for the latter, if ethical and technical problems could be overcome. A third approach would examine the relationship between central command and peripheral feedback at places where they are anatomically juxtaposed: for example, in the intermediate zone of the cerebellar cortex. Are motor cerebral cortex, sensory cerebral cortex and limb somatosensory feedback *each* capable of initiating a change in interpositus output? Or is an output generated under some special conditions when and only when *all* inputs are active? Or does one input *bias* or *condition* the other *triggering* inputs? Could such a bias-plus-trigger circuit qualify as a comparator? Finally, the question raised by Poseidonios in the third century as to whether the cerebellum has a specific role in (motor) learning again comes up (1, 30) and must be settled by some kind of experiment.

SUMMARY

Despite all that is now known about cerebellar circuitry, little is known of what the constituent cells specifically add to the circuits in which they are arranged, or what the cerebellum specifically contributes to posture and movement.

In an attempt to learn more about the natural properties of cerebellar output, its synthesis, and its possible uses by the rest of the nervous system, Evarts' methods have been used to record the discharge of single neurons in the cerebellum of awake monkeys as they perform conditioned movements and postures.

As for properties of the cerebellar output, this approach has given a measure of the discharge frequency at which these neurons operate. The variation in pattern of discharge from one cell to the next and from one movement to another suggests specificity of the relationship of cell to movement—but not the nature of the specificity. Timing of the changes that occur in relation to volitional movement suggest that dentate plays an early role in the initiation of movement and that interpositus may play a later role—even after the onset of movement.

As for the synthesis of cerebellar output, evidence is offered that mossy fibers initiate the first changes in nuclear cell output and that these changes are then opposed by mounting inhibition from Purkinje cells, which work to restrain the nuclear cell change. Such a mechanism might be used in differentiating, filtering, and learning a mossy fiber input, as well as a number of other applications.

As for the various possible uses of cerebellar output that are suggested by these and other studies, several approaches seem likely of securing answers.

REFERENCES

1. Arbib, M. A., Franklin, G. F. and Nilsson, N. Some ideas on information processing in the cerebellum. *Proc. Summer School of Math. Models of Neuronic Networks,* Ravello, Italy, June 4-19, 1967.
2. Arduini, A. and Pompeiano, O. Microelectrode analysis of the rostral portion of the nucleus fastigii, *Arch. ital. Biol.,* 95, 56-70, 1957.
3. Armstrong, D. M. and Harvey, R. J. Responses of a spino-olivo-cerebellar pathway in the cat. *J. Physiol.* (Lond.), 194, 147-168, 1968.
4. Bell, C. C. and Dow, R. S. Cerebellar Circuitry. *Neurosciences Res. Program Bull.,* 5, 121-222, 1967.
4b. Brookhart, J. M., Moruzzi, G. and Snider, R. S. Spike discharges of single units in the cerebellar cortex. *J. Neurophysiol.,* 13, 465-486, 1950.
5. Crill, W. E. Unitary multi-spiked responses in cat inferior olive nucleus. *J. Neurophysiol.,* 33, 199-209, 1970.
6. Chan-Palay, V. The recurrent collaterals of Purkinje cell axons: a correlated study of the rats cerebellar cortex with electron microscopy and the Golgi method. *Z. Anat. Entwickl.-Gesch.,* 134, 200-234, 1971.
7. Chan-Palay, V. and Palay, S. Interrelations of basket cell axons and climbing fibers in the cerebellar cortex of the rat. *Z. Anat. Entwickl.-Gesch.,* 132, 191-227, 1970.
8. Chan-Palay, V. and Palay, S. The synapse en marron between Golgi II neurons and mossy fibers in the rat's cerebellar cortex. *Z. Anat. Entwickl.-Gesch.,* 133, 274-287, 1971.
9. Chan-Palay, V. and Palay, S. Tendril and glomerular collaterals of climbing fibers in the granular layer of the rats cerebellar cortex. *Z. Anat. Entwickl.-Gesch.,* 133, 247-273, 1971.

10. Dow, R. S. Cerebellar action potentials in response to stimulation of the cerebral cortex in monkeys and cats. *J. Neurophysiol.*, 5, 121-136, 1942.
11. Eccles, J. C., Ito, M. and Szentagothai, J. *The Cerebellum as a Neuronal Machine.* Springer, New York, 335 pp., 1967.
12. Eccles, J. C., Llinas, R. and Sasaki, K. The mossy fibre-granule cell relay and its inhibitory control by Golgi cells. *Exp. Brain Res.*, 1, 82-101, 1966.
13. Eccles, J. C., Llinas, R. and Sasaki, K. Parallel fiber stimulation and responses induced thereby in the Purkinje cells of the cerebellum. *Exp. Brain Res.*, 1, 17-39, 1966.
14. Eccles, J. C., Llinas, R. and Sasaki, K. The excitatory synaptic action of climbing fibers on the Purkinje cells of the cerebellum. *J. Physiol.* (Lond.), 182, 268-296, 1966.
15. Evarts, E. V. Relation of discharge frequency to conduction velocity in pyramidal tract neurons. *J. Neurophysiol.*, 28, 216-228, 1964.
16. Evarts, E. V. Pyramidal tract activity associated with a conditioned hand movement in the monkey. *J. Neurophysiol.*, 29, 1011-1027, 1966.
17. Evarts, E. V. A technique for recording activity of subcortical neurons in moving animals. *Electroenceph. Clin. Neurophysiol.*, 24, 83-86, 1968.
18. Evarts, E. V. and Thach, W. T. Motor mechanisms of the CNS: cerebrocerebellar interrelations. *Ann. Rev. Physiol.*, 31, 451-498, 1969.
19. Fetz, E. and Finochio, D. B. Operant conditioning of specific patterns of neural and muscular activity. *Science*, 174, 431-435, 1971.
20. Granit, R. and Phillips, C. G. Excitatory and inhibitory processes acting upon individual Purkinje cells of the cerebellum in cats. *J. Physiol.* (Lond.), 133, 520-547, 1956.
21. Herrick, C. J. Origin and evolution of the cerebellum. *Arch. Neurol. Psychiat.*, 11, 621-652, 1924.
22. Holmes, G. The cerebellum of man. *Brain*, 62, 1-30, 1939.
23. Hubel, D. H. Tungsten microelectrodes for recording from single units. *Science*, 125, 549-550, 1957.
24. Ito, M. The cerebello-vestibular interaction in cats vestibular nuclei neurons. *Symp. Vestibular Mechanisms*, Miami, 1968, in press.
25. Ito, M. and Simpson, J. I. Discharges in Purkinje cell axons during climbing fiber activation. *Brain Research*, 31, 215-219, 1971.
26. Ito, M., Yoshida, M. and Obata, J. Monosynaptic inhibition of the intracerebellar nuclei induced from the cerebellar cortex. *Experientia* (Basel), 20, 295-296, 1964.
27. Jansen, J. and Brodal, A. *Aspects of Cerebellar Anatomy*, Grundt-Tanum, Oslo, 1954.
28. Jansen, J., Jr. and Fangel, C. Observations on cerebro-cerebellar evoked potentials in the cat. *Exp. Neurol.*, 3, 160-173, 1961.

29. Mano, N. Changes of simple and complex spike activity of cerebellar Purkinje cells with sleep and waking. *Science,* 170, 1325-1327, 1970.

30. Marr, D. A theory of cerebellar cortex. *J. Physiol.* (Lond.), 202, 437-470, 1969.

31. Mortimer, J. A. and Evarts, E. V. Latency differences in cerebellar Purkinje and nuclear cell activity in association with startle responses. *Fed. Proc.,* 902, 1972.

31b. Murphy, M. G. and O'Leary, J. L. Neurological deficit in cats with lesions of the olivo-cerebellar system. *Arch. Neurol.,* 24, 145-157, 1971.

32. Szentagothai, J. and Rajkovits, J. Uber den Ursprung der Kletterfasern des Kleinhirns. *Z. Anat. Entwickl.-Gesch.,* 121, 130-141, 1959.

33. Tarnecki, R. and Konorski, J. Patterns of responses of Purkinje cells in cats to passive displacements of limbs, squeezing, and touching. *Acta Biol. Exp.* (Warszawa), in press.

34. Thach, W. T. Somatosensory receptive fields of single units in cat cerebellar cortex. *J. Neurophysiol.,* 30, 675-696, 1967.

35. Thach, W. T. Discharge of Purkinje and cerebellar nuclear neurons during rapidly alternating arm movements in the monkey. *J. Neurophysiol.,* 31, 785-797, 1968.

36. Thach, W. T. Discharge of cerebellar neurons related to two maintained postures and two prompt movements. I. Nuclear cell output. *J. Neurophysiol.,* 33, 527-536, 1970.

37. Thach, W. T. Discharge of cerebellar neurons related to two maintained postures and two prompt movements. II. Purkinje cell output and input. *J. Neurophysiol.,* 33, 537-547, 1970.

38. Thach, W. T. Cerebellar output: properties, synthesis, and uses. *Brain Research,* 40, 89-97, 1972.

39. Wolbarsht, M. L., MacNichol, E. F. and Wagner, H. G. Glass insulated platinum microelectrodes. *Science,* 132, 1309-1310, 1960,

Chapter XIII

LONG-TERM SPONTANEOUS ACTIVITY OF INDIVIDUAL CEREBELLAR NEURONS IN THE AWAKE AND UNRESTRAINED CAT

JAMES G. McELLIGOTT

THE NUMBER OF studies on the electrophysiology of the cerebellar cortex has grown significantly within the past few years (7, 17). Nevertheless, there has been a considerable lack of experimentation in the unanesthetized and intact preparation, with the exception of the studies performed by Thach (32, 33, 34). His experiments on the monkey have been directed towards describing the role of Purkinje and cerebellar nuclear cells with regard to movement. More recently there have also been a number of studies on firing patterns of cerebellar neurons during sleep-wakefulness cycles (14, 18, 19).

One of the purposes in this series of experiments was to investigate the spontaneous firing patterns of cerebellar neurons in the unanesthetized and intact cat over relatively long periods. Techniques have been developed to record the extracellular potentials of individual neurons using fine wire electrodes that are permanently implanted in the chronic animal (26, 27). Similar

It is a pleasure to thank Dr. W. Ross Adey for his support during the term of these experiments and for his critical evaluation of the manuscript. I would also like to thank Dr. C. Batini and Dr. R. Kado for their critical comments, Vern Foust for programming assistance, Jackie Payne for preparation of the figures, and Loretta McKenna for typing the manuscript.

This work was carried out at the Space Biology Lab of the Brain Research Institute and Department of Anatomy at U.C.L.A. Support was obtained from NASA Grant NGR 05-007-195 and U.S. Air Force Grant F44620-70-C-0017 to the Space Biology Laboratory, and USPHS NIH Grant NSO 2501 to the Data Processing Laboratory of the Brain Research Institute, as well as from the UCLA Brain Information Service, a member of the NINDS neurological network, flexible fine wires have also been used in the cerebellum (5) and reticular formation (28) of acute preparations to secure stable extracellular records. The implantations in this study were maintained for twelve to eighteen months, and extracellular recordings from several neurons in each animal were obtained. The potentials from an individual neuron can be recorded for periods ranging from several hours to days in the freely moving animal. Combining this technique with radio telemetry, it has been possible to make single cell recordings on the totally unrestrained animal (22, 23).

In the experiments presented here, two types of cells have been encountered. One of these had firing patterns not previously reported. This report describes the firing patterns of these cells during periods of spontaneous activity when the animal was awake and resting quietly. A subsequent report describes the changes in these firing patterns of one of these neuron types when sensory stimulation is presented to the animal (21).

Methods

Electrode Implantation

Implantations were performed on fifteen cats anesthetized with sodium pentobarbital (35 mg/kg) and placed in a stereotaxic instrument. Small insulated fine wire electrodes (dia. 25 μ) of either stainless steel (Johnson-Matthey Metals, London) or nickel-chromium (Wilbur B. Driver, Los Angeles) were prepared by cutting pieces of wire from the spool with scissors (5, 26, 27). There was no other special preparation of the electrode tip.

Usually a number of these wires (four to seven) were bunched together with their tips vertically displaced over a 0.5 mm range. This cluster of wires was attached to a rigid supporting rod with wax and extended about 15 mm beyond the end of the rod. This rod was fastened to a standard electrode carrier. After craniotomy and folding back of the underlying dura mater, a small puncture was made in the pia and the electrodes were stereotaxically directed to cortical structures in the intermediate zone of lobes V and VI about 10 mm below the exposed surface. After gelfoam was placed on the cortical surface around the wires, they were rigidly attached to the skull with dental cement and then soldered to a thirty-four pin female Winchester plug. Upon removal of the supporting rod, additional cement was used to seal the hole and attach the plug to the skull. Usually two clusters of wires were implanted bilaterally in this manner. Anterior and posterior sagittal skull screws served as an electrical ground. After about a week of postoperative recovery, both testing and recording sessions were initiated and continued during a twelve to eighteen month period.

Recording Equipment and Data Acquisition

The neural spike potentials were fed via connecting cables (Microdot) into differential, high impedance FET amplifiers and Tektronix 122 preamplifiers. Alternately, neural spikes were transmitted via a small telemetry device that had been incorporated into the male connector plug and placed on the animal's head. The method of telemetering neural spike data has been described elsewhere (22, 23). Generally, the reference electrode was one of the other nonactive fine wire electrodes in the cluster. In all cases, neural spikes were recorded over a bandwidth of 400 Hz to 10 kHz (3 db). These spikes, as well as the pulses which they generated in a Schmitt trigger, and a digital time code were recorded on magnetic tape by an Ampex recorder (FR-1300). Often the neural spikes were photographed directly by a Grass camera (Model C4) from a Hewlett Packard oscilloscope (#132A), or from a Tektronix storage oscilloscope (#564) with a Polaroid camera. At times, the neural data were placed directly on a Honeywell Visocorder (#1706).

Experimental Paradigm

In the experiment to be described in this paper, the animal was placed in a box (1.1 m × 0.6 m × 0.5 m) having a one way transparent glass mirror. The laboratory room was darkened to facilitate viewing of the animal through the glass. The animal was unrestricted except for the connecting cable and when the telemetry device was used there was complete freedom of movement within the box. Two 25 watt bulbs provided an overall illumination of 22.5 footcandles. Ambient noise was at a level of 62 db (re SPL) and emanated mainly from recording equipment in the laboratory.

The firings of cells were monitored by the experimenter via a set of earphones. Spontaneous firings were recorded with the animal awake and sitting, or lying quietly in the box. In all cases, the animals were well habituated to the experimental box and the situation.

Computer Analysis

The magnetically taped data were then digitalized and analyzed by the SDS 9300 (Scientific Data Systems) computer of the Brain Research Institute. Digitizing rates as high as 16,000 and 10,667 samples/sec with concomitant bin widths of 62.5 and 94 μsec were used.

Fortran programs, for the analysis of neural spike data stored in the computer, were accessed via the SLIP console system (2). For the Group I bursting cell, these programs fell into two categories, depending upon the particular type of intervals with which they dealt. These intervals were either in the interburst (long intervals between bursts) or the intraburst (short intervals within bursts) class. Programs in the former category include interval histograms (*i.e.*, interburst interval histograms), interburst auto- and cross-correlograms. Programs in the latter category include the probability distribution histogram, which graphically illustrates for a particular neuron the percent of times a burst will contain a given number of spikes. There are also intraburst interval histograms, one of which is formed for each order of magnitude of a burst. The number of spikes in a burst determines the order of magnitude. These histograms are formed with the first spike of the burst occurring at the origin and the subsequent spikes in the burst occurring at their respective times along the abscissa or time axis. From these individuals intraburst histograms, the timing of spikes within bursts of different orders of magnitude can be determined. These programs were also used to evaluate the burst-like firing of the Group II cell. In addition, standard interval histograms and auto-correlograms were also used to evaluate this cell when it fired with a train of single spikes.

Histology

The animals were sacrificed under pentobarbital anesthesia by perfusion with normal saline and 10 percent formalin via the common carotid arteries. An anodal current of 10 μA for 30 sec was passed through the electrodes. The Prussian blue staining technique was used for location of the tips of the stainless steel wire and the dimethylglyoxime method for nickel was used for the nickel-chromium wire. The brain was fixed in 10 percent formalin and frozen serial sections 50 μ thick were stained with carbol fuchsin for the stainless steel wire or thionin for the nickel-chromium wire.

RESULTS

Extracellular potentials from individual cerebellar neurons have been recorded in the unanesthetized and unrestrained cat for periods ranging from a few hours to five days. During this time the neural spike potential manifests a constant amplitude between 30-100 μv (pp) superimposed on a 5-10 μv (rms) level of background neural activity. This and a stable wave form are two of the criteria used for determining that the potential emanates from the same neuron. When the spike potential of a single unit is about to disappear, there is a noticeable increase or decrease in amplitude over a period of hours to days, followed by the subsequent loss of the neural spike. The background activity remains relatively constant during this entire period. After several days or weeks, another extracellular potential may emerge above the background activity and can be recorded. When this happens on the same electrode, it is difficult to say if this is the reappearance of the cell previously recorded or an entirely new one. Inasmuch as there are a number of fine wires clustered together and implanted in each animal, it has been possible to record the potentials from two neurons simultaneously. It should be noted also that on many electrodes no extracellular potentials are ever seen.

Data will be presented that were obtained from twenty-two neurons recorded at four different sites in three cats. In all instances, the recording area was in the intermediate zone of lobes

V and VI of the cerebellar cortex, confirmed by the histology. Individual cerebellar cell types could not be ascertained from the histology due to the relatively large size of the electrode tip. Two different groups of cells have been recorded. Group I contains seventeen neurons that fired only in a burst or rapid succession of spikes. Group II contains five neurons that emitted bursts similar to those in Group I but also fired in trains of single spikes between the bursts.

I. *Group I Neurons*

A. Long intervals between bursts (Interburst).

    The long intervals between bursts of the Group I neurons form

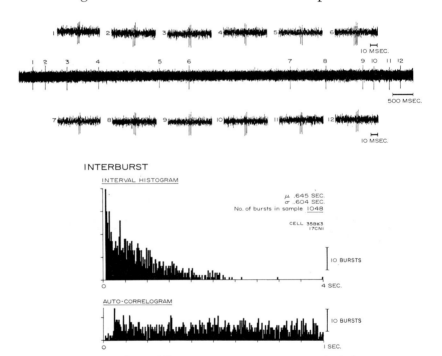

Figure 13.1. Top: The middle trace is a continuous record of the extracellular potentials from a Group I bursting cell (time base = 500 msec). The numbered traces above and below this are identical with their equivalents in the middle trace. They are presented on a faster time base (10 msec) to show the burst-like firing of the cell.

Bottom: The two plots represent the interburst interval histogram and interburst autocorrelogram. They describe the characteristics of the long intervals between bursts.

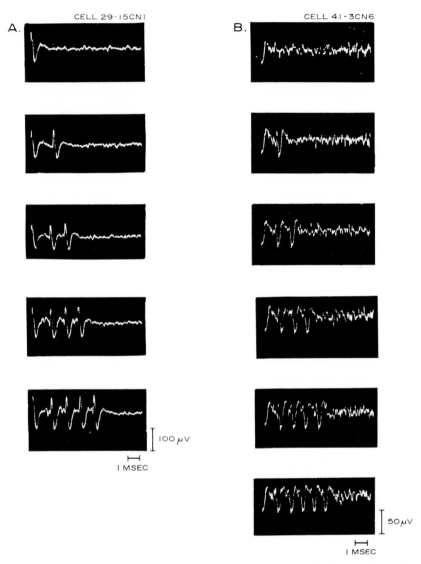

Figure 13.2. Two examples of the Group I bursting cell. The cell on the left (A) emitted from one to five spikes per burst. The cell on the right could produce up to six spikes. For each of the cells, the wave form and amplitude of all of the spikes in any burst were identical.

interburst interval histograms that have Poisson-like distributions (Fig. 13.1). For all cells investigated, the mean intervals for these distributions were 0.6 to 0.7 sec with a range from 0.4 to 1.2 sec. The coefficient of variation (standard deviation/mean interval) was about 0.8 and ranged from 0.75 to 1.2. The longest recorded intervals between bursts were about 15 sec. At the other extreme, these intervals can be as short as 50 msec and in some instances three bursts occurred within a 100 msec period. These cells tend to emit bursts randomly. The flat auto-correlation histograms that have been obtained in all cases testify to this (Fig. 13.1).

B. Characteristics of spikes and intervals within the burst (Intraburst).

The amplitude of the extracellular spike potentials within a burst appeared to be of equal amplitude and similar wave form. There was no decrement in amplitude for subsequent spikes within the burst (Fig. 13.2). These measurements were made over an 8 Hz to 10 kHz, as well as the 400 Hz to 10 kHz bandpass. The number of spikes per burst varied randomly from burst to burst, and there appeared to be no relation between the number of spikes in a burst and the duration of the long interval just preceding the burst. Six spikes was the maximum seen in any particular burst. Generally most cells emitted one to four spikes whereas bursts of five and six spikes were less common. Furthermore, each individual cell had its own probability distribution for the number of spikes per burst. Figure 13.3 (I, II, III and IV) depicts distributions for four different neurons. They were obtained from spontaneous firing of a neuron over a period, and then the bursts were sorted according to the number of spikes. Repeated sampling of a bursting cell shows that these probability distribution histograms were consistent and did not change their distributions radically. This is graphically illustrated for two separate neurons in Figure 13.3 (III: A, B, C, D and IV: A, B, C, D). For each neuron, these samples were taken during a single experimental session over several hours when the animal was awake and resting quietly. In the probability distribution histogram, the Kolmogorov-Smirnov non-parametric test (K-S) was applied to determine if two histograms were significantly different from

PROBABILITY DISTRIBUTION HISTOGRAM OF SPIKES
PER BURST OF FOUR DIFFERENT NEURONS

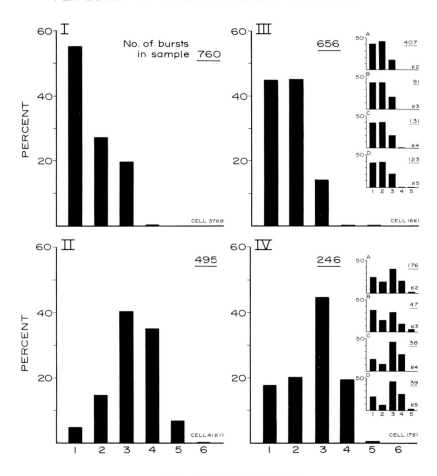

NO. OF SPIKES/BURST

Figure 13.3. The probability distribution histograms of four different
Group I cells (I, II, III, IV). This histogram represents the percentage
of times the cell emits a burst containing a certain number of spikes during
spontaneous firing periods. Repeated successive sampling shows that individual neurons have a consistent probability distribution histogram. This
is presented for two separate cells in III (A, B, C, D) and IV (A, B, C, D).
These successive samples were taken during periods that spanned several
hours. The number of bursts that were used to form the histogram is
given in the upper right hand corner in each case.

each other. Arbitrarily a significant difference was judged to be present if p < .0005. The various distributions for the two different neurons (Fig. 13.3: I, II, III, IV) were all found to be different from each other at this level. Moreover, for the two neurons where several independent samples were taken (Fig. 13.3: III: A, B, C, D and IV: A, B, C, D), no significant difference was found. The smallest difference within each group was greater than the 0.1 level and most were at the 0.8 level of probability.

Another feature of the bursting cell is that the spikes within the burst are highly regular. Recordings of thousands of bursts from an individual cell show that there is a preferred timing sequence in the firing pattern. This property becomes even more evident if we sort the bursts into individual intraburst interval histograms according to the order of magnitude of a burst (i.e., number of spikes/burst). In each case, first spike in the burst occurs at the origin or time zero of the histogram (Fig. 13.4). Subsequent spikes in the burst fall along the abscissa. Note that no histogram can be formed where there is only one spike per burst. The cumulative intraburst interval histogram is the sum of the individual ones. In general, most of the respective spikes fall within one bin width of each other on the individual histograms (bin width = 94 μsec). Thus, individual histograms, which were formed by hundreds of bursts, demonstrated the extremely stable timing of the spike production from burst to burst. The neuron in Figure 13.4A is a typical example of this and represents all but one of the Group I bursting cells recorded. This one exception is presented in Figure 13.4B. For this particular cell, the respective spikes in the accumulated bursts tended to form a normal distribution with a greater variance about their means.

The timings of the spikes manifested a relatively stereotyped pattern. Within any burst the longest interval was the first with successive intervals becoming progressively shorter. A similar relationship existed between first intervals. Shorter first intervals were found as the number of spikes per burst increased. Therefore, for a particular bursting neuron, the first interval of a doublet (two spikes/burst) was the longest, whereas the shortest intervals were the later intervals of a higher order burst. Thus, it is evident that the higher order bursts possessed the fastest rates of

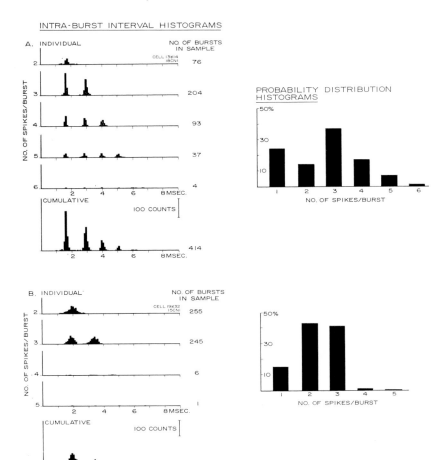

Figure 13.4. Intraburst interval histograms for two different Group I cells (A and B). These histograms are formed by having the first spike in a burst occur at the origin with subsequent spikes in the burst occurring along the time axis. Individual histograms are formed for each order of magnitude of a burst. The order of magnitude is determined by the number of spikes per burst. The cumulative histogram is the sum of the individual ones. Note that no histogram can be formed when there is only one spike per burst. The intraburst firing patterns presented for the first cell (A) are typical for sixteen cells; those of (B) are typical for only the one cell presented. The corresponding probability distribution histograms for these two cells (A and B) are presented to the right of their respective histograms.

spike production. This gradual shortening of the intervals is graphically (Fig. 13.5) and numerically (Table 13.1) illustrated. Figure 13.5 is a three dimensional representation of the stereotyped firing patterns of a Group I burster obtained from the individual intraburst interval histograms. The height above the plane is the amount of time that the respective intervals are shorter than the longest intraburst interval recorded for that cell. In all cases, this is the interval in a doublet burst. The points for this plot come from Table 13.1B and the confidence boundaries from Table

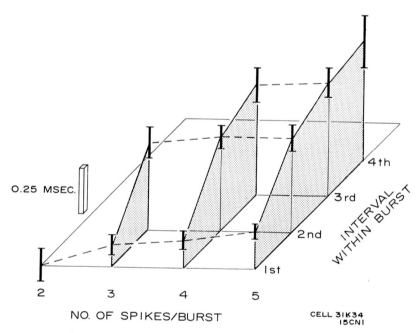

Figure 13.5. A three dimensional representation of the stereotype firing pattern of the Group I cell that is obtained from the individual intraburst interval histograms. This is a graphical picture of the numerical data presented in Table I (B and C). The height above the plane is the amount of time in milliseconds that the respective intraburst intervals are shorter than the interval within a doublet burst. This is generally the longest intraburst interval recorded. Note that there is a gradual shortening for the latter intervals within a burst and for the corresponding intervals in bursts of different orders of magnitude. In the case presented only the various first intervals shorten significantly. The confidence bars represent plus and minus one standard deviation.

TABLE 13.1

	No. of Spikes Per Burst				Interval Within the Burst
	2	3	4	5	
No. of bursts in sample	131	304	191	52	
Mean duration of burst (msec)	1.72	2.85	3.81	4.92	
A. Intraburst interval length (msec)				1.08	4th
			1.13	1.11	3rd
		1.25	1.21	1.21	2nd
	1.72	1.60	1.57	1.52	1st
B. Intraburst interval shortening (msec)				−.64	4th
			−.59	−.61	3rd
		−.47	−.51	−.51	2nd
	−.00	−.12	−.15	−.20	1st
C. Standard deviation (msec)				.141	4th
			.092	.081	3rd
		.084	.060	.075	2nd
	.088	.056	.049	.044	1st

This table deals with the intervals within bursts according to the number of spikes in the burst and the position of the particular interval within the burst. The first part of the table gives the number of bursts in that sample as well as the mean duration of the burst in that sample. Subsequent parts of the table depict respectively: A. The length of the various intervals within bursts of different orders of magnitude. The timings in milliseconds are derived from the individual intrabursts histogram. B. The amount of time that the respective intervals are shorter than the interval in a doublet burst. This doublet interval is the longest intraburst interval recorded. Thus, this table is obtained by subtracting 1.72 msec from each individual entry in (A). C. The standard deviation associated with the various intraburst intervals.

13.1C. Shorter intervals are represented by greater heights above the plane. The general contour of this figure is similar for all the Group I cells.

Repeated samples taken over several hours indicate that this timing behavior for any one bursting cell was very stable. In a small number of cases, the later intervals in a higher order burst (quintuplet or sextuplet) did not follow this orderly sequence and were of equal or longer duration than prior intervals within the burst. Estimates for this timing sequence within bursts were obtained from the individual intraburst interval histograms and also by direct measurements from photographs and from the face of the storage oscilloscope.

Individual cells have different rates of burster spike production. These timing differences are small, and there is a great deal of overlap among the cells. The longest first intervals obtained from different neurons ranged from 1.5 to 2.2 msec. Most of the cells possessed values in the 1.7 to 1.9 msec range. The shortest intervals seen (last interval of a quintuplet or sextuplet) ranged from 1.2 to 1.0 msec. When different bursting neurons were compared, there appeared to be no relationship between the rate of burster spike production and the probability distribution histogram. Thus, cells that had a propensity to produce higher order bursts did not have faster rates of spike production than those which produced lower order bursts more often.

The combination of this individual burst timing sequence for each cell with its probability distribution histogram is another criterion by which individual bursting cells can be distinguished from one another.

C. Spontaneous firing of bursting neurons for extended periods.

It was possible to record the activity of four bursting neurons for periods of three or more days. During each experimental session, the animal appeared to be in the same behavioral state, *i.e.*, awake and resting quietly. Samples of the extracellular potentials during a five day period indicated that the spike potentials originated from the same neuron (Fig. 13.6). The probability distribution histogram, which is an estimate of the propensity for a neuron to produce bursts of a given number of spikes, manifested a certain stability for an individual neuron from day to day. There were slight changes in this distribution histogram, but such alterations had also been seen during the course of one experimental session. In the example cited in Figure 13.6, only on the fifth day was there a marked shift in the probability distribution histogram. The K-S statistical test showed that this was different from that of the other days at the .0005 level. In addition, the timings of the spikes within the bursts did not change appreciably over several days. Furthermore, the mean interval between the bursts also remained quite stable during the period.

D. Simultaneous recording of two neurons.

In seven cases, the spike potentials from a pair of bursting

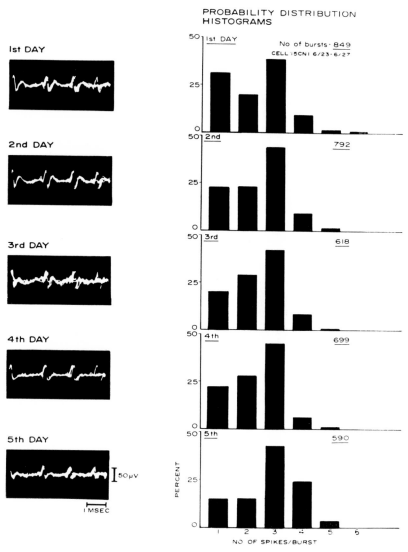

Figure 13.6. Left: Extracellular potentials of a Group I cell recorded over a five day period. Each record contains five superimposed traces triggered on the first spike in the burst.

Right: The probability distribution histogram for the cell on each of the five days. The number of bursts that contributed to the histogram is given in the upper right hand corner in each case.

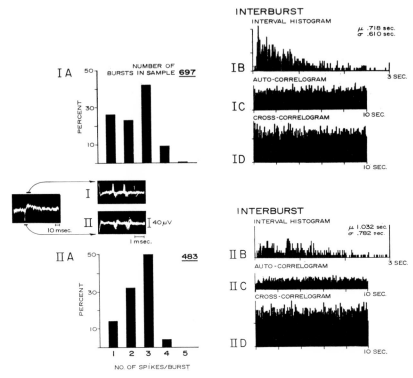

Figure 13.7. This composite figure represents the recordings and various histograms describing the firing patterns for two Group I cells recorded simultaneously on the same electrode. The record at the extreme left shows the potentials from the two cells when they fired close together. I. Ten superimposed traces of a burst triggering on the first (positive-going) cell. II. Ten superimposed traces triggering on the second (negative-going) cell. IA and IIA. The probability distribution histograms for first and second cells respectively. IB and IIB. Interburst interval histograms for the first and second cells respectively. IC and IIC. Interburst autocorrelogram for the first and second cells respectively. ID and IID. Interburst cross correlogram. The cross correlogram in ID is formed by using the first cell as reference and looking at the firing of the second cell with respect to it. Time zero is at the left hand side of the axis. The cross correlogram in IID is formed in a similar manner but the second cell is the reference.

cerebellar neurons were recorded simultaneously. In four cases, these cells were present on two different electrodes whose tips were separated by 200 to 400 μ. In only one of the three cases where two Group I bursters appeared on the same electrode could adequate separation of the two cells be made. In this one case, the first cell manifested a negative potential and the second cell had positive-going spikes. Separation of the pair could be easily made by setting appropriate positive and negative voltage levels on two window amplifiers (Fig. 13.7).

The firing of two bursting neurons seemed to have little relationship with each other. Cross correlations of the long intervals

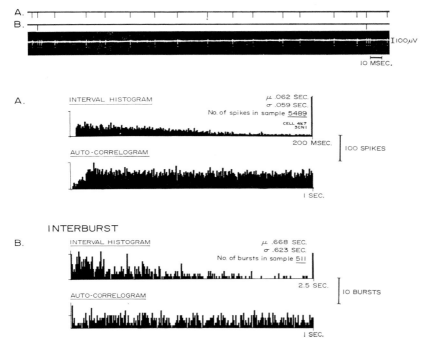

Figure 13.8. The photographic record at the top depicts the firing pattern of a Group II cell. The interval histogram and autocorrelogram in (A) were formed primarily from the single spike firings. The interburst interval histogram and autocorrelogram deal with the long intervals between bursts after the single spike firings are deleted. The two traces (A and B) above the photographic record show how these two groups of intervals are formed.

between the bursts for all pairs of neurons are virtually flat, and there is no evidence of inhibition or facilitation of one neuron upon another (Fig. 13.7: I D and II D). Also, there appeared to be no relation between the number of spikes in a burst by one cell and the number in a concurrent burst of the second cell.

II. Group II Cells of the Cerebellar Cortex

Group II cells fired in trains of single spikes that were inter-digitated with a burst-like firing of spikes. Five neurons of this type were examined. The mean interval for the single spike firings varied from 20 to 80 msec with standard deviations in the range of 30 to 50 msec. All auto-correlograms for single spike firings were virtually flat (Fig. 13.8A).

After deleting the trains of single spike firings, the periods between the bursts form Poisson distributions with a mean interval around 0.7 sec and standard deviations of about 0.8 sec. These interburst periods also formed flat auto-correlograms.

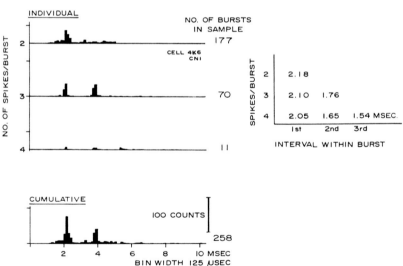

Figure 13.9. The intraburst interval histograms for a Group II cell. It is formed in a manner similar to that for the Group I cell. The table on the right gives the length of the various intervals within bursts of different order of magnitude. It is derived directly from the individual intraburst interval histograms.

For this entire group, four spikes was the maximum produced for any burst. The characteristics of burster firing for these neurons were markedly similar to those in Group I (Fig. 13.9). The timing of the spikes was highly regular within a burst. The longest interval occurred in bursts containing only two spikes (doublet). The first interval in the burst became shorter as the number of spikes per burst increased. Successive intervals within a burst also became progressively shorter.

DISCUSSION

The seventeen Group I cells reported in this paper manifested a firing pattern that has previously not been reported. These recordings made in the unanesthetized and unrestrained cat showed that this neuron fired about once a second and only in a burst of spikes. Due to the unusual nature of these patterns one of the main objects of this study was to investigate the spontaneous activity of these neurons over long periods of time.

This Group I neuron manifested a great deal of stability over periods ranging from hours to days. During the periods of spontaneous activity, each of the cells had a propensity to emit bursts of a given number of spikes. Furthermore, the regular and stereotype timing of the spikes within the bursts did not change. The mean interval of the long periods between the bursts also remained stable. Although these properties remained constant for an individual neuron, different values were obtained for other bursting cells. Thus, these three properties can be considered to be independent parameters by which a particular Group I bursting neuron could be identified.

There is no direct evidence in the experiments performed to indicate which of the five possible cell types of the cerebellar cortex gives rise to the particular firing pattern of the Group I burster. Usually it is possible to imply cell type from the depth of the recording electrode below the surface of the cortex or by stimulation of fiber tracts. These parameters were not used for the electrodes are chronically implanted and recordings are made over a long period. It is probable that slight but significant movements of the electrode take place. In addition, exact histological confirmation of individual cells was not possible due to the relatively large size of the electrode tip identification mark.

Anatomical Considerations

Electrodes usually record the potentials from the larger diameter cells (35). Thus, the Purkinje cell (dia. 30 μ) emerges as the best candidate to have been recorded with the Golgi (20-30 μ) and basket (20 μ) cells following closely behind (7).

The average distance between similar type cell bodies is also an important factor because in three instances the potentials of two Group I bursters were simultaneously recorded on the same electrode. Previous reports state that the distance over which an extracellular potential can be measured is in order of 100 to 200 μ (3, 24). Bishop (3) indicates that this figure is probably greater for large diameter microelectrodes.

The granule cell is the most densely packed cell in the cerebellum with extremely small intercellular distances (11), but it also possesses the smallest cell body size (dia. 9-10 μ). The mean distance between adjacent Purkinje cells is 50 μ in the transverse direction and 50-100 μ longitudinally. The basket cells are slightly closer together for the ratio of basket to Purkinje cells is 1.2 to 1. On the other hand, there is only one Golgi cell for every ten Purkinje neurons (7).

Therefore, considering cell body size and packing density, the Purkinje and basket cells emerge as the most likely neurons to have been recorded.

Spike Firing Patterns

The Group I cell fires only in bursts and so its firing pattern can be described by two discrete sets of intervals, namely, those within (intra-) and those between (inter-) the bursts. The Group II cell fires in trains of single spikes that interdigitate with burst-like firing. The single spikes and the bursts of this type cell were treated separately (Fig. 13.8).

Comparison of the intra- and interburst intervals of Group I cells with those of Group II shows a remarkable similarity. Both types emit bursts randomly at very low firing rates. They form Poisson-like interburst interval histograms with similar mean intervals and standard deviations (Figs. 13. 1, 7 and 8). Furthermore, each produces a highly regular burst of spikes. The shortening of successive intervals within a burst and the more rapid rate of spike production for higher order bursts are also characteristic of both types. In addition, the spikes within a burst of a Group I cell are of equal amplitude and similar wave form. This is also true for the Group II cell.

Most of the previous reports on spontaneous firing patterns have dealt with the Purkinje cell. These studies have been carried out in either the intact and unanesthetized animal (14, 18, 19, 32, 33, 34), decerebrate preparation (4, 5, 10, 13, 25, 30) or under barbiturate (1, 8, 25) or chloralose (4, 5, 15, 29) anesthesia. There have been no reports of firing patterns that resemble those of the Group I burster. On the other hand, there are marked qualitative and quantitative similarities between these previous reports and those of the Group II cell. This becomes evident when the burst-like firing of the Group II cell is equated with the climbing fiber response and single spikes with that of the mossy fiber response. The climbing fiber response (7), the inactivation response (13), and the complex spike (4, 32) that are mentioned by various investigators, are considered to be manifestations of the same event. In a similar manner, the mossy fiber response (7) and the simple spike (32) are equated.

Whereas the climbing fiber response can generally be distinguished from that of the mossy fiber by the wave form of the potentials, the distinction made in the Group II cell is in terms of the natural grouping and timings of the spikes. The amplitude and wave form of a single spike of the Group II cell is identical with that of a spike produced within a burst.

Therefore, from both the anatomical considerations and the firing patterns, it seems reasonable to consider the Group II neuron to be a Purkinje cell, the burst to represent a response to the climbing fiber input and the single firing, a response to the mossy fiber-granule cell input. Furthermore, the Group I burster could also be a Purkinje cell that fired only in the climbing fiber mode.

There are several possible ways in which only the climbing fiber response of the Purkinje cell could occur. Firstly, there are reports that if the electrode is placed in the dendritic arborization of the Purkinje cell, only the climbing fiber response is recorded

(12, 31). Thus, the Group I neuron could have also been producing simple spikes derived from the mossy fiber input system that went unrecorded due to the position of the electrode in the dendritic tree of the Purkinje cell.

Secondly, it is possible that the electrode has damaged the cell. Eccles et al. (8, 9) and Thach (31) have reported that after damaging a Purkinje cell the climbing fiber response was still present, whereas the mossy fiber response was eliminated. It should be emphasized, however, that the Group I burster was not an isolated phenomenon. Seventeen such cells were recorded from three different sites. These cells otherwise appeared in good physiological condition for they manifested consistent and stable firing patterns sometimes over a period of several days. Furthermore, the following paper will demonstrate subtle changes in the firing patterns of the Group I burster that are produced by sensory stimulation (21).

Thirdly, the possibility arises that the burst of spikes emitted by the Group I cell are axonal and arise from the climbing fiber, per se. This is suggested by the fact that the spikes in a burst are of equal amplitude. Previous studies (7) have shown that the climbing fiber response of a Purkinje cell body is a prolonged depolarization upon which is superimposed a burst of spikes declining in amplitude. It is interesting to note that the Group II cell also has spikes of equal amplitudes within its bursts. Furthermore, it seems unlikely that axonal spikes could be recorded in a freely moving animal for long periods of time with an electrode having a tip diameter of 25 μ. A comparison with results of others must take into consideration the differences between this electrode and the more commonly used microelectrodes. These microelectrodes have a tip size of 1 or 2 μ and can be located relatively close to the cell membrane. In this study the electrodes with their 25 μ tip cross section approximates the diameter of the soma of a cell. Thus, this electrode tip is probably farther away from the cell and integrates the signal over a wider area. Therefore a direct comparison of wave form for these two different electrode types may not be possible.

Finally, there could be profound effects on a number of Purkinje cells which are due to anesthetics and the decerebrate preparation. This particular question has given rise to a number of recent reports (4, 6, 16, 24). Bloedel and Roberts (4) have reported results on Purkinje cell activity that are not in agreement with other previous reports (7). They suggest that the discrepancy is due to the barbituate depression on the tonic activity that normally impinges on the Purkinje cell. By a simple analogy, the firing pattern of a Group I burster is possible in the unanesthetized animal. On the other hand, Group I cells have not been observed in other reports on unanesthetized and intact animals (14, 18, 19, 32, 33, 34). It may be significant in this regard that the earliest a Group I burster appeared on any electrode was 4 months after implantation.

Mechanism of Burst Production

The mechanism by which the spikes are produced within a burst is indeed a very stable one. For any individual neuron, the regularity and stereotyped timing of these spikes over long periods of time attest to this. Prolonged depolarizations of a cell's membrane can give rise to a rapid production of spikes and the potential of the membrane can determine the rate of spike production (20). The timing pattern could be accounted for by the form of the depolarization wave. The extreme synchrony of the spikes from burst to burst could be due to a relatively stereotyped depolarization wave. The particular timing of the spikes within a burst, namely, the shortening of the later intervals, would indicate that these spikes are generated on the rising phase of this depolarization. Bursts of a higher order of magnitude (*i.e.*, more spikes per burst) maintain the same pattern of firing but have comparatively shorter intervals. A more rapid increase in the depolarization would produce this. The fact that the first interval of a higher order burst is significantly shorter than the first interval of a burst containing less spikes must be taken into account (Fig. 13.5). This would indicate that the rate of initial depolarization itself is a factor in determining the number of spikes per burst.

If the Group I bursting cell is indeed a Purkinje cell and its firing pattern is a real phenomenon and not just an artifact of the experiment, then current theories must make provision for Purkinje cells which fire only in the climbing fiber mode. In the absence of more exact histological confirmation any conclusion must remain tentative. Nevertheless it has been shown that in the unanesthetized cat the Group I cells possess an extremely stable burst-producing mechanism and that individual cells have a propensity for emitting bursts of a given number of spikes. These properties are maintained over relatively long periods of time. Implications of this and the fact that sensory stimulation can affect the burst firing pattern will be treated in the following paper (21).

SUMMARY

Extracellular potentials from two different groups of cells were recorded from the cerebellar cortex of the unanesthetized and intact cat during spontaneous firing periods. The neurons in Group I (seventeen cells) fired only in a burst of highly regular spikes. Those in Group II (five cells) produced bursts but also fired in trains of single spikes.

The Group I cells fired randomly about 1/sec and each firing was a burst of one to six spikes. Each of these cells had a distinct probability distribution as to the number of spikes produced within each burst. This distribution was relatively constant over long periods of time during a single experimental session and also during several days when the animal was in the same behavioral state, i.e., awake and resting quietly. The timing of the spikes within the bursts was extremely stable. The first interval in the burst is the longest with subsequent intervals becoming progressively shorter. The greater the number of spikes in a burst, the shorter the respective intervals.

The Group II cells manifested similar burst characteristics in all respects but, in addition, fired in trains of single spikes that occurred between the bursts. The mean intervals for the single firings varied from 20 to 80 msec.

From anatomical considerations and spike firing patterns, it was concluded that the Group II cell was a Purkinje cell. The burst represented a response to a climbing fiber input, and the single firing to a mossy fiber input. The possibility exists that the Group I cell was a Purkinje cell that fired only in response to climbing fiber input.

REFERENCES

1. Bell, C. C. and R. J. Grimm. Discharge properties of Purkinje cells recorded on single and double microelectrodes. *J. Neurophysiol.* 32:1044-1055, 1969.

2. Betyar, L. A user-oriented time-shared online system. *Comm. of A.C.M.* 10:413-419, 1967.

3. Bishop, P. O., W. Burke and R. Davis. The interpretation of the extracellular response of single lateral geniculate cells. *J. Physiol.* (London) 162:451-472, 1962.

4. Bloedel, J. R. and W. J. Roberts. Functional relationship among neurons of the cerebellar cortex in the absence of anesthesia. *J. Neurophysiol.* 32:75-84, 1969.

5. Brookhart, J. M., G. Moruzzi and R. S. Snider. Spike discharges of single units in cerebellar cortex. *J. Neurophysiol.* 13:465-486, 1950.

6. Eccles, J. C., D. S. Faber and H. Tábořiková. The action of a parallel fiber volley on the antidromic invasion of Purkyně cells of cat cerebellum. *Brain Res.* 25:335-356, 1971.

7. Eccles, J. C., M. Ito and J. Szentagothai. *The Cerebellum as a Neuronal Machine.* New York: Springer, 1967.

8. Eccles, J. C., R. Llinás and K. Sasaki. The excitatory synaptic action of climbing fibers on Purkinje cells of the cerebellum. *J. Physiol.* (London) 182:268-296, 1966.

9. Eccles, J. C., R. Llinás, K. Sasaki and P. E. Voorhoeve. Interaction experiments on the responses evoked in Purkinje cells by climbing fibers. *J. Physiol.* (London) 182:297-315, 1966.

10. Ferin, M., R. A. Grigorian and P. Strata. Mossy and climbing fiber activation on the cat cerebellum by stimulation of the labyrinth. *Exp. Brain Res.* 12:1-17, 1971.

11. Fox, C. A. and J. W. Barnard. A quantitative study of Purkinje cell dendritic branchlets and their relationship to afferent fibers. *J. Anat.* 91:299-313, 1957.

12. Fujita, Y. Activity of dendrites of single Purkinje cells and its relationship to so-called inactivation response in rabbit cerebellum. *J. Neurophysiol.* 31:131-141, 1968.

13. Granit, R. and C. G. Phillips. Excitatory and inhibitory processes acting upon individual Purkinje cells of the cerebellum in cats. *J. Physiol.* (London) 133:520-547, 1956.

14. Hobson, J. A. and R. W. McCarley. Spontaneous unit activity of cat cerebellar Purkinje cells in sleep and waking. *Psychophysiol.* 7: 311, 1970.

15. Khanbabyn, M. V. Cerebellar unit responses to visual stimuli. *Neurosci. Transl.* 14:58-62, 1970.

16. Latham, A. and D. H. Paul. Effects of sodium thiopentone on cerebellar neurone activity. *Brain Res.* 25:212-215, 1971.

17. Llinás, R. *Neurobiology of Cerebellar Evolution and Development.* Chicago: Am. Med. Assoc. of Educ. Res. Found., 1969.

18. Mano, N. Changes of simple and complex activity of cerebellar Purkinje cells with sleep and waking. *Science* 170:1325-1327, 1970.

19. Marchesi, G. F. and P. Strata. Climbing fibers of cat cerebellum: Modulation during sleep. *Brain Res.* 17:145-148, 1970.

20. Martinez, F. E., W. E. Crill and T. T. Kennedy. Electrogenesis of cerebellar Purkinje cell responses in cats. *J. Neurophysiol.* 34:348-356, 1971.

21. McElligott, J. G. Bursting Cells in the Cerebellar Cortex of the Unanesthetized and Unrestrained Cat during Sensory Stimulation. In M. I. Phillips (Ed.), *Brain Unit Activity During Behavior,* Charles C Thomas, Pub., Springfield, Ill. 224-243, 1973.

22. McElligott, J. G. A Telemetry System for the Transmission of Single and Multiple Channel Data from Individual Neurons in the Brain. In M. I. Phillips (Ed.) *Brain Unit Activity During Behavior,* Charles C Thomas, Pub., Springfield, Ill. 53-66, 1973.

23. McElligott, J. G., R. T. Kado and J. R. Zweizig. A miniaturized telemetry device for the transmission of the electrical activity of single nerve cells in the brain. *Proc. Nat'l Telemetering Conf.,* 207-210, 1969.

24. Mountcastle, V. B., P. W. Davies and A. L. Berman. Response properties of neurons of cat's somatic sensory cortex to peripheral stimuli. *J. Neurophysiol.* 20:374-407, 1957.

25. Murphy, J. T. and N. H. Sabah. Spontaneous firing of Purkinje cells in decerebrate and barbiturate anesthetized cats. *Brain Res.* 17:515-519, 1970.

26. O'Keefe, J. and H. Bouma. Complex sensory properties of certain amygdala units in the freely moving cat. *Exp. Neurol.* 23:384-398, 1969.

27. Olds, J. Operant conditioning of single unit responses. *Proc. XXIII Intern. Congr. Physiol. Union* 4:372-380, 1965.

28. Scheibel, M., A. Scheibel, A. Mollica and G. Moruzzi. Convergence and interaction of afferent impulses on single units of reticular formation. *J. Neurophysiol.* 18:309-331, 1955.

29. Talbott, R. E., A. L. Towe and T. T. Kennedy. Physiological and histological classification of cerebellar neurons in chloralose-anesthetized cats. *Exp. Neurol.* 19:46-64, 1967.

30. Tarnecki, R. and J. Konorski. Patterns of responses of Purkinje cells in cats to passive displacements of limbs, squeezing and touching. *Acta Neurobiol. Exp.* 30:95-119, 1970.

31. Thach, W. T. Somatosensory receptive fields of single units in cat cerebellar cortex. *J. Neurophysiol.* 30:675-696, 1967.

32. Thach, W. T. Discharge of Purkinje and cerebellar nuclear neurons

during rapidly alternating arm movement in the monkey. *J. Neurophysiol.* 31:785-797, 1968.

33. Thach, W. T. Discharge of cerebellar neurons related to two maintained postures and two prompt movements. I. Nuclear cell output. *J. Neurophysiol.* 33:527-536, 1970.

34. Thach, W. T. Discharge of cerebellar neurons related to two maintained postures and two prompt movements. II. Purkinje cell output and input. *J. Neurophysiol.* 33:537-547, 1970.

35. Towe, A. L. and G. W. Harding. Extracellular microelectrode sampling bias. *Exp. Neurol.* 29:366-381, 1970.

Chapter XIV

BURSTING CELLS IN THE CEREBELLAR CORTEX OF THE UNANESTHETIZED AND UNRESTRAINED CAT DURING SENSORY STIMULATION

JAMES G. McELLIGOTT

THE CEREBELLUM IS most widely known for its proprioceptive role in the control of motor behavior. Its role in other functions has also been recognized. Numerous reports have indicated that natural stimulation of different sensory systems conveys information to the cerebellar cortex. Apart from proprioception (24, 26, 27), a sampling of previous work indicates that sensory input from auditory (2, 10, 15, 16, 17, 20, 21, 28, 29), visual (10, 13, 14, 15, 21, 29), somatosensory (1, 4, 10, 22, 23, 24, 25), and vestibular (9) systems reaches the cerebellum.

These reports have described either macropotentials of evoked responses or the spike potentials of individual neurons as they related to sensory stimulation. With the exception of Thach's studies on movement and proprioception (26, 27), these experiments have been conducted on anesthetized or decerebrate preparations.

The preceding paper (18) described the spontaneous firing of

It is a pleasure to thank Dr. W. Ross Adey for his support during the term of these experiments and for his critical evaluation of the manuscript. I would also like to thank Vern Foust for programming assistance, Jackie Payne for preparation of the figures, and Jody Diacovo for typing the manuscript. This work was performed at Space Biology Lab, Brain Research Institute and the Department of Anatomy, U.C.L.A. Support was obtained from NASA Grant NGR 05-007-195 and U.S. Air Force Grant F44620-70-C-0017 to the Space Biology Laboratory, and USPHS NIH Grant NSO 2501 to the Data Processing Laboratory of the Brain Research Institute, as well as from the UCLA Brain Information Service, a member of the NINDS neurological network.

bursting neurons (Group I cell) that emitted a burst of spikes randomly about once a second. These bursts contained one to six identical spikes that occurred at stereotyped and extremely regular intervals. From indirect evidence it was concluded that there is a high probability that this is a Purkinje cell and the burst represented the response to climbing fiber input. Several possibilities were considered to explain why there were no single spikes or responses to input via the mossy-parallel fiber input system.

This report is concerned with the activity of these neurons during auditory and visual stimulation in the unanesthetized and unrestrained cat. Investigations were directed toward examining how information about stimuli is coded by these neurons.

METHODS

Implantations of small fine wire electrodes (dia. 25 μ) were performed on fifteen cats. The animals used in this study were the same as in the previous paper (18). The methods of implantation and recording of neural spike data were identical to those described. However, several changes and additions for this study were made. Of the seventeen Group I bursting cells recorded in the previous paper, eleven were tested with sensory stimulation in this study.

Sensory Stimulation

Sensory stimulation was presented to the animal in a testing box (1.1 m × 0.6 m × 0.5 m), with ambient illumination of about 22.5 ft-candles. Ambient noise level was about 62 db (re SPL) and emanated mainly from recording equipment. When the door of the box was closed, the animal could be viewed through one way transparent mirror glass. Clicks (1 msec duration) with an intensity 1 to 40 db above the ambient noise level were presented via a speaker within the box. The clicks were delivered at constant or varied rates ranging from 1/13.5 sec to 4/sec. These clicks were generated by a series of Textronix wave form (#162) and pulse (#161) generators and audio amplifier. Their intensity was measured with a General Radio sound level meter (#1565-A), and based on peak excursion of the meter. Due to their short duration, this is probably an underestimate of the true peak intensity in decibels (re SPL) (6). Flashes (10 μsec duration) were presented by a Grass stimulator (PS-2). The intensity of the flash was in the low to medium ranges of the instrument (setting 1 to 4). Both speaker and photostimulator were never closer than 0.7 meters to the animal. In some experiments with well habituated animals, the door to the box was left open and the animal could view the experimenter and equipment in the dimly lit laboratory.

Stimuli were presented in blocks of about one hundred. Each block consisted of a click or flash at fixed intensity and repetition rate. During a single session, many blocks of stimuli were delivered over several hours in all stimulus combinations.

Correlates of Bursting with Sleep Stages

To evaluate possible changes in cell bursting pattern with sleep stages, clicks were presented continuously at constant intensity (15 db above ambient) and rate (1/2.5 sec) for several hours, covering a sequence of sleep-wakefulness cycles. The EEG (0.5 to 50 Hz bandwidth) was recorded differentially between two fine wire electrodes in the cerebellum or monopolarly using the skull screws as electrical ground. Three stages in the sleep-wakefulness cycle were categorized as: Awake Phase (AW)—eyes open, behaviorally alert and desynchronized EEG; Slow Wave Sleep Phase (SWS)—eyes closed, reclining position, slow waves and/or spindles in the EEG; Paradoxical or Rapid Eye Movement Phase (REM)—rapid eye movements, periods of muscular twitching of limbs, head or body and desynchronized EEG.

Analysis of Data

Spike intervals were converted to digital form with an SDS-9300 computer and the intervals analyzed (18). Poststimulus histograms were employed to investigate the characteristics of the bursts produced by Group I cells as they related to the various parameters of stimulation. Response percentages, probability distribution histograms, and individual intraburst interval histograms were computed for various periods after the stimulus. For example, the parameters of the bursts recorded during the 0 to 100 msec poststimulus response period were determined. These were compared with bursts at later poststimulus periods and during spontaneous firing.

The response percentage is the percent of occurrence of a single burst in the period 0 to 100 msec after stimulus presentation. This may exceed 100 percent since it is possible for a single stimulus to evoke two distinct bursts in this period. A response percentage for later poststimulus periods was calculated in the same way. If the later poststimulus periods exceeded 100 msec, then the respective response percentages were divided by the appropriate number of 100 msec segments in that period. This response percentage is directly related to the mean firing rate since it expresses the probability of recording a burst of spikes during any 100 msec period.

The probability distribution histogram (PDH) is displayed as a bar graph of the percent of times that a Group I neuron emits a burst containing a given number of spikes. A composite probability distribution histogram is made up of two or more PDHs, with a PDH formed for each of the various time periods after the stimulus.

A separate intraburst interval histogram was calculated for each order of magnitude of a burst. The number of spikes in a burst determines the order of magnitude. These histograms are displayed with the first spike of the burst occurring at the origin and subsequent spikes located at their respective times on the abscissa. The timing of spikes within bursts of different orders of magnitude was thus determined. The intraburst interval histograms for each time period after a stimulus, was used to determine if there were timing differences within a burst due to sensory stimulation. Other transforms, such as the interburst interval histogram, auto-correlogram and cross-correlogram described in the previous paper (18), were also formed.

RESULTS

Group I bursting cells fire randomly at very low discharge rates (mean interval 0.7 sec) with highly regular and stereotyped bursts containing one to six identical spikes. Each of the bursting cells has a distinct probability distribution of the number of spikes in each burst. The probabilities remain relatively constant and stable for a given neuron over a period of a few hours to several days when recorded during the same behavioral state, *i.e.,* awake and resting quietly. In addition, the timing of the spikes within a burst is extremely stable. The longest interval recorded within

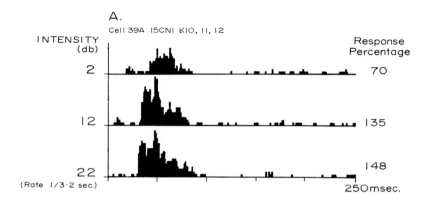

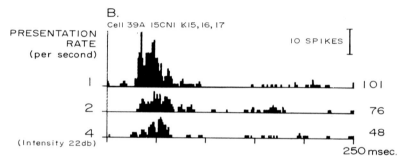

Figure 14.1. Poststimulus histograms (PSH) were formed for a Group I bursting cerebellar neuron that was driven by auditory stimulation. Each PSH represents the responses to a block of one hundred stimulus presentations.

A. Each of the first three histograms was obtained for a different stimulus intensity. The intensity is given in decibels (db) above the ambient noise level. In these cases, the repetition rate of the auditory click was kept constant at one stimulus every 3.2 sec (1/3.2 sec).

B. Each of the next three histograms was formed for different rates of stimulus presentation. Here the intensity of the click was kept constant at 22 db above ambient. The response percentage to the right of each PSH is the percent of times that a single burst of spikes occurs in the 0-100 msec period after stimulus presentation. This figure sometimes exceeds 100 percent since it is possible for an individual stimulus to evoke two distinct bursts. From these PSHs and the response percentages, it is evident that a stimulus is more effective in evoking a response as the intensity increases and/or the repetition rate decreases.

Cell 39A 15CN1 K12

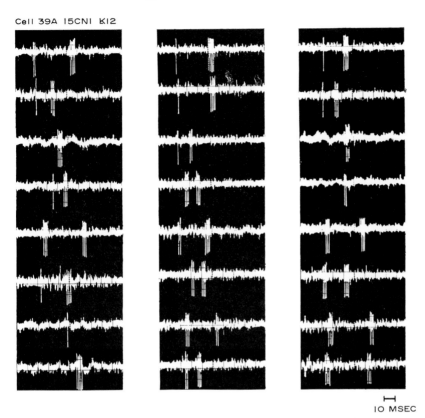

10 MSEC

Figure 14.2. Each of these twenty-four traces represents the response evoked from the same cell by an auditory click presented at a repetition rate of 1/3.2 sec and intensity of 22 db above ambient. Individual traces are 100 msec in duration and are triggered by the stimulus. For this particular neuron under these stimulus conditions, there was a high probability that a single stimulus would evoke two distinct bursts.

a burst is about 2.1 msec. and the shortest about 1.0 msec. The first interval within a burst is the longest with subsequent intervals successively shorter. Furthermore, the greater the number of spikes in a burst, the shorter the respective intervals in the burst.

Bursts of Group I Cells Evoked by Auditory Stimulation

In nine bursting cells, a click produced a burst of spikes with a latency of 20 to 100 msec. The majority of bursts occurred between 40 and 60 msec. In general, repeated stimulation over many

A. POST STIMULUS HISTOGRAM

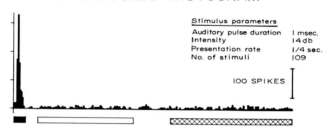

Stimulus parameters

Auditory pulse duration	I msec.
Intensity	I4db
Presentation rate	I/4 sec.
No. of stimuli	I09

IOO SPIKES

B. PROBABILITY DISTRIBUTION HISTOGRAM

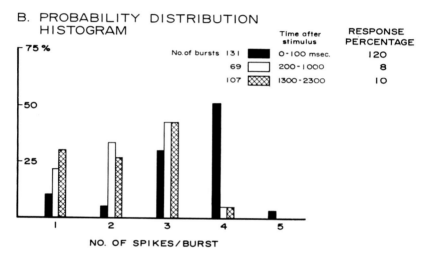

			Time after stimulus	RESPONSE PERCENTAGE
No.of bursts	I3I	■	O-IOO msec.	I20
	69	☐	200-IOOO	8
	IO7	▨	I300-2300	IO

NO. OF SPIKES/BURST

Figure 14.3. A. A poststimulus histogram (0-2300 msec) was formed for a Group I bursting neuron that was driven by auditory stimulation presented at an intensity of 14 db above ambient and at a rate one every fourth second (¼ sec).

B. A composite of three probability distribution histograms (PDH) is presented together. Each separate PDH represents the percent of times (ordinate) that a Group I neuron emits a burst containing a given number of spikes (abscissa). In this case a different PDH is formed for each of the three time periods after the stimulus (*i.e.*, 0-100 msec, 200-1000 msec, and 1300-2300 msec). The response percentage for the three periods is presented to the right of this histogram. For the 0-100 msec period, this figure represents the percent of times a single burst follows an individual stimulus. This number can exceed 100 percent for at times an individual stimulus produces two distinct bursts. The response percentage for the hundreds and even thousands of presentations produced the same type of response without habituation. However, each click did not produce a burst of spikes. A response was judged to be present if a single burst of spikes occurred within the 0-100 msec poststimulus period. Thus, the response percentage was determined as a measure of the effectiveness of a stimulus. The presence or absence of a response varied without obvious relationship to small changes in resting behavior.

The reliability of a response increased as the intensity of the stimulus increased. Figure 14.1A shows the relationship of stimulus intensity to firing of a typical auditory bursting neuron in the post-stimulus histograms and associated response percentages.

In addition, this response percentage decreased as the presentation rate increased. Rates greater than 1/sec produced a sharp decrement in the response (Fig. 14.1B). When stimuli were presented at very slow rates (1/10 sec and 1/13.5 sec), the percent of responses obtained for a block of 100 stimuli did not differ from that obtained when the presentation rate was 1/2 sec. This was found to be true for all cells responding to auditory stimulation.

Not all auditory bursting cells responded an equal percent of the time to stimuli of similar repetition rates and intensity. When the most effective stimuli were used, the response percentages of some cells varied from 10 percent to 70 percent above the spontaneous firing rate. Moreover, in all but one of the cells a stimulus could produce two distinct bursts separated by intervals of 7 to 50 msec. (Fig. 14.2). In these, the response percentage was greater than 100 percent because this parameter was defined as the percentage of times that a single burst of spikes occurs in the 0-100 msec. period after stimulus presentation. A stimulus presented at high intensity and slow repetition rates was the most effective in producing double bursts.

---

later poststimulus periods is formed in a similar manner. Since the later poststimulus periods exceeded 100 msec in duration, the respective response percentages were divided by the appropriate number of 100 msec segments in that period. Thus, the response percentage is the probability of recording a burst of spikes during any 100 msec period. The PDH indicates that the bursts evoked by the auditory click in the 0-100 msec period contain on the average more spikes per burst than during later poststimulus periods.

Changes in Number of Spikes Per Burst Evoked by Auditory Stimulation

As noted previously (18), during spontaneous activity each Group I bursting cell has a distinct probability distribution histogram or propensity to emit bursts containing a specific number of spikes. Bursts evoked by clicks in the 0-100 msec poststimulus period typically contained more spikes than at later poststimulus periods (> 100 msec.), or during nonstimulated periods. The composite probability distribution histogram (Fig. 14.3) demonstrates this. The composite probability distribution histogram and associated response percentages are described in the Methods. This increased percentage of higher order bursts is also enhanced by slow rates of presentation (< 1/sec) and/or by increasing the intensity of the stimulus (Fig. 14.4). This was found in all but one bursting neuron driven by clicks.

Therefore, it is evident that the Group I burster can respond to an increase in stimulus effectiveness in several ways. For weakly effective stimuli, the bursting neuron responds by a slight increase in the number of bursts (response percentage) obtained in the 0-100 msec. post-stimulus period. As the stimulus effectiveness increases, there is a further increase in the response percentage and also increased percentage of higher order bursts (*i.e.*, bursts with more spikes). For the strongest stimuli, these neurons respond by a progressive increase in the number of bursts and higher order bursts, and also by emitting two distinct bursts for each stimulus presented. Not all neurons exhibit this complete response pattern for they can be only weakly driven even by the most effective stimulus.

It was noted that the response percentage of the later poststimulus periods (> 100 msec.) was equivalent to the firing rate during nonstimulated or spontaneously active periods. This response percentage is directly related to mean firing rate since this percentage expresses the probability of recording a burst of spikes during any 100 msec period. In addition, the probability distribution histograms for these later poststimulus periods were identical to each other and also to those histograms obtained during

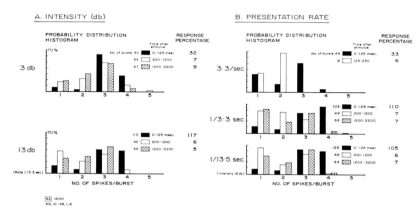

Figure 14.4. Each composite probability distribution histogram (PDH) and associated response percentage were formed in the same manner as described for that in Figure 14.3.

A. These two PDHs were formed for two different stimulus intensities (3 db and 13 db) above ambient, while the presentation rate was held constant (1/3.5 sec).

B. These three composite PDHs were formed for three different rates of stimulus presentations (3.3/sec, 1/3.3 sec, and 1/13.5 sec), a constant stimulus intensity (16 db) above ambient. It is evident that as the intensity of the stimulus increases and/or the repetition rate decreases there is an increase in the number of bursts during the 0-125 msec period. Furthermore, these bursts will contain more spikes.

spontaneously active periods (p > 0.1, Kolmogorov-Smirnov non-parametric test).

Typically, later poststimulus periods (> 100 msec) were from 200 msec to 1 sec in duration and were necessary to obtain an adequate sample size at the low firing rates in these periods. It is possible that there were fluctuations in the probability distribution histogram and response percentage during shorter poststimulus time segments which were obliterated by averaging over these relatively long periods.

In a few analyses, the poststimulus period was divided into 100 msec. segments, and the probability distribution histogram and response percentage were computed for each. In general, no differences were seen in these two parameters when the various 100 msec. epochs were compared with each other and with those of nonstimulated and spontaneous firing periods.

Timing of Spikes Within a Burst During Auditory Stimulation

Previously it had been found that during spontaneous activity, spike potentials within bursts manifested extremely stable and precise timings (18), based on the individual intraburst interval histograms. The respective spikes in bursts of equal orders of magnitude generally fell within one bin width (94 μsec. or 125 μsec.) of each other when digitizing rates of 10, 667 or 8000 samples/sec. were used. Thus, the jitter of a spike within a burst has been estimated to be in the order of 100 μsec.

Samples of bursts to auditory stimulation were taken from the 0-100 msec poststimulus period and the individual intraburst histograms calculated. Histograms were also prepared for bursts from later poststimulus periods ($>$ 100 msec), as well as during nonstimulated spontaneously active periods. The spike timings within equal magnitude bursts during the various periods were compared. No differences were detected in spike timings when bursts evoked by auditory stimulation and those obtained during the later periods ($>$ 100 msec.) were compared.

Visual Stimulation

Among the group of seven bursting cells tested, a response was evoked from six cells by a flash of light. The characteristics of the bursts to visual stimulation were similar to those from auditory stimulation.

A light flash produced a burst of spikes with a 20 to 100 msec. latency. The response persisted without habituation. Again each and every stimulus did not produce a response and the percentage of times a response was present varied from cell to cell, and in two cells increased with decreasing rates of stimulus presentation and/or increase in intensity. In three of the cells responding to visual stimulation, there were increased higher order bursts during the 0-100 msec. period. As with cells driven by auditory stimulation, no intraburst spikes timing differences were seen between bursts evoked in the 0-100 msec. poststimulus period and those recorded during later poststimulus periods. It was not possible to produce any double bursts with visual stimulation.

Simultaneous Recording of Two Bursting Cells During Sensory Stimulation

In two instances, a pair of bursting cells were recorded simultaneously from two different electrodes during sensory stimulation. The electrodes were in close proximity with a tip separation of about 200 to 400 μ.

In one pair, the first burster did not respond to either visual or auditory stimulation; the other cell was primarily a visual burster. In the other pair, both cells were driven by auditory stimulation. The response to auditory stimulation of each cell differed. Also, while one cell responded with increased higher order bursts, the other did not.

The flat cross correlogram histogram of the two cells during spontaneously active nonstimulated periods indicates no obvious interaction between them. Similar histograms obtained during periods of auditory stimulation show peaks normally distributed about the origin. This is expected, since both cells are time linked to the auditory stimuli.

Long Term Sensory Stimulation During Sleep-Wakefulness Cycles

In one experiment, clicks (1/2.5 sec, 15 db above ambient) were presented continuously over a four hour session. Previously, the animal had been exposed to this type of situation and numerous other stimulus presentations. After a short interval of less than fifteen minutes, the cat appeared to pay little overt attention to the clicks and assumed a resting position. The firing pattern of a Group I bursting neuron was recorded as the animal passed through various sleep-wakefulness cycles. The response to the stimulation was similar to that obtained from other auditory bursters. In addition, the response persisted without habituation for the entire session, and no change in the response was detected that might be due to the different states of sleep and wakefulness.

Figure 14.5 presents the various poststimulus histograms, prob-

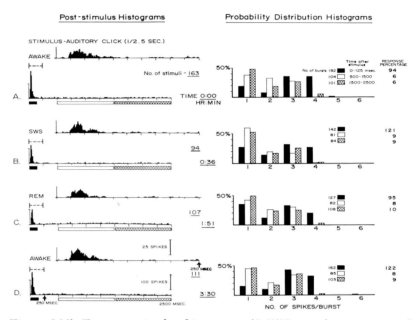

Figure 14.5. Four poststimulus histograms (0-2500 msec) are presented for a Group I bursting neuron driven by auditory stimulation. The supplemental poststimulus histograms associated with each of these represents an expanded version of the first 250 msec. Each set of PSHs was obtained successively at the time (hr:min) indicated to the right of the histogram while the animal was in a different stage of sleep or wakefulness. The composite probability distribution histograms and response percentages are presented to the right of the respective PSHs. The method of forming the probability distribution histogram and response percentages is described in the caption of Figure 14.3. During this experiment the auditory click was presented continuously at a rate of 1/2.5 sec. This figure shows that there is no habituation to the click presented continuously over a three and one-half hour period and that the response is not affected by different sleep states.

ability distribution histograms and response percentages for four selected periods during the experiment. They are typical of all others. Although no gross changes appeared in the poststimulus histograms, the response percentage of the 0-125 msec. period varied randomly from about 80 percent to 120 percent without any relation to sleep state. In only one case, when the animal was awake and grooming, was there a decrease to 36 percent. The response percentages for all later poststimulus periods (> 125 msec.) were in the 6 percent to 10 percent level, which is equivalent to the spontaneous firing rate.

Analysis of the probability distribution histograms shows that the ability of this bursting neuron to produce an increase in higher order bursts (quadruplets) to stimulation continued undiminished for the entire session. Furthermore, it was not influenced by the sleep periods, and no differences in the timing of the spikes within bursts of equal orders of magnitude were noticed for the entire session.

DISCUSSION

A conclusion in the preceding study (18) was that the bursts of the Group I cells are most likely the climbing fiber responses of the Purkinje neuron. Moreover, firing patterns in the awake cat during quiet resting behavior were stable for periods of several hours to a few days. For an individual cell, there were no long term changes in the mean interval between bursts, the timing of the spikes within the bursts and the probability that a cell would emit bursts containing a given number of spikes.

The experiments described here have shown that it is possible to evoke a response by auditory and/or visual stimulation from a number of these Group I bursters. These cells respond by emitting a burst 40 to 60 msec after stimulus presentation. Every stimulus does not evoke a burst of spikes, however.

These Group I bursting neurons manifest a response hierarchy to stimulation. As the effectiveness of the stimuli increases, the cells respond first by increased probability that an individual stimulus evokes a burst of spikes. There is then an increase in percentage of higher order bursts (*i.e.*, more spikes per burst) in the response period. Finally, for the most effective stimulus (high intensity and slow repetition rate), an individual presentation will sometimes produce two distinctive bursts generally less than 50 msec apart. In no instances is the timing of the spikes within the bursts affected by stimulation.

For slow continuous presentation rates, this response persists for hours without habituation. In fact, it is not affected by the various sleep-wakefulness states of the animal.

A number of results obtained in this study are in basic agreement with previous experiments on anesthetized preparations. Natural auditory and visual stimulation were used to elicit evoked responses or alterations in single cell activity. These studies demonstrated that increases in stimulation rate (> 1/sec) cause a decrement in the response (13, 14, 15) and that the magnitude of the response is directly related to stimulus intensity (10, 14). Similar results have also been obtained in other studies where natural somatosensory (10, 25) and vestibular (9) stimulation were employed.

In particular, Shofer and Nahvi (20) found increased Purkinje cell firing to click and attributed it to mossy fiber afferents. They found that the irregular and recurrent climbing fiber responses was temporally unrelated to the acoustic stimulus. In addition, the Purkinje cell response to click or flash that Freeman (10) measured was a short burst of spikes followed by a long period of spike suppression. He concluded that both mossy and climbing fibers participate in this response. In both these reports (10, 20), the response latency (about 20 msec.) was shorter than that reported here. Khanbabyn (13) found both a spontaneously active and a silent group of cerebellar neurons that responded to visual stimulation. The response of the spontaneously active group consisted of an initial increase and then inhibition of background activity. The silent cell emitted one or more bursts with a latency 27 to 50 msec after the stimulus. Using the depth of the electrode tip as a criterion, Khanbabyn concludes that 60 percent of the silent neurons were either stellate or basket cells and 20 percent were Purkinje neurons. It is difficult to compare these reports and the responses tested here, due to the lack of detail about the characteristics of the burst. It would seem that the Group I bursting cell most resembles the silent cell measured by Khanbabyn.

It is well to consider the findings of Freeman (10) whose results appear at variance with those reported here. He states that responses to different inputs do not reveal any evidence of stimulus coding other than variations in latency of the burst response. In particular, he has found little or no variability with respect to the pattern of response, total number of spikes per burst and duration of the initial burst. This is in contrast to the results reported here which reveal that there are no latency changes but that there are changes in the number of spikes per burst and the burst duration. It is doubtful that the burst response described by Freeman and that reported in this study are the same phenomenon. Aside from the significant difference in response latencies, the bursts measured by Freeman do not appear to be the stereotyped and synchronous bursts of Group I cells. Furthermore, no intraburst interval in the Group I cell has been found to exceed 2 to 3 msec (18), whereas those reported by Freeman can range from 10 to 60 msec or more [see Fig. 2 (10)]. These significant differences could be caused by the effects of anesthetics or the existence of two subclasses of neurons.

The basic contention of this paper is that a number of Group I bursting neurons, tentatively identified as Purkinje cells, respond to sensory input with a climbing fiber response. There are also other reports that natural somatosensory (25), vestibular (9), and proprioceptive (24) stimuli produced individual and multiple climbing fiber responses.

We have demonstrated that the parameters of stimulation influence not only the probability of a burst response from an individual neuron but also the number of spikes in a burst. Due to the stereotyped and regular timing of spikes within bursts of different orders of magnitude, the duration of a burst is proportional to the number of spikes in a burst. For example, in the previous paper (18), a particular cell was described which could emit up to five spikes per burst. For bursts ranging from two to five spikes, the average duration of each is 1.72 msec, 2.85 msec, 3.91 msec and 4.92 msec, respectively [Table 13.I (18)]. If all spikes in a burst are transmitted down the Purkinje cell axon to the target neuron, then this response could act as a variable duration gating mechanism. Thus, a period of extended inhibition could appear in the cerebellar nuclear cell at some critical period. The effect is enhanced when two such bursts in rapid succession are elicited by the stimulus. It has been reported that multiple spikes of a climbing fiber response do travel down the Purkinje cell axon (12).

Several hypotheses regarding the function of the climbing fiber response have been formulated. Harmon et al. (11) and also Murphy and Sabah (19) have proposed that the response acts as a resetting mechanism on the Purkinje cell. Bloedel and Roberts (3) have stated that it is not the climbing fiber response per se that is important but the prolonged suppression that follows. Eccles et al. (7, 8) have stipulated that the climbing fiber functions to sample from instant to instant the integrated excitatory-inhibitory state of the Purkinje cell and operates as a detailed patterned sampling device. This is reflected by the number of spikes in the climbing fiber response.

The data presented here and in the previous paper (18) may fit certain aspects of the hypothesis of Eccles. It has been established that an individual Group I bursting neuron has a propensity to emit bursts of a given number of spikes. This has been illustrated by the various probability distribution histograms that remain relatively constant over long periods of time. An appropriate stimulus changes the probability distribution and causes the cell to emit on the average more spikes per burst than it normally does. Furthermore, as the effectiveness of the stimulus increases, there is a greater number of these higher order bursts.

There are currently no other reports on the long term activity of cerebellar neurons in the unanesthetized and intact cat during sensory stimulation. Measurements of the evoked response in the cerebellum under similar conditions manifest no habituation (2). This agrees with the lack of habituation at the single cell level that was reported here (Fig. 14.5). It is interesting that clicks of similar intensity and repetition rate do not produce habituation in auditory relay nuclei from the periphery to the inferior colliculus (30). Figure 14.5 also demonstrates that this response is unaffected by the various sleep-wakefulness cycles.

The bursting cells described in this paper represent a homogenous group that manifested stable properties over long periods of time. This includes the propensity for the individual cells to produce bursts of a given number of spikes and to generate spikes in a regular and stereotyped manner. Sensory stimulation can modulate and vary the number of spikes within a burst. Thus, these cells act as a variable duration gate upon their target neurons and information about the stimulus is represented by a pulse code. Since the spikes are produced in very rapid succession, the result must be a very powerful synaptic input on the target cell.

SUMMARY

The experiments described have shown that it is possible to evoke a response by auditory stimulation from a number of cerebellar bursting neurons in the unanesthetized and unrestrained cat. These neurons, assumed to be Purkinje cells, fire spontaneously about 1/sec, emitting a burst of one to six identical spikes. Upon presentation of a stimulus, a burst will generally occur in the 40 to 60 msec. poststimulus period. Every stimulus does not evoke a burst of spikes, however. More intense stimulation and/or slower presentation rates increase the probability of obtaining a response. Furthermore, the bursts emitted by an individual neuron in the poststimulus response period contain typically more spikes per burst than those recorded at later poststimulus periods or during spontaneous firing periods. In no instance is the timing of the spikes within the bursts affected by the stimuli.

These bursting neurons manifest a response hierarchy to stimulation. As the effectiveness of the stimulus increases, the cells respond firstly by an increase in the probability that a burst of spikes will follow the stimulus. There will then be an increase in the number of higher order bursts (*i.e.*, more spikes per burst) during the response period. For the most effective stimulus (high intensity and slow presentation rate), a single stimulus will produce two distinct bursts that are generally less than 50 msec. apart. Neurons that are only weakly driven by even the most effective stimulus do not display this complete response repertoire. A number of bursting neurons respond in a like manner to visual stimulation.

In one experiment, clicks delivered continuously at slow rates evoked a response that persisted for hours without habituation. Indeed, the response was not affected by the various sleep-wakefulness states of the animal.

These cells act as a variable duration gate upon their target neurons and information about sensory stimuli is represented by a pulse code.

REFERENCES

1. Batini, C. and R. Pumain. Activation of Purkinje neurons through climbing fibers after chronic lesions of the olivo-cerebellar pathway. *Experientia* 24:914-916, 1968.
2. Berlucchi, G., J. B. Munson and G. Rizolatti. Changes in click-evoked responses in the auditory system and the cerebellum of free-moving cats during sleep and waking. *Arch. Ital. Biol.* 105:118-135, 1967.
3. Bloedel, J. and W. Roberts. Action of climbing fibers in cerebellar cortex of the cat. *J. Neurophysiol.* 34:17-31, 1971.
4. Brookhart, J. M., G. Moruzzi and R. S. Snider. Spike discharges of single units in the cerebellar cortex. *J. Neurophysiol.* 13:465-486, 1950.
5. Crill, W. E. Delayed depolarization and repetitive firing in cat inferior olive neurons. *XXIV Internat. Congr. Physiol. Sci. Abstr.*, p. 96, Washington, D.C., 1968.
6. Dunlop, C. W., W. R. Webster and R. H. Day. Amplitude changes of evoked potentials at the inferior colliculus during acoustic habituation. *J. of Aud. Res.* 4:159-169, 1964.
7. Eccles, J. C., M. Ito and J. Szentágothai. *The Cerebellum as a Neuronal Machine*. New York: Springer, 1967.
8. Eccles, J. C., R. Llinás and K. Sasaki. The excitatory synaptic action of climbing fibers on the Purkinje cells of the cerebellum. *J. Physiol.* 182:268-296, 1966.
9. Ferin, M., R. A. Grigorian and P. Strata. Mossy and climbing fiber activation in the cat cerebellum by stimulation of the labyrinth. *Exp. Brain Res.* 12:1-17, 1971.
10. Freeman, J. A. Responses of cat cerebellar Purkinje cells to convergent inputs from cerebral cortex and peripheral sensory systems. *J. Neurophysiol.* 33:697-712, 1970.
11. Harmon, L. D., R. T. Kado and E. R. Lewis. Cerebellar Modelling Problems. In: *To Understand Brains* . . . , edited by L. D. Harmon. Prentice-Hall: Englewood Cliffs, N.J. (In press.)
12. Ito, M. and J. I. Simpson. Discharges in Purkinje cell axons during climbing fiber activation. *Brain Res.* 31:215-219, 1971.
13. Khanbabyn, M. V. Cerebellar unit responses to visual stimuli. *Neurosci. Transl.* 14:58-62, 1970.
14. Koella, W. P. Some functional properties of optically evoked potentials in cerebellar cortex of the cat. *J. Neurophysiol.* 22:61-77, 1959.
15. Levy, C., J. D. Loeser and W. P. Koella. The cerebellar acoustic response and its interaction with optic responses. *Electroenceph. clin. Neurophysiol.* 13:234-242, 1961.

16. Maruyama, N., H. Kagitomi, H. Shinoda, A. Higuchi, Y. Kanno and M. Morimoto. Electric responses to sound stimulation from the cerebellum in cat. *Acta. Med. et Biol.* 4:317-324, 1957.

17. Maruyama, N. and T. Kawasaki. Unitary responses to tone stimulation recorded from the cerebellar cortex in the cat. *XXIII Internat. Congr. Physiol. Sci. Abstr.*, p. 372, Tokyo, 1965.

18. McElligott, J. G. Long term spontaneous activity of individual cerebellar neurons in the awake and unrestrained cat. In M. I. Phillips (Ed.) *Brain Unit Activity During Behavior*, Charles C Thomas, Pub., Springfield, Ill.

19. Murphy, J. T. and N. H. Sabah. Cerebellar Purkinje cell responses to afferent inputs. I. Climbing fiber activation. *Brain Res.* 25:449-467, 1971.

20. Shofer, R. J. and M. J. Nahvi. Firing patterns induced by sound in single units of the cerebellar cortex. *Exp. Brain Res.* 8:327-345, 1969.

21. Snider, R. S. and A. Stowell. Receiving areas of the tactile, auditory and visual systems in the cerebellum. *J. Neurophysiol.* 7:331-357, 1944.

22. Suda, I. and T. Amano. An analysis of evoked cerebellar activity. *Arch. Ital. Biol.* 102:156-182, 1964.

23. Talbott, R. E., A. L. Towe and T. T. Kennedy. Physiological and histological classification of cerebellar neurons in chloralose-anesthetized cats. *Exp. Neurol.* 19:46-64, 1967.

24. Tarnecki, R. and J. Konorski, J. Patterns of responses of Purkinje cells in cats to passive displacements of limbs, squeezing and touching. *Acta Neurobiol. Exp.* 30:95-119, 1970.

25. Thach, W. T. Somatosensory receptive fields of single units in cat cerebellar cortex. *J. Neurophysiol.* 30:675-696, 1967.

26. Thach, W. T. Discharge of Purkinje and cerebellar nuclear neurons during rapid alternating arm movements in the monkey. *J. Neurophysiol.* 31:785-797, 1968.

27. Thach, W. T. Discharge of cerebellar neurons related to two maintained postures and two prompt movements. II. Purkinje cell output and input. *J. Neurophysiol.* 33:537-547, 1970.

28. Wickelgren, W. O. Effect of state of arousal on click-evoked responses in cats. *J. Neurophysiol.* 31:757-768, 1968.

29. Wickelgren, W. O. Effects of walking and flash stimulation on click-evoked responses in cats. *J. Neurophysiol.* 31:769-776, 1968.

30. Wickelgren, W. O. Effect of acoustic habituation on click-evoked responses in cats. *J. Neurophysiol.* 31:777-784, 1968.

Chapter XV

NEUROCHEMICALLY DEFINED NEURONS: BEHAVIORAL CORRELATES OF UNIT ACTIVITY OF SEROTONIN-CONTAINING CELLS

D. J. McGINTY

SEROTONIN (5HT) SATISFIES most of the criteria that have been established to identify neurotransmitters in the brain. In a specific neural system 5HT is localized and released by excitation of that system (1, 3, 20, 33, 46). It is found in synaptosomes (50, 66) and the requisite enzymatic machinery for synthesis and degradation are present (13). In addition, microiontophoretic application of 5HT alters the excitability of certain neurons (47, 52). The following report of the unit spike activity of 5HT containing neurons is the first description of monoaminergic unit activity in behaving animals.

Serotonin appears to play a role in the neural control of sleep and a variety of waking behavioral processes. For example, depletion of brain 5HT by inhibition of synthesis (43) has been shown to modify sleep (22, 45, 61), perception of pain (57), social and sexual behavior (30, 53), and arousal and emotionality (31, 56). 5HT also has been implicated in the mechanisms underlying the psychotomimetic actions of lysergic acid diethylamide (LSD) (2, 35, 62), in morphine addiction (58, 60) and in psychotic depression (12, 18). However, behavioral processes such as these involve the neural integration of many behavioral elements including drive, sensory perception, cognition, motor expressions

The author wishes to thank R. M. Harper and Mary Fairbanks for their assistance. This research was supported by USPHS Grant MH 10083 and by the U. S. Veterans Administration. Computational assistance was furnished by the Data Processing Laboratory of the Brain Research Institute, UCLA, which is supported by USPHS Grant NS-02501.

and specific affective states such as pleasure or fear. 5HT may play a role in one or more of these elements of complex behaviors.

The determination of the exact role of 5HT, that is, the isolation of the mode of 5HT action among these interacting elements of integrated behavior, is difficult to achieve with behavioral, pharmacological, or neurochemical techniques. The extension of our knowledge requires that we determine the exact occasions of the release of 5HT at nerve terminals in relation to specific behavioral elements. Since quantal release of transmitter from neurons is thought to occur only when action potentials invade the presynaptic terminals, monitoring of unit activity of neurochemically identified systems allows us to determine the occasions of transmitter release.

Swedish investigators have developed a histochemical technique for localizing 5HT and other monamines in the brain (20, 29, 39). 5HT is found in a restricted group of neurons whose somata reside in the raphe nuclei in the midline of the brainstem. These neurons distribute axons and terminals within the brainstem, down the spinal cord, and to several regions in the forebrain (33). The dorsal raphe nucleus of the caudal midbrain tegmentum is an important source of ascending axons (34). This compact homogeneous group of cells was chosen for our initial studies of unit activity of 5HT containing neurons in behaving animals.

The present report describes the activity of dorsal raphe neurons, with particular emphasis on correlations with the states of sleep and wakefulness. Koella (44) and Jouvet (40) have proposed a role for 5HT in slow wave sleep (SWS).* Depletion of 5HT causes a reversible suppression of sleep (22, 45, 61), while intracarotid injections of 5HT produce electroencephalographic (EEG) synchronization which is normally associated with SWS. Furthermore, electrolytic lesions of the raphe nuclei, which result in loss of brain 5HT, are followed by a suppression of sleep

---

* The stages of sleep are described in detail in Chapter IX of this volume. Sleep in mammals consists of two distinct phases, slow wave sleep—SWS (spindle-burst sleep, quiet sleep), and rapid eye movement sleep—REM (paradoxical sleep, active sleep).

(40). Of particular interest to the present study is the role of 5HT in the control of certain monophasic wave spiking activity of the lateral geniculate nucleus which may occur in the *absence of eye movements* (LGn waves).[†] This wave activity normally occurs only during and just preceding rapid eye movement (REM) sleep and is representative of the phasic activity of REM sleep (see Chapter VI). Dement (25) has shown that LGn waves may occur in the waking state after depletion of 5HT.

Previous studies of raphe neurons have been carried out in anesthetized rats by Aghajanian and coworkers (2, 4, 32) and by Couch (19). They have described slow rhythmically firing neurons which are suppressed by systemic injections of LSD. The present study extends these findings to behaving animals and demonstrates changes in firing rates during sleep states.

METHODS

Single units were recorded from the brains of adult cats with chronically implanted 62 μ microwires using the technique described by Harper and McGinty in Chapter VI of this volume. The dorsal raphe nucleus (AP 0 to 2, H 1, midline) was approached through the cerebellum with a microwire bundle and microdrive inclined caudally 35° from the vertical to avoid the bony tentorium. As this nucleus provides a narrow target, the stereotaxic technique must be used with care.

When stable single units were isolated by the descending electrodes, a continuous recording including a complete sleep cycle was carried out. In some experiments the effect of drugs or certain stimuli were tested as described in the results. Sleep and waking states were identified on the basis of EEG, eye movement, and neck muscle recordings using standard criteria (49, 55). Recordings of lateral geniculate nucleus slow wave activity were obtained from bipolar stainless steel electrodes (.01 in.) with uninsulated tips separated by about 1.5 mm vertically. In most recording sessions two or more neurons were studied simultaneously.

---

† Similar LGn waves may occur in some cats in association with eye movements in both waking and REM sleep. In the present report the term *LGn waves* refers to waves occurring in the absence of eye movements.

The results presented here are documented primarily by polygraph recordings with individual spikes indicated by pen deflections produced by a pulse height analyzer. This type of record proved to be useful in the present study because of the slow firing of these neurons and the primary significance of the relation between spike activity and polygraphic recordings of EEG and LGn activity. Statistical properties of raphe neurons will be described elsewhere (McGinty and Harper, in preparation).

Characteristics of Dorsal Raphe Unit Activity

These results are based on recordings from thirty-six neurons in the vicinity of the dorsal raphe nucleus, including twenty-eight which shared several basic characteristics. This homogeneous group of twenty-eight neurons will be designated in this paper as the "S1" class to denote a presumed serotoninergic function with the knowledge that this label is tentative. This paper will describe the characteristics of these twenty-eight S1-class neurons.

S1 spikes were generally small (50-150 μ V) initially negative or initially positive biphasic potentials recorded in low level background activity. A sample recording is shown in Figure 15.1. The regularity of firing in this sample as well as the pause in firing correlated with the LGn wave was typical of S1 neurons. The latter phenomena are described in detail below. An electrode location can be seen in the photomicrograph in Figure 15.2. Neurons of the S1 class were found in both medial and lateral divisions of the dorsal raphe nucleus.

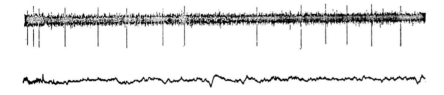

Figure 15.1. Top: Spontaneous extracellular spike activity of a dorsal raphe neuron during slow wave sleep. Spikes occurred rhythmically at about one per second. Bottom: Simultaneous recording of LGn EEG activity. The raphe unit does not fire prior to the LGn wave. Record from Varian electrostatic recorder. Calibration is five seconds.

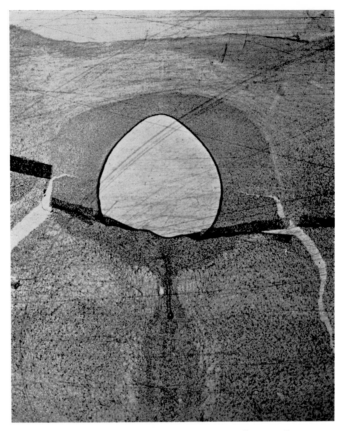

Figure 15.2. Photomicrograph showing Prussian Blue mark at termination of the descent of microwire electrode bundle at the ventral part of the dorsal raphe nucleus. Typical S1-class raphe units were recorded from this site and above. Carbofuxin stain.

Sleep and Waking States

In the quiet waking state all S1 neurons exhibited a regular firing pattern at rates of 0.5-4 spikes per second. Examples are shown in Figures 15.1 and 15.3. In our sample of thirty-six neurons in the vicinity of the dorsal raphe nucleus, S1 neurons were operationally defined as those units exhibiting firing rates within this range. These neurons have *never* been observed to show bursting or rapid acceleration of firing rates. The stability of raphe unit activity during wakefulness also will be discussed below.

S1 class neurons showed consistent firing rate changes in relation to shifts between W, QS and REM. The most striking event was a marked depression or cessation of firing during REM. This change is seen in Figure 15.3. In addition, most neurons

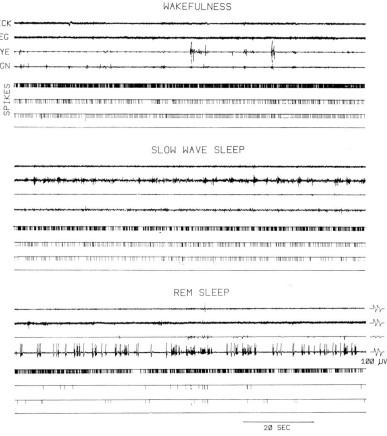

Figure 15.3. Polygraphic recording with activity of three neurons showing raphe unit activity during three states: W, SWS, and REM sleep. The bottom two neurons are typical S1 raphe neurons, showing slight slowing of firing in SWS and striking slowing of firing in REM. Note the rhythmicity of firing during W, especially in the bottom recording. "Spikes" shown in this figure and in Figures 15.5-15.8 are lengthened pulses produced by a spike height discriminator.

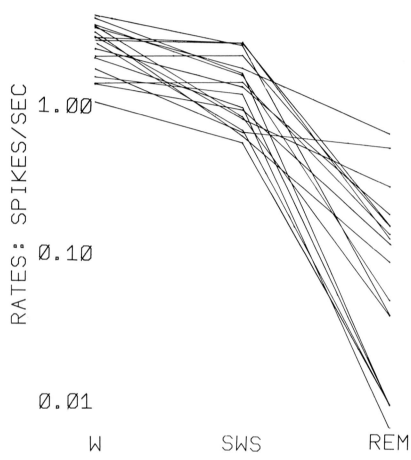

Figure 15.4. Rates of eighteen typical S1 raphe neurons during W, SWS, and REM on log scale from one cat. The rates during wakefulness in this type of neuron were restricted to a narrow range. This range was subsequently chosen to define the S1 class of neurons. Mean rate during REM is about one tenth second. Rates are based on ten ten-second samples from each state for each neuron. SWS samples were taken in the absence of LGn waves.

showed a small reduction in firing rate in SWS. These rate changes are shown on a log scale for eighteen individual S1 neurons from one cat in Figure 15.4. Note that half of these units fired less than once every ten seconds during REM. The rate changes between SWS and REM were significant in seventeen of these eighteen neurons while the changes between wakefulness and SWS were significant in thirteen (2-tailed *t* test, p < .05). Similar rate changes were found in the entire sample of twenty-eight S1 neurons. Many rate changes between W and QS, although small, were significant because of the absence of variability in firing rate within each state.

The record of the end of a REM period, shown in Figure 15.5, illustrates two additional characteristics of S1 neurons. First, during short epochs within the REM period marked by cessation of LGn waves, firing of S1 units became regular momentarily. Thus, firing was negatively correlated with the occurrence of LGn waves, although S1 unit spikes occasionally *followed* an LGn wave. Second, S1 units often resumed firing at the end of a REM period prior to other signs of REM termination. Thus, resumption of regular firing of S1 units often predicted the end of a REM period.

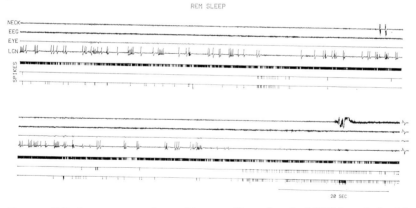

Figure 15.5. Continuous polygraphic recording of end of REM period with three raphe neurons of which bottom two are typical S1 neurons. Note that end of REM period is heralded by resumption of regular S1 unit firing. The temporary interruption of the train of LGn waves during REM was also marked by resumption of firing.

Changes in firing rate during sleep states were *not* associated with changes in firing patterns, such as bursting, as have been reported for most brain neurons. The regular pattern is maintained in SWS and, on those few occasions when repetitive unit firing is seen, during REM.

Relation to LGn Wave Activity

LGn waves occur during SWS, usually beginning one to two minutes before the onset of a REM period, but occasionally in isolated groups or preceding an arousal reaction. The firing of S1 units usually slowed or stopped prior to the occurrence of these SWS-LGn waves. Indeed, it was often possible to predict the occurrence of LGn spikes by noting interruptions of S1 spiking. An example is shown in Figure 15-1. Although LGn spikes were usually preceded by S1 unit slowing, it must be noted that unit slowing sometimes occurred without LGn spiking.

PCPA Treated Cats

Parachlorophenylalanine (PCPA) produces a reversible blockade of biosynthesis of 5HT by inhibition of the rate-limiting step, the hydroxylation of tryptophan (conversion to 5-hydroxytryptophan, 5HTP). 5HT is gradually depleted during a forty-eight to seventy-two hour period. Catecholamine levels are reduced only slightly (43). Both SWS and, in the cat, REM are reduced beginning twenty-four to forty-eight hours after PCPA treatment (22, 45); the sleep loss follows a time course similar to that of brain 5HT levels. Both sleep and 5HT levels are restored by administration of 5HTP (45, 59). As noted above, Dement (25) has reported that LGn waves occurring in the absence of eye movements show an altered distribution in PCPA-treated cats. Beginning twenty-four to forty-eight hours after treatment, these LGn waves which are normally restricted to REM and pre-REM SWS periods begin to occur during wakefulness.

We report here some preliminary observations on the effects of 5HT depletion by PCPA and repletion by 5HTP on unit activity of 5HT-containing cells. We have confirmed the observations of sleep suppression and the appearance of waking LGn spikes. These replications indicate the effectiveness of PCPA treatment in our study, in lieu of measurements of brain 5HT levels in val-

BASELINE: 48 H AFTER PCPA

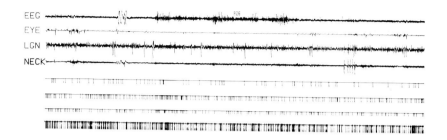

3 H AFTER 5HTP

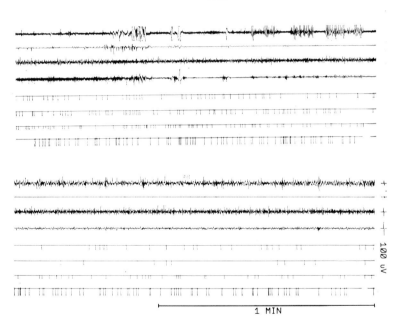

1 MIN

Figure 15.6. Effects of 5HT depletion and repletion on raphe unit firing. Polygraphic recording with four raphe neurons. Top three are typical S1 neurons as defined by rate range during W (.5-4/s). Forty-eight hours after PCPA (two daily doses subcutaneously, one hundred fifty mg/kg) LGn waves are observed in wakefulness. Waking spikes are preceded by raphe unit slowing (additional examples are seen in Fig. 7). Repletion of 5HT by 5HTP (25 mg/kg, IP) results in slowing of raphe units and suppression of LGn waves. Slowing after 5HTP is seen during both W (middle sample) and SWS (lower sample).

uable unit recording preparations. The questions we posed concerned (1) the effect of altered brain 5HT levels on S1 unit firing, and (2) the relationship between unit activity and waking LGn waves.

These preliminary studies concerning the first question indicate that 5HT depletion produces no dramatic change in S1 unit activity rate or pattern. However, some units appeared to increase firing rate during the first 48 hours, although this change may have resulted from the increased behavioral arousal produced by PCPA. Waking S1 unit activity also appeared to be slightly more variable in rate, with frequent pauses in firing that are rare in untreated animals. We are presently quantifying these observations.

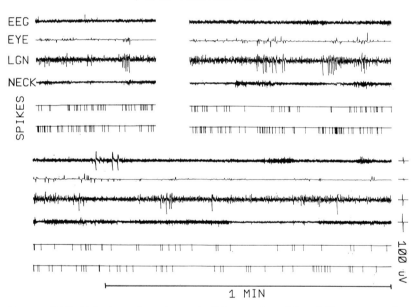

PCPA–TREATED CAT

Figure 15.7. Relation of raphe unit firing and waking LGn waves after 5HT depletion. Three sample recordings made forty-eight to seventy-two hours after PCPA (two daily doses: one hundred fifty mg/kg sub Q). Note bursts of waking LGn waves are preceded by slowing of raphe units. Waking LGn waves were often, though not invariably, seen to occur in the absence of eye movements, as in normal REM sleep. Close examination of the record indicated that eye movements often closely *followed* LGn waves.

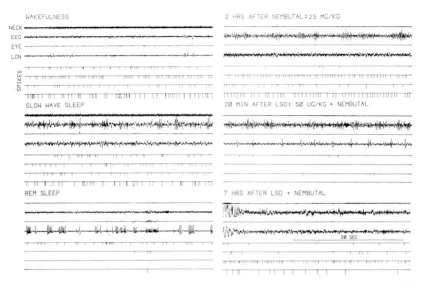

Figure 15.8. Effects of LSD on raphe units. Polygraphic recordings with four typical S1 raphe units. Left: Normal firing rates during W, SWS, and REM. Right: Same neurons after Nembutal, and Nembutal plus LSD. LSD resulted in a dramatic slowing of raphe bursts in the anesthetized cat. Recovery of firing was incomplete after seven hours. Nembutal by itself caused a slight slowing of S1 units, comparable to that seen in normal SWS. The top unit appeared to be less suppressed during REM sleep and more suppressed by Nembutal than other units.

While the effect of 5HT depletion was not conclusive, the effect of rapidly increasing 5HT levels with the administration of 5HTP was clear. As shown in Figure 15.6, increasing brain 5HT produced a slowing of S1 unit firing. This slowing was independent of behavioral state.

Waking LGn waves, appearing forty-eight to seventy-two hours after PCPA treatment, were preceded by slowing or cessation of firing of S1 units. Some examples are shown in Figure 15.7 LGn waves occur in the waking cat, in most cases, when the cat: (a) ceases behavioral activity and assumes a resting, sitting, or lying posture, and (b) exhibits EEG synchronization associated with a *drowsy* state. These two events, behavioral quiescence and EEG synchronization, are also associated with S1 unit slowing in untreated animals. We cannot yet answer the fascinating question as to whether or not S1 unit slowing preceding LGn waves is more pronounced in treated than in normal animals.

Effects of LSD

Aghajanian and his associates have reported that in anesthetized rats raphe unit activity is suppressed by LSD (2). We have confirmed this observation in identified S1 units in cats. We found that the relatively low doses of LSD employed by these workers in rats were effective only in suppressing S1 unit activity in cats only in combination with an anesthetic. We have not tested higher doses. We noted that the suppression of S1 unit firing by LSD plus Nembutal was associated with the occurrence of LGn spikes. An example is shown in Figure 15.8. This observation suggests that the hallucinogenic action of LSD may be closely related to the hallucinogenic activity of PCPA. These observations are consistent with the long standing hypothesis that LSD acts by "antagonizing" 5HT (2, 35, 62). The mechanism of "antagonism" suggested by these data is the suppression of the release of 5HT (but, see Discussion).

Waking Behavior

Proposals that 5HT is involved in control of behavioral processes such as perception of pain, habituation, and social behavior led us to search for further behavioral correlates of changes in S1 unit activity. We have examined responses to simple sensory stimulation, complex stimuli such as kittens or baby rats, and painful stimuli. We are struck by the regularity and stability of S1 unit firing and the absence of clear rate changes during these tests. No phasic bursts of activity or long silent periods have been observed. The changes which do occur are subtle, brief increases in interspike intervals or slight changes in rate. Since S1 units are often very rhythmic in their firing, such subtle changes may be important. Quantitative studies will be required to discover any systematic correlations with discrete behaviors.

These general observations do allow us to suggest one interpretation. S1 units do not exhibit the changes in firing pattern which make them suitable for conveying discrete message as in the case of sensory or motor pathways. They are more suited to modulate slower changing baseline conditions such as drive, affective states or arousal.

DISCUSSION

Our interpretation that certain neurons, herein denoted as S1 neurons, are the 5HT-containing neurons of the dorsal raphe nucleus is based on three results. First, recordings from histologically verified electrode tracts within the dorsal raphe nucleus provided S1 type neurons, while recording from tracts more than 0.5 mm laterally did not. The fact that 80 percent of recorded units from dorsal raphe sites exhibited similar properties suggestive of a homogeneous type of neuron is consistent with the anatomical homogeneity of this nucleus. Second, the rate and pattern of firing in our units were identical to that observed by Aghajanian and his associates with conventional small-tipped microelectrodes in anesthetized rats (2, 4, 32). Third, the suppression of firing of S1 neurons by LSD in the anesthetized animal also is in agreement with the results of Aghajanian et al. (2) and, according to these investigators, is observed exclusively in raphe neurons among the neurons of the midbrain. The state independent response of S1 neurons to 5HTP is also consistent with the interpretation that we are recording from 5HT-containing neurons. A discussion of the general validity of our unit recording technique may be found in Chapter VI of this volume.

The S1 neurons described here shared several properties. Each of these neurons exhibited slow and regular firing activity. Virtually all of these neurons fired more slowly in REM sleep than in SWS and more than two-thirds fired more slowly in SWS than in W. In addition, the majority exhibited slower firing prior to the occurrence of LGn spikes in SWS periods preceding REM. Finally, no S1 neurons exhibited phasic acceleration of firing or bursting under any conditions. These properties may be used to define S1 class neurons. Additionally, studies in progress indicate that S1 unit firing is suppressed by both LSD and 5HTP. Other groups of 5HT-containing neurons may share some or all of these properties.

The interpretation of the behavioral significance of these data rests on the assumption that S1 unit activity is correlated with the release of 5HT at nerve terminals. This assumption is supported

by the observation that electrical stimulation of raphe nuclei results in the release of 5HT at nerve terminals (1, 46). There is
also evidence that the depletion of 5HT after synthesis inhibition is dependent on nerve impulse flow. Depletion fails to occur
caudal to a spinal transection (7). Further, depletion of spinal
5HT following synthesis inhibition may be accelerated by electrical stimulation of raphe nuclei in the medulla (21).

5HT and Sleep

The present data suggest that the release of 5HT is consistently decreased during slow wave sleep. Several investigators, notably
Jouvet and Koella, have suggested that 5HT brings about or facilitates SWS. This latter hypothesis is supported by the observation of insomnia after brain 5HT depletion (22, 45, 61) and SWS
facilitation after brain 5HT elevation (40). The definite resolution of this discrepancy depends upon further investigation of the
effects of 5HT receptor stimulation. However, some reasonable
speculations are offered here to guide future studies.

The studies supporting a facilitatory role of 5HT in sleep may
be reinterpreted as follows. 5HT depletion by PCPA causes the
appearance of S1 unit slowing during wakefulness and the in-
trusion of waking LGn waves. As previously suggested by Dement (25), the waking waves appear to be correlated with
arousal of the cats. 5HT depletion also results in the exag-
geration of certain waking behaviors including sexual behavior
(30), grooming (54), aggressiveness and hallucinatory activity
(30). Thus, sleep may be prevented by the release of incompatible behaviors. It is noteworthy that, during chronic PCPA
treatment, sleep eventually returns to normal although brain 5HT
levels remain depressed (25). This explanation emphasizes an
abnormal disruptive influence on sleep rather than a normal
suppression of a sleep initiating mechanism.

The SWS facilitation produced by 5HTP may also be reinterpreted. 5HTP causes a marked slowing of S1 neurons. This suppression of 5HT neural unit firing also has been observed in
anesthetized rats after elevation of 5HT levels by monoamine
oxidase inhibiters (4). These observations suggest that a feedback control mechanism compensates for elevated 5HT levels by

reduced unit firing. Similar feedback control mechanisms have been demonstrated in other monoaminergic systems and implicated in effects of LSD. When 5HTP is administered systemically, an experience to which the nervous system is not adapted, the feedback control mechanism which detects 5HT levels may be stimulated *more* than the synaptic regions. The latter are quite protected by the close apposition of presynaptic and postsynaptic membranes. Thus, the reduction in unit firing may *overcompensate* for the increased 5HT pool. The same explanation may account for the EEG synchronization produced by application of 5HT to the IVth ventricle (44). We would predict that such application would suppress S1 unit firing and result in reduced 5HT release in remote terminals.

The comments above suggest alternative explanations for previous experiments supporting the role of 5HT in sleep. The present data are also subject to additional interpretations:

1. 5HT-containing neurons in other raphe nuclei may exhibit different patterns of firing rate changes during sleep and wakefulness. Some 5HT neurons may increase firing during SWS.

2. The postsynaptic effects of 5HT may not be correlated with rate of 5HT release because of systematic variations in postsynaptic sensitivity to 5HT or rate of 5HT inactivation.

3. The release of 5HT produced by each presynaptic impulse may vary greatly and may be greater during periods of SWS. Thus, although unit activity is reduced during SWS, 5HT may be increased.

The latter two possibilities can be assessed when we develop techniques to measure 5HT receptor stimulation directly.

REM Sleep

The depression of raphe unit firing during REM contrasts sharply with changes in unit activity in other brain sites (see Chapter IX of this volume for a review of changes in unit activity during REM). No other brain neurons, except motoneurons (by indirect tests), exhibit complete suppression of firing during REM. No other neurons exhibit state specific changes in

REM, that is, changes in firing which occur only during REM sleep. These observations indicate 5HT plays some critical role in REM sleep. We have noted that the slowing of 5HT neurons is the earliest known physiological sign of the approach of REM sleep. These correlational data suggest the hypothesis that the cessation of 5HT release brings about some critical physiological changes that characterize REM. Of course, we cannot exclude the possibility that some unknown elements cause both the depression of raphe unit firing and other properties of REM sleep. However, a number of observations offer indirect support for this hypothesis. These observations include (1) the interactions between 5HT, LGn waves, and REM, (2) the effects of REM deprivation, (3) the effects on REM of certain manipulations that augment 5HT levels, and (4) the effects of 5HT on spinal reflex transmission. These observations are reviewed below.

LGn waves appear to reflect a critical process during REM. An important physiological function for REM is indicated by the fact that REM deprivation is followed by a compensatory rebound increase in the amount of REM (24, 26, 54). Deprivation of REM sleep which minimizes loss of waves minimizes the rebound following deprivation, while maximizing deprivation of LGn waves maximizes the rebound (25). The number of LGn waves is remarkably stable from day-to-day (40). Thus, LGn waves seem to reflect, quantitatively, a function of REM.

5HT appears to inhibit the occurrence of LGn waves. S1 unit slowing precedes the occurrence of LGn waves appearing during REM, isolated LGn waves and waking LGn waves. The release of LGn waves during waking after depletion of 5HT also supports this hypothesis. Since LGn waves represent a critical parameter of REM sleep and that waves appear to occur after slowing of 5HT release, this slowing of release may be a primary function of REM sleep. It should be noted that the tonic aspects of REM may occur with diminished or absent LGn waves after treatment with PCPA or reserpine (23). Thus, the tonic and phasic aspects of REM may not be controlled by the same mechanism.

Certain similar behavioral changes are produced by REM deprivation and depletion of 5HT by PCPA. Both manipulations may produce hypersexuality (26, 30), increased aggressiveness

(30, 51), and lowered seizure thresholds (5, 16). Thus, although the testing procedures for observing the changes after the two treatments differed, it appears that REM deprivation produces some of the effects of 5HT depletion. This observation leads to a second corollary hypothesis. A function of REM may be to restore levels of 5HT, perhaps within the active pool in nerve terminals. In direct support of this hypothesis is the finding that REM deprivation produces increased utilization of 5HT (38).

This hypothesis also is supported by observations on certain diverse manipulations that produce a decrease or deprivation of REM with little or no subsequent compensatory rebound. These manipulations include ECS (17), treatment with imipramine (36), and monoamine oxidase inhibitors (40, 63). All of these have in common an augmentation of 5HT levels or synthesis (14, 28, 41, 48). Thus, manipulations which increase 5HT appear to reduce the requirement for REM. However, since these same manipulations affect catecholamines, a clear interpretation is not yet possible.

Finally, 5HT may modulate changes in reflex modulation during REM. Elevation of spinal 5HT levels increases motoneuron excitability (6, 10, 11). This cessation of 5HT release could result in a well known REM related depression of motoneuron excitation directly or by releasing some inhibitory system. It should be noted, however, that an inhibitory influence of 5HT on reflex excitability has also been noted (15, 27).

While animal studies have implicated 5HT in the control of SWS, pharmacological manipulations of 5HT in humans have suggested a role in REM. The human studies suggest that increasing 5HT augments REM. Administration of 5HTP augments REM sleep and rapid eye movement intensity but not SWS (65). On the other hand, PCPA treatment reduces REM but not SWS (64). The difference between results with animals and humans has not been explained. The present results appear to be incompatible with the human data as with the animal studies.

5HT as a Transmitter

The list of criteria for a transmitter in the brain includes the demonstration that exogenous transmitter and released transmitter have the same postsynaptic consequences in a specific synapse. The present data provide an indirect form of such evidence for 5HT as a modulation of LGn waves. Changes in 5HT levels by depletion and repletion have the same effects on LGn waves as transmitter release correlated with nerve activity. This particular evidence will be stronger when one knows the specific postsynaptic events resulting in LGn spikes.

SUMMARY

Neurons of the dorsal raphe nucleus containing 5HT were studied in order to estimate the release of 5HT from nerve terminals during behavioral states. Most neurons recorded in this site shared six properties: (1) slow firing (0.5-4/s during wakefulness), (2) rhythmic firing, (3) total absence of bursts of firing, (4) slowing or cessation of firing during REM sleep compared with slow wave sleep, (5) slight slowing of firing during slow wave sleep compared to wakefulness, and (6) slowing of firing immediately prior to occurrence of LGn waves during slow wave sleep. No clear rate changes during waking behaviors were discovered.

Depletion of brain 5HT by PCPA resulted in insomnia and the occurrence of LGn spikes in wakefulness but little overall change of raphe unit firing. However, waking LGn spikes were preceded by raphe unit slowing. Repletion of 5HT by 5HTP slowed raphe unit firing and facilitated sleep. LSD also suppressed raphe unit activity in low doses in combination with Nembutal.

The slowing of raphe unit firing during sleep contradicts current theories suggesting a facilitatory role for 5HT in sleep. It is speculated that cessation of 5HT release during REM sleep may restore active 5HT pools. A regulatory role in the control of waking behaviors may be played by 5HT.

REFERENCES

1. Aghajanian, G. K., J. A. Rosecrans, and M. H. Sheard. Serotonin: Release in the forebrain by stimulation of midbrain raphe. Science 156:402-403, 1967.

2. Aghajanian, G. K., W. E. Foote, and M. H. Sheard. Lysergic acid diethylamide: Sensitive neuronal units in the midbrain raphe. Science 161:706-708, 1968.

3. Aghajanian, G. K., F. E. Bloom, and M. H. Sheard. Electron microscopy of degeneration within the serotonin pathway of rat brain. Brain Res. 13:266-273, 1969.
4. Aghajanian, G. K., A. W. Graham, and M. H. Sheard. Serotonin-containing neurons in the brain: Depression of firing by monoamine oxidase inhibitors. Science 169:1100-1102, 1970.
5. Alexander, G. J., and L. M. Kopeloff. Metrazol seizures in rats: Effect of p-chlorophenylalanine. Brain Res. 22:231-235, 1970.
6. Andén, N.-E. Discussion of serotonin and dopamine in the extrapyramidal system. Adv. Pharmac. 6A:347-349, 1968.
7. Andén, N.-E., K. Fuxe, and T. Hökfelt. The importance of the nervous impulse flow for the depletion of the monoamines from central neurons by some drugs. J. Pharmac. 18:630-632, 1966.
8. Andén, N.-E., H. Corrodi, K. Fuxe, and T. Hökfelt. Increased impulse flow in bulbospinal noradrenaline neurons produced by catecholamine receptor blocking agents. Eur. J. Pharmac. 2:59-64, 1967.
9. Andén, N.-E., H. Corrodi, K. Fuxe, and T. Hökfelt. Evidence for a central 5-hydroxytryptamine receptor stimulation by lysergic acid diethylamide. Br. J. Pharmac. 34:1-7, 1968.
10. Anderson, E. G., R. G. Baker, and N. R. Banna. The effects of monoamine oxidase inhibitors on spinal synaptic activity. J. Pharmac. exp. Ther. 158:405-415, 1967.
11. Anderson, E. G., and T. Shibuya. The effects of 5-hydroxytryptophan and I-tryptophan on spinal synaptic activity. J. Pharmacol. exp. Ther. 153:352-360, 1966.
12. Ashcroft, G. W., and D. F. Sharman. 5-Hydroxyindoles in human cerebrospinal fluid. Nature 186:1050-1051, 1960.
13. Bogdanski, D. F., H. Weissbach, and S. Udenfriend. The distribution of serotonin, 5-hydroxytryptophan decarboxylase, and monoamine oxidase in brain. J. Neurochem. 1:272-278, 1957.
14. Carlsson, A., H. Corrodi, K. Fuxe, and T. Hökfelt. Effect of antidepressant drugs on the depletion of intraneuronal brain 5-hydroxytryptamine stores caused by 4-methyl-α-ethyl-meta-tyramine. Eur. J. Pharmacol. 5:357-366, 1969.
15. Clineschmidt, B. V., and E. G. Anderson. The blockade of bulbospinal inhibition by 5-hydroxytryptamine antagonists. Exp. Brain Res. 11:175-186, 1970.
16. Cohen, H. B., and W. C. Dement. Sleep: Changes in threshold to electroconvulsive shock in rats after deprivation of the paradoxical phase. Science 150:1318-1319, 1965.
17. Cohen, H. B., and W. C. Dement. Suppression of rapid eye movement phase in the cat after electroconvulsive shock. Science 154:396-398, 1966.
18. Coppen, A., D. M. Shaw, and A. J. Malleson. Changes in 5-hydroxy-

tryptophan metabolism in depression. Brit. J. Psychiat. 111:105-107, 1965.

19. Couch, James R., Jr. Responses of neurons in the raphe nuclei to serotonin, norepinephrine and acetylcholine and their correlation with an excitatory synaptic input. Brain Res. 19:137-150, 1970.

20. Dahlstrom, A., and K. Fuxe. Evidence for the existence of monoamine-containing neurons in the central nervous system: I. Demonstration of monoamines in the cell bodies of brain stem neurons. Acta Physiol. Scand. Suppl. 232, 62:1-55, 1964.

21. Dahlstrom, A., K. Fuxe, D. Kernell, and G. Sedvall. Reduction of the monoamine stores in the terminals of bulbospinal neurones following stimulation in the medulla oblongata. Life Sci., Oxford, 4: 1207-1212, 1965.

22. Delorme, F., J. L. Froment, and M. Jouvet. Suppression du sommeil par la p. chloromethamphetamine et la p. chlorophenylalanine. C. R. Soc. Biol. 160:2347-2351, 1966.

23. Delorme, F., M. Jeannerod, and M. Jouvet. Effects remarquables de la réserpine sur l'activité EEG phasique ponto-géniculo-occipitale. C. R. Soc. Biol. 159:900, 1965.

24. Dement, W. C. The effect of dream deprivation. Science 131: 1705-1707, 1960.

25. Dement, W. C. The biological role of REM sleep (circa 1968). In A. Kales (Ed.) *Sleep, Physiology and Pathology.* Lippincott, Philadelphia, 1969, pp. 245-265.

26. Dement, W., P. Henry, H. Cohen, and J. Ferguson. Studies of the effect of REM deprivation in humans and in animals. In S. S. Kety, E. V. Evarts, and H. L. Williams (Eds.) *Sleep and Altered States of Consciousness.* Williams and Wilkins, Baltimore, 1967, pp. 456-468.

27. Engberg, I., and R. W. Ryoll. The inhibitory action of noradrenaline and other monoamines on spinal neurons. J. Physiol. 185:298-322, 1966.

28. Essman, W. B. Electroshock-induced retrograde amnesia and brain serotonin metabolism: Effect of several antidepressant compounds. Psychopharmacologia (Berl.) 13:258-266, 1968.

29. Falck, B., N. A. Hillarp, G. Thieme, and A. Torp. Fluorescence of catecholamines and related compounds condensed with formaldehyde. J. Histochem. Cytochem. 10:348-354, 1962.

30. Ferguson, J., S. Henriksen, H. Cohen, G. Mitchell, J. Barchas, and W. Dement. "Hypersexuality" and behavioral changes in cats caused by administration of p-chlorophenylalanine. Science 168: 499-501, 1970.

31. Fibiger, H. C., and B. A. Campbell. The effect of para-chlorophenylalanine on spontaneous locomotor activity in the rat. Neuropharmacol. 10:25-32, 1971.

32. Foote, W. E., M. H. Sheard, and G. K. Aghajanian. Comparison of effects of LSD and amphetamine on midbrain raphe units. Nature 222:567-569, 1969.

33. Fuxe, K. Distribution of monoamine nerve terminals in the central nervous system. Acta Physiol. Scand. Suppl. 247, 64:30-84, 1965.

34. Fuxe, K., T. Hökfelt, and U. Ungerstedt. Localization of indolealkylamines in central nervous system. Advanc. Pharmacol. 6:235-251, 1968.

35. Gaddam, J. H. Antagonism between lysergic acid diethylamide and 5-hydroxytryptamine. J. Physiol. 121:15, 1953.

36. Hartmann, E. Convusion threshold: Effect of conditions which alter D-pressure. Paper Presented at 9th Ann. Meeting of Assoc. for the Psychophysiological Study of Sleep, Boston, Mass., March, 1969.

37. Hartmann, E. The sleep-dream cycle and brain serotonin. Psychonom. Sci. 8:295-296, 1967.

38. Hery, F., J.-F. Pujol, M. Lopez, J. Macon, and J. Glowinski. Increased synthesis and utilization of serotonin in the central nervous system of the rat during paradoxical sleep deprivation. Brain Res. 21: 391-403, 1970.

39. Hillarp, N.-A., K. Fuxe, and A. Dahlstrom. Demonstration and mapping of central neurons containing dopamine, noradrenaline, and 5-hydroxytryptamine and their reaction to psychopharmeca. Pharm. Rev. 18:727-741, 1966.

40. Jouvet, M. Mechanisms of the states of sleep: A neuropharmacological approach. In S. S. Kety, E. V. Evarts, and H. L. Williams (Eds.) *Sleep and Altered States of Consciousness.* Williams and Wilkins, Baltimore, 1967, pp. 86-126.

41. Kato, L., G. Gozsy, P. B. Roy, and V. Groh. Histamine, serotonin, epinephrine, and norepinephrine in the rat brain following convulsions. Int. J. Neuropsychiat. 3:46-51, 1967.

42. Khazan, N., and F. G. Sulman. Effect of imipramine on paradoxical sleep in animals with reference to dreaming and enuresis. Psychopharmacologia (Berl.) 10:89-95, 1966.

43. Koe, B. K., and A. Weissman. P-chlorophenylalanine: A specific depletor of brain serotonin. J. Pharmac. exp. Ther. 154:499-516, 1966.

44. Koella, W. P., A. Feldstein, and J. S. Czicman. The effect of para-chlorophenylalanine on the sleep of cats. Electroenceph. clin. Neurophysiol. 25:481-490, 1968.

45. Koella, W. P., and J. Czicman. Mechanism of the EEG synchronizing action of serotonin. Amer. J. Physiol. 211:926-934, 1966.

46. Kostowski, W., E. Giacalone, S. Garattini, and L. Valyelli. Electrical stimulation of midbrain raphe: Biochemical, behavioral, and bioelectric effects. Eur. J. Pharmac. 7:170-175, 1969.

47. Krnjevic, K., and J. W. Phillips. Action of certain amines on cerebral

cortical neurons. Brit. J. Pharmacol. Chemotherap. 20:471-490, 1963.

48. Lin, R. C., N. H. Neff, S. H. Ngai, and E. Costa. Turnover rates of serotonin and norepinephrine in brain of normal and pargyline-treated rats. Life Sci. 8:1077-1084, 1969.

49. McGinty, D. J., and M. B. Sterman. Sleep suppression after basal forebrain lesions in the cat. Science 160:1253-1255, 1968.

50. Michaelson, I. A., and V. P. Whittaker. The subcellular localization of 5-hydroxytryptamine in guinea pig brain. Biochem. Pharmacol. 12:203-211, 1963.

51. Morden, B., R. Conner, G. Mitchell, W. Dement, and S. Levine. Effects of rapid eye movement (REM) sleep deprivation on shock-induced fighting. Physiol. Behav. 3:425-432, 1968.

52. Roberts, M. H., and D. W. Straughan. An excitatory effect of 5-hydroxytryptamine on single cerebral cortical neurons. J. Physiol. 188:27, 1967.

53. Seigel, J., and T. Gordon. Paradoxical sleep: deprivation in the cat. Science 148:978-979, 1965.

54. Shillito, Elizabeth E. The effect of parachlorophenylalanine on social interaction of male rats. Br. J. Pharmacy 38:305-315, 1970.

55. Sterman, M. B., T. Knauss, D. Lehmann, and C. D. Clemente. Circadian sleep and waking patterns in the laboratory cat. Electroenceph. clin. Neurophysiol. 19:509-517, 1965.

56. Stevens, D. A., O. Resnick, and D. M. Krus. The effects of p-chlorophenylalanine, a depletor of brain serotonin, on behavior: I. Facilitation of discrimination learning. Life Sci. 6:2215-2220, 1967.

57. Tenen, S. S. The effects of p-chlorophenylalanine, a serotonin depletor, on avoidance acquisition, pain sensitivity, and related behavior in the rat. Psychopharmacologia 10:204-219, 1967.

58. Tenen, S. S. Antagonism of the analgesic effect of morphine and other drugs by p-chlorophenylalanine, a serotonin depletor. Psychopharmacologia 12:278-285, 1968.

59. Undefriend, S., H. Weissbach, and D. G. Bogdanski. Increase in tissue serotonin following administration of its percursor, 5HTP. J. Biol. Chem. 224:803-810, 195.

60. Way, E. L., H. H. Loh, and F. Shen. Morphine tolerance, physical dependence, and synthesis of brain 5-hydroxytryptamine. Science 162:1290-1292, 1968.

61. Weitzman, E. D., M. M. Rapport, P. McGregor, and J. Jacoby. Sleep patterns of the monkey and brain serotonin concentration: Effect of p-chlorophenylalanine. Science 160:1361-1363, 1968.

62. Wooley, D. W., and E. Shaw. A biochemical and pharmacological suggestion about certain mental disorders. Science 119:587-588, 1954.

63. Wyatt, R. J., D. J. Kupfer, J. Scott, D. S. Robinson, and F. Snyder. Longitudinal studies of the effect of monoamine oxidase inhibitors on sleep in man. Psychopharmacologia (Berl.) 15:236-244, 1969.

64. Wyatt, R. J., K. Engelman, D. J. Kupfer, J. Scott, A. Sjoerdsma, and F. Snyder. Effect of parachlorophenylalanine on sleep in man. Electroenceph. clin. Neurophysiol. 27:529-532, 1969.

65. Wyatt, R. J., V. Zarcone, K. Engelman, W. C. Dement, F. Snyder, and A. Sjoerdsma. Effects of 5-hydroxytryptophan on the sleep of normal human subjects. Electroenceph. clin. Neurophysiol. 30: 505-509, 1971.

66. Zieher, L. M., and E. De Robertis. Subcellular localization of 5-hydroxytryptamine in cat brain. Biochem. Pharmac. 12:596-598, 1963.

Chapter XVI

A MULTIDIMENSIONAL APPROACH TO THE STUDY OF UNIT ACTIVITY IN FREELY MOVING ANIMALS

B. L. JACOBS

ALTHOUGH THE TECHNIQUE of recording the extracellular electrical activity of single units has been used to great advantage in the study of sensory and motor systems, one is struck by the lack of conceptual developments derived from unit studies of brain areas primarily involved in motivational or cognitive function.* In contrast to sensory and motor systems, where we often have excellent *a priori* information concerning the afferent and/or behavioral correlates of unit activity, one must begin the study of integrative mechanisms, at the neuronal level, with a paucity of presumptive empirical correlates. For example, lesion, stimulation, and evoked potential studies have told us a good deal about the function of the lateral geniculate body and the red nucleus, but we have gained little definitive information from these techniques concerning the role of the lateral hypothalamus or basolateral amygdala. Since the behavioral importance of many of these brain areas remains obscure, elucidation of the functional significance of individual neurons within brain structures concerned with integrative processes requires undertaking an open-minded, free ranging, exploratory approach unconstrained by dogma. This necessitates the collection of data in a variety of ex-

Based on a dissertation submitted in partial fulfillment of the requirements for the Ph.D. degree at the University of California, Los Angeles. Supported by USPHS Grant MH-10083, the U. S. Veterans Administration, and a N.I.M.H. predoctoral fellowship (1 FO1 MH47388-01). I would like to thank Dr. D. J. McGinty for his assistance in the preparation of this chapter.

* In the present context, *motivational* and *cognitive* are subsumed under the term *integrative* and is operationally defined as any brain area outside of the classical sensory or motor systems.

perimental situations in freely moving animals, which in turn necessitates that units be studied over long periods of time; this has become technically feasible only within the last few years. Failure to study these units under a variety of conditions leaves us with a situation analogous to the blind men who stated that the object before them was a wall, a spear, or a rope, depending on whether they happened to touch the elephant's side, tusk or tail. Similarly, investigators of single unit activity have been unable to give meaningful representations of the nature, or function, of integrative cells because they gathered their data from only one point of view, *e.g.*, studying sleep, or conditioning, or sensory responsiveness, etc.

In order to remedy this situation, a multidimensional approach to the study of unit activity was employed in the series of experiments described in this chapter. Thus, the activity of each unit was studied under a variety of conditions. In this way, the results of one experiment do not stand in a vacuum, rather they provide a theoretical jumping off point for subsequent research. As more and more data are collected, one obtains a fuller picture of the nature of the cells under study. It is only by piecing together many bits of information that we can hope to gain an understanding of structures with complex functions such as those in the limbic system, association cortex, diencephalon, and brain stem reticular formation. This approach also avoids drawing conclusions tainted by the pitfalls and biases indigenous to each individual paradigm, since these idiosyncracies cancel each other out as *noise* when experiments performed under a variety of conditions are summed together to form a total picture.

In a second strategy employed in the present study, an attempt was made to record from a restricted anatomical locus in the hope that this would provide data on a relatively homogeneous group of neurons; the rationale being that this would decrease the variability of the data and thereby make any meaningful results stand out. Although we often use one term to describe all the cell bodies in one general area, *e.g.*, the hypothalamus or the amygdala, we know that individual nuclei often derive, ontogenetically or phylogenetically, from different tissue or from structures subserving quite separate functions. Hence, when it was decided to investigate the integrative nature of the amygdala[†] at the neuronal level, the microelectrodes were implanted only in the magnocellular portion of the basal amygdaloid nucleus (in the cat, an area containing predominantly cell bodies of 25-35 μ dia).

Literature Review

Previous investigations of amygdala unit activity have been confined to studying the effects of sensory stimulation and direct stimulation of the peripheral and central nervous system. Machne and Segundo (24), using curarized cats, reported that touch, proprioceptive stimuli and sciatic stimulation had the most pronounced effect on amygdala unit activity, while few cells responded to clicks or light flashes. They also reported that inputs from several modalities often converged upon a single cell. Wendt and Albe-Fessard (39) reported that amygdala units were quite responsive to electric shocks applied to the paws of a chloralosed cat.

The first investigation of amygdala unit activity in a freely moving animal was done by Sawa and Delgado (35). They presented both simple and complex stimuli to cats and reported that a *meow* was the most effective stimulus; smoke and touch were also effective. Inputs from several modalities were also found to converge upon a single unit.

Creutzfeldt et al. (5), using curarized cats, reported that amygdala cells were difficult to "pick up" and that their spontaneous discharge rate was quite low. Most cells were responsive to olfactory stimulation (smoke), while few showed a specific response to sciatic stimulation. Auditory and tactile stimuli were almost without effect and no cells responded to visual stimulation. There was very little convergence of inputs.

Finally, in a recent study, O'Keefe and Bouma (30) reported finding cells in the basolateral amygdala of freely moving cats that were responsive to complex stimuli, especially those in the auditory modality (*e.g.*, low pitched human voice and a bird chirp).

[†] For a discussion of the amygdala as an integrative structure, see reviews by Gloor (13) and Goddard (14).

What conclusions can we draw from these studies? Inputs for all sensory modalities reach the amygdala. The most provocative stimulus, at least in freely moving cats, appears to be complex auditory inputs such as *meows*. Many amygdala cells receive inputs from a number of modalities; this convergence may be taken as

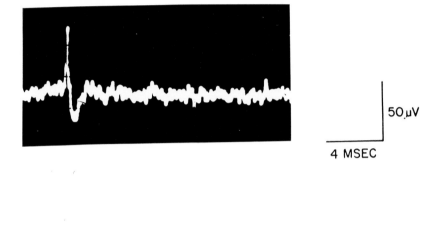

50 μV

4 MSEC

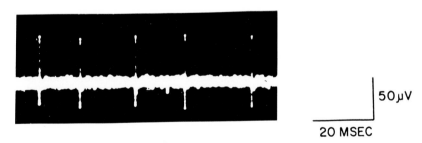

50 μV

20 MSEC

Figure 16.1. Photographs of oscilloscopic traces of amygdala discharges. Top: single spike at fast oscilloscope sweep speed. Bottom: burst of five spikes at slower sweep speed. Reprinted by permission of Academic Press Inc., New York, from a paper by B. L. Jacobs and D. J. McGinty, *Exper. Neurol.* 33:1-15, 1971.

evidence in support of the notion that the amygdala performs an integrative function. It is clear from this brief review that the only aspect of amygdala unit activity that has been studied is the response of these cells to various stimuli. Therefore, in the present series of experiments, unit activity was studied during sleep and waking; in association with an EEG rhythm indicative of a state characterized by inhibition of phasic motor activity; in response to reinforcing electrical stimulation of the brain; during a conditioned state of fear; and in response to a variety of sensory stimuli. These data have been presented or published in greater detail elsewhere (16, 17, 19, 20, 21).

Method

The methods employed have been described in previous publications (18, 20), and are described in full detail in a separate chapter in the present volume (see chapter by Harper and McGinty). Briefly stated, standard techniques were used to record the electroencephalogram, electrooculogram, and neck electromyogram in ten adult cats. Unit activity was recorded from 65 μ dia nichrome wires which were implanted in bundles of ten each in the magnocellular portion of the basal amygdaloid nucleus (A 11.0; L 9.5; H-5.0). Data were analyzed both on line and from magnetic tape by means of an electronic counter and a small laboratory computer. Figure 16.1 exemplifies the quality of the recordings obtainable through the use of this technique.

Experiment 1

Unit activity was recorded from the magnocellular basal amygdaloid nucleus during sleep and wakefulness (20). Previous studies of unit activity during sleep-wakefulness have been confined to sensory, motor and central core structures, and their rostral extensions.

The animals were placed in a sound attenuating behavioral chamber and allowed to go through at least one complete sleep-waking cycle, *i.e.*, quiet waking (QW), slow wave sleep (SWS) (indicated by cortical EEG spindle bursts of at least 200 μV), and paradoxical sleep (PS) (indicated by low voltage fast EEG, flattened neck EMG, rapid eye movements). Data analysis con-

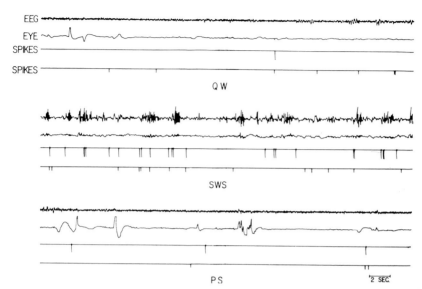

Figure 16.2. Unit activity of two amygdala cells during sleep and waking. Polygraphic recordings of electroencephalogram (EEG), electrooculogram (EOG), and spike discharges during quiet waking (QW), slow wave sleep (SWS) and paradoxical sleep (PS). The spikes are the triggered standard pulse output of a spike height discriminator. Both cells discharged at very low rates during QW and PS. Note the increased clustering of spikes during SWS. Reprinted by permission of Academic Press Inc., New York, from a paper by B. L. Jacobs and D. J. McGinty, *Exper. Neurol.* 33:1-15, 1971.

sisted of comparing mean cell discharge rates during at least eight 10 sec epochs in each of the three states.

The most important results of the present study may be summarized as follows: a) The majority of cells (39/61) discharged at significantly higher ($p < .01$ level used for all rate comparisons) rates during SWS than in either PS or QW. Figure 16.2 illustrates two such cells. b) In only ten of sixty-one cases was the discharge rate in PS greater than that in SWS (seven cells discharged fastest in QW, and the other five of the sixty-one cells were equally fast in two or three states). c) No increase in discharge rate was observed in association with the phasic activity of PS. In fact, 39 percent of the cells showed a significant decrease (two tailed t tests, $p < .01$) in rate during eye movements.

All of these results are contrary to those reported in studies of other brain loci.

Cells which discharged fastest in SWS were generally slow firing cells (Md = 0.5 spikes/sec in SWS), while those cells which were fastest in QW or PS were faster firing cells (Md = 1.8 spikes/sec in SWS). The difference in the distributions of the mean rates of the cells in these two groups is significant (Mann-Whitney U = 215; n_1 = 17, n_2 = 44; p < .01, two-tailed test) indicating that the cells were sampled from different populations and may have represented different functional groups. Furthermore, most cell discharge rates were decreased by the presentation of an arousing stimulus (0.5 sec duration, 110 db white noise) and those that were increased by arousal were typically cells that discharged faster in QW than in SWS. This may be a further indication that the low rate and the higher rate cells are from separate cell populations.

Amygdala units displayed an interesting characteristic during PS; they often increased in rate in association with a 12-16 hz EEG rhythm recorded over the sensorimotor cortex. In the waking animal the occurrence of this rhythm, the so-called sensorimotor rhythm (SMR) (33), is always correlated with the absence of overt behavior (33, 38, 40). The same is true of its occurrence during PS, that is, this rhythm is only seen in the absence of phasic EMG changes or rapid eye movements (37). Of the thirty-three cells recorded during periods of sensorimotor rhythm in PS, twelve showed significant rate increases and none decreased in rate (p < .02, two tailed t tests were used to compare rates during periods of sensorimotor rhythm, of at least 80 μV amplitude, in PS, with control periods of equal length during PS). All of these twelve cells discharged fastest in SWS which is another indication that they may represent a functionally distinct group from those cells which are fastest in PS or QW.

To what can we attribute the divergency of the present results from those of previous experiments on sensory, motor, and central core structures (*e.g.*, 1, 8, 9, 10, 12, 15, 25, 26, 34)? These latter studies generally report that: the unit discharge rate is higher during PS than during either SWS or QW; with few exceptions, the neuronal activity of a specific structure is lowest during

SWS; and finally, an enhancement of cell discharge rate often accompanies the phasic activity of PS (*i.e.,* rapid eye movements). One possibility is that the present results are characteristic of all structures located within the limbic system. There is some support for this from two previous studies of cells in the hippocampus, the only other limbic neurons studied during sleep and waking. In the first study, all six cells recorded from the dorsal hippocampus of rats discharged faster in SWS than in PS (28). In the second study, although dorsal hippocampal cells in cats discharged fastest in PS, the phasic movements of PS were not accompanied by an increase in the rate of firing (29).

A second explanation is that these data are characteristic of forebrain structures whose function is inhibitory with respect to behavior. There is a good deal of evidence which indicates that the area in and around the magnocellular basal amygdaloid nucleus is important in behavioral inhibition. Lesion and stimulation studies have shown its importance in the inhibition of feeding (11, 23), in the inhibition of aggression (6, 7), and in the production of slow waves or SWS (3, 4, 22, 27). Experiments on other structures thought to be involved in behavioral inhibition also support this hypothesis. Cells in the ventromedial hypothalamus of cats discharged faster in SWS than in PS or arousal (18, 32). Similarly, the two studies, cited above, which deal with hippocampal unit activity and sleep also lend support. This *inhibitory* hypothesis would account for the increased discharge rate observed both during SWS and during those aspects of PS in which the sensorimotor rhythm is seen. It would also account, in a reciprocal fashion, for the decreased firing during arousal and during the phasic aspects of PS.

In attempting to test which, if either, of these two hypotheses is true, one would have to employ these as *a priori* hypotheses and conduct independent experiments based on them. Following this line of reasoning, one would study unit activity during sleep-wakefulness in limbic structures other than the amygdala, and in non-limbic structures presumed to be involved in behavioral inhibition.

In conclusion, these results support the notion that the basal amygdala plays a role in certain types of behavioral inhibition.

Evidence was also presented indicating that there is a group of cells in this area that could be considered functionally homogeneous on the basis of the similarity of their activity during sleep and waking.

Experiment 2

Based on the previous experiment which found that amygdala unit activity was enhanced during the inhibition of phasic motor activity in the sleeping animal, *i.e.*, during SWS and in the presence of the SMR during PS, the present experiment (16, 19) studied amygdala unit activity during behavioral inhibition in the awake animal. As stated above, the SMR is seen only in the absence of overt behavior. Furthermore, occurrence of phasic motor activity *blocks* the SMR (33, 38); and recent data indicate that both heart rate and respiratory rate are decreased during the SMR (2, 40). Therefore, comparing amygdala unit discharge rate during SMR with contiguous periods when SMR is absent from the EEG record provides some measure of amygdaloid involvement in one type of behavioral inhibition.

This experiment began by allowing the animal to go through one sleep-waking cycle and then classifying the cells as either S (fastest during SWS) or F (fastest during QW or PS). The purpose of this was to see if the hypothesis that there are two functionally distinct groups of cells in the basal amygdala could be profitably extended to data of the present experiment.

Spontaneous occurrences of the SMR (recorded from jewelers' screws threaded into the skull over the somatosensory cortex) were detected by means of an EEG frequency analyzer (peak frequency 13.5 Hz). SMR recordings of at least 80 μV amplitude were reinforced through the presentation of a rewarding electrical stimulation to the lateral hypothalamus. This operant conditioning procedure resulted in the production of trains of SMR lasting for up to forty seconds. Data analysis consisted of comparing the discharge rates during ten epochs of SMR with the rates during ten contiguous epochs of low voltage fast EEG activity of equal length.

Ten cells were classified as S type and seven as F type. Eight cells significantly increased in discharge rate during SMR (median rate = 1.6 spikes/sec) when compared to the rate during QW in the absence of SMR (median rate = 0.3 spikes/sec; p < .01, two-tailed t test). All eight of these were S cells (Figure 16.3 illustrates two cells that increased their discharge rate in the presence of SMR). Of the seven F cells, two significantly decreased in

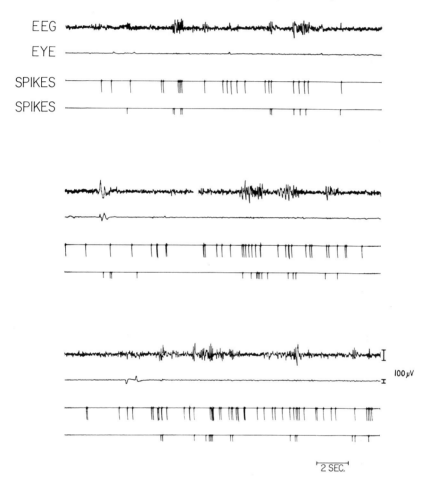

Figure 16.3. Increase in unit activity during the conditioned production of the sensorimotor rhythm (SMR). This shows two cells that significantly increased in rate of discharge in the presence of SMR (of at least 80 μV amplitude). See legend for Figure 16.2 for further details. *Reprinted by permission of Elsevier Publishing Co., Amsterdam, from a paper by B. L. Jacobs and D. J. McGinty, Brain Res. 36:431-436, 1972.*

discharge rate during SMR and none increased. Median rates of discharge for these seven cells during QW and SMR were 7.8 and 8.7 spikes/sec, respectively. There is a significantly different (p < .004, Fisher exact probability test) distribution of the number of cells which increased and decreased during SMR between S and F cells.

Consistent with the hypothesis that the basal amygdala plays an active role in behavioral inhibition, the neuronal activity of the predominant cell type in this area (over 60 percent of the cells studied were S type) was found to be positively correlated with SMR. These data also point out the advantage of analyzing unit activity according to some preconceived schema, in this case, the pattern of activity across sleep-wakefulness.

Experiment 3

This experiment studied the effects of the rewarding brain stimulation used in the previous experiment upon basal amygdaloid unit activity (17). In addition to the brain stimulation (500 msec trains of 3-4 V, 0.5 msec duration pulses at a frequency of 100 Hz delivered to the lateral hypothalamus) that the animal received by producing high amplitude SMR in the course of the SMR conditioning experiment, a number of these same stimuli were randomly applied at the end of the experiment.

Data analysis consisted of poststimulus histograms consisting of unit activity during the two seconds (400, 5 msec. bins) following stimulus offset (sixty stimulus presentations were used). Using such a long poststimulus period allowed enough data to be gathered on these slow firing cells to perform statistical analyses. A further analysis compared the mean rate of discharge during the two second poststimulus period in the SMR condition with the spontaneous discharge rate during two second periods of low voltage fast activity in neighboring segments. Two tailed t tests using thirty samples in each of the latter two conditions were used for statistical comparisons.

Data were obtained from the same seventeen cells studied in the previous experiment. In general, the results may be summarized as follows: S cells (fastest in SWS) decreased in rate in response to brain stimulation. Six of ten of these cells showed statistically significant decreases in rate in response to brain stimulation and none significantly increased in rate. All of these six cells showed a decreased tendency toward firing in the first 100 msec. following stimulus offset. F cells (fastest in PS or QW) increased in rate in response to brain stimulation. Three of seven of these cells showed statistically significant rate increases and only one cell significantly decreased in rate. The increased discharge rate was largely manifested in the first 500 msec post-stimulus. A statistical analysis of the data indicated that brain stimulation had a significantly different effect on S cells than it did on F cells ($p < .03$, Fisher exact probability test).

Random presentations of the brain stimulation produced no significantly different effect on unit activity than did the brain stimulation in the SMR conditioning phase. There was, however, a tendency for the magnitude of the former changes to be smaller than the latter changes.

These data once again point out the advantage of classifying cells according to some basic characteristic prior to data analysis. The decrease in discharge rate of the S cells following rewarding brain stimulation is similar to the decrease seen following an arousing stimulus (see Experiment 1). This is not unexpected since the brain stimulation desynchronizes the cortical EEG as does any arousing stimulus. Decreased amygdaloid unit activity consequent to the presentation of a rewarding brain stimulus is consistent with the theories of Olds (31) and Stein (36) who hold that the amygdala exerts tonic inhibitory control over the anatomical substrate of the reward system, the medial forebrain bundle.

Experiment 4

Basal amygdaloid unit activity was studied in a situation in which a food deprived animal inhibited or suppressed feeding in response to a conditioned stimulus (17). This provided an independent examination of amygdaloid involvement in behavioral inhibition.

Prior to initiation of data collection for each cell, the animal was allowed to go through a sleep-waking cycle in order to classify the cell as S type or F type. All animals were three days food deprived. In the conditioning phase of the experiment, the animal was given a minimum of thirty paired presentations of a 10 sec duration, 1 kHz tone, and a strong 0.5 sec duration air puff. The air puff was of sufficient strength to cause the animal to withdraw and crouch in the corner. In the testing phase, which immediately followed the conditioning phase, a mixture of chicken and tuna was placed in a bowl directly beneath the air hole. Approximately 10-20 sec after the animal, still three days food deprived, began eating, the 1 kHz tone was presented for ten seconds. The animal typically stopped eating within a few sec. after tone onset. The next trial began when the animal spontaneously resumed eating.

Data analysis consisted of comparing the mean discharge rate during the 10 sec tone of ten *suppression* trials with the preceding 10 sec period during eating. Two tailed t tests were used throughout.

None of the eight S cells were augmented in rate during the 10 sec tone. In fact, five of these cells significantly decreased in discharge rate during this stimulus. Three of five of the F cells significantly increased in rate and one cell decreased in rate during the tone. Figure 16.4 illustrates an S cell whose firing was completely suppressed during the period when the tone was on. Note that the EEG recorded from the marginal lead abruptly desynchronizes with the onset of the tone and begins to show some synchrony again following tone offset. Following tone offset, four out of eight S cells significantly increased in firing rate when compared to the rate during the tone. During this period, the animal would remain at a distance from the food dish and stare at it intently. SMR was frequently recorded from the coronal EEG lead during this period (see Fig. 16.4).

These results indicate that increased basal amygdaloid unit activity is not a necessary concomitant of all types of behavioral inhibition. It may be that the amygdala participates in states of behavioral inhibition that are accompanied by EEG slow waves, and that inhibition accompanied by low voltage fast EEG activity, *e.g.*, a fear state, does not require amygdaloid participation. An important aspect of the present experiment lends support to this hypothesis. Four out of eight S cells increased in discharge rate following tone offset, but while the animal was still inhibiting

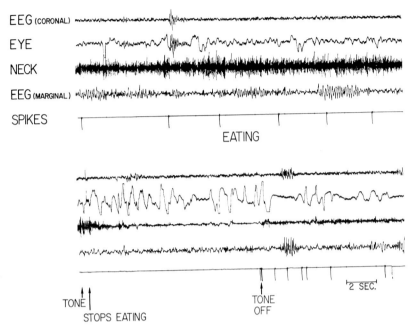

EEG (CORONAL)

EYE

NECK

EEG (MARGINAL)

SPIKES

EATING

TONE

STOPS EATING

TONE
OFF

2 SEC.

Figure 16.4. Unit activity during conditioned suppression. Note that the cell is totally silent while the tone is on and that it begins firing again soon after tone offset. Note also the decrease in neck EMG while the tone is on. Synchronous EEG activity can be seen soon after tone offset while the animal is still inhibiting eating. See legend for Figure 16.2 for further details.

eating. This tonic state of inhibition was accompanied by EEG slow waves, *i.e.*, SMR. Thus the basolateral amygdala may be important in sustaining this type of inhibition, but not in its initiation.

Experiment 5

The final experiment in this series (21) studied the influence, on basal amygdaloid units, of various simple stimuli (clicks, tones, white noise, flashlight beam, chamber lights on and off, and flashes) and complex stimuli (olfactory stimuli, somesthetic and proprioceptive stimuli, meows, cat howls, *kitty*, dog barks, squeals, whistles, hisses, cat food, white rat, kitten, and hand and voice threat by the experimenter). I was particularly interested in observing whether S cells responded in any way characteristically different from F cells.

The sensory responsiveness of fifty-six cells was studied; sleep-waking data indicated that thirty-six cells from this sample were of the S type, while the remaining twenty were F type. Ten cells were found to respond selectively to complex sensory stimuli, and nine of these were S cells (the tenth cell was not studied during sleep). A cell which responded selectively to a meow is displayed in Figure 16.5. Table 16.1 presents descriptive data for the response of these ten cells. Note that many of the stimuli to which these cells were selectively responsive could be described as environmentally significant. For example, cells were found that responded selectively to the movement of an albino rat, a cat howl, and the rustling of wood chips. Note also, that six out of ten of these cells were selectively responsive to complex auditory stimuli.

Of the twenty cells that discharged at their highest spontaneous rate during either QW or PS, none were selectively responsive to complex stimuli, and only one responded to a simple stimulus. Thus, there is a significantly higher probability (p < .02, Fisher exact probability test) that a cell which responds selectively to a

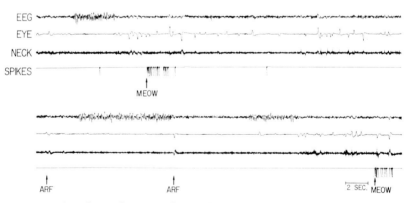

Figure 16.5. Polygraphic recordings showing a cell that responded selectively to a *meow* sound. Note that the cell had virtually no spontaneous activity and that a barking sound had no effect. See legend for Figure 16.2 for further details. *Reprinted by permission of Elsevier Publishing Co., Amsterdam, from a paper by B. L. Jacobs and D. J. McGinty, Brain Res.* 36:431-436, 1972.

TABLE 16.1

VARIOUS INDICES OF CELLS WHICH RESPOND SELECTIVELY
TO COMPLEX AFFERENT INPUT

Cell	Eliciting Stimuli	Mean Rate of Response (spikes/sec)	Mean Duration of Response (sec)	Spontaneous Mean Rate During QW (spikes/sec)
1	Room door opening and closing	10.2	1.8	0.1
2	Turn head or upper body to right	14.0 tonic 43.1 bursts	tonic 0.2	0.1
3	"Kitty," "meow," sight of rat	"kitty" 5.3	3.0	0.0
4	Cat howl	11.9	2.0	0.0
5	Rat moving about chamber	4.0 tonic 14.7 bursts	tonic 0.4	0.0
6	Howl, bark, "meow," rat	howl 5.5	1.0	0.0
7	Rustling of wood chips	7.3	1.1	0.0
8	Smoke, formalin, tuna	3.2 tonic	tonic	0.0
9	Experimenter threatens cat with hand	5.0	2.0	0.2
10	Clang of garbage can cover	25.0	0.4	—

Reprinted by permission of Elsevier Publishing Co., Amsterdam, from a paper by B. L. Jacobs and D. J. McGinty, *Brain Res* 36:431-436, 1972.

complex stimulus will come from the population of slow firing cells which discharge fastest in SWS (S cells) rather than from the faster firing cells which discharge fastest in QW or PS (F cells).

Briefly, the general response characteristics of the two classes of cells are as follows. S cells either decreased in discharge rate or were unresponsive to a variety of stimuli (*e.g.*, tones, white noise, light flashes, olfactory stimuli). On the other hand, although F cells did not respond selectively to any complex stimuli, they did respond with an increase in discharge rate to a variety of stimuli. Therefore, the response profile of a cell across sleep-waking was a good predictor of the cell's general response to afferent input.

These results are similar to previous studies which reported that amygdala units are responsive to complex sensory stimuli, especially those in the auditory modality (30, 35). Finally, the fruitfulness of categorizing cells prior to data analysis is perhaps most clearly seen in the present experiment; all of the cells that responded selectively to complex sensory stimuli were cells which discharged at their highest rate during SWS, *i.e.*, S cells.

DISCUSSION

The predominant type of unit found in the magnocellular portion of the basal amygdaloid nucleus may be characterized as follows: low spontaneous discharge rate in all states of sleep-waking, with the highest rate in SWS; increased rate of firing in association with behavioral inhibition, and decreased in response to a variety of arousing stimuli; *tuned* to discharge selectively in response to a particular complex sensory stimulus. The similarity of response characteristics of these cells across a variety of situations suggests that they may comprise a functionally homogeneous group of cells. Finally, the response profile of a cell across sleep-waking was found to be a good predictor of the cell's activity in a variety of paradigms.

Reaching these conclusions would have been impossible if these cells had not been studied through the application of a multidimensional approach. For example, results of the sleep-wakefulness experiment gave rise to hypotheses concerning behavioral inhibition, which were confirmed in the awake animal in a subsequent experiment. When the hypothesis of amygdaloid involvement in behavioral inhibition was extended to a conditioned suppression paradigm, however, the negative results caused a modification of this working hypothesis.

Continuing this multipronged attack, studies are currently under way on the effect of stimulation of the raphé nuclei on amygdaloid unit activity. This is particularly relevant since most of the serotonin containing cell bodies are found in the raphé, and since the amygdala is a serotonin rich structure. Thus, the raphé neurons appear to send out long axons which terminate in the amygdala. Future experiments will include the study of serotonin depleting drugs and psychotomimetic drugs on amygdala unit activity.

REFERENCES

1. Bizzi, E., O. Pompeiano and I. Somogyi. Spontaneous activity of single vestibular neurons of unrestrained cats during sleep and wakefulness. *Arch. Ital. Biol.* 102:308-330, 1964.
2. Chase, M. H. and R. M. Harper. Respiratory and cardiac patterns associated with conditioned EEG activity of the sensorimotor cortex. *Physiologist* 12:195, 1969.
3. Clemente, C. D. and M. B. Sterman. Cortical synchronization and sleep patterns in acute restrained and chronic behaving cats induced by forebrain stimulation. *Electroenceph. Clin. Neurophysiol.* Suppl. 24:172-187, 1963.
4. Clemente, C. D. and M. B. Sterman. Basal forebrain mechanisms for internal inhibition and sleep. In S. S. Kety, E. V. Evarts, and H. L. Williams (Eds.). *Sleep and Altered States of Consciousness.* Williams and Wilkins, Baltimore, 1967, pp. 127-147.
5. Creutzfeldt, O. D., F. R. Bell and W. R. Adey. The activity of neurons in the amygdala of the cat following afferent stimulation. In W. Bargmann and J. P. Schade (Eds.) *Progress in Brain Research*, Vol. 3. Elsevier, New York, 1963, pp. 31-49.
6. Egger, M. D. and J. P. Flynn. Effects of electrical stimulation of the amygdala on hypothalamically elicited attack behavior in cats. *J. Neurophysiol.* 26:705-720, 1963.
7. Egger, M. D. and J. P. Flynn. Further studies on the effects of amygdaloid stimulation and ablation on hypothalamically elicited attack behavior in cats. In W. R. Adey and T. Tokizane (Eds.). *Progress in Brain Research.* Vol. 27. Elsevier, New York, 1967, pp. 165-182.
8. Evarts, E. V. Activity of neurons in visual cortex of the cat during sleep with low voltage fast EEG activity. *J. Neurophysiol.* 25: 812-816, 1962.
9. Evarts, E. V. Temporal patterns of discharge of pyramidal tract neurons during sleep and waking in the monkey. *J. Neurophysiol.* 27: 152-171, 1964.
10. Findlay, A. L. R. and J. N. Hayward. Spontaneous activity of single neurons in the hypothalamus of rabbits during sleep and waking. *J. Physiol.* 201:237-258, 1969.
11. Fonberg, E. and J. M. R. Delgado. Avoidance and alimentary reactions during amygdala stimulation. *J. Neurophysiol.* 24:651-664, 1961.
12. Gassel, M. M., P. L. Marchiafava and O. Pompeiano. Activity of the red nucleus during deep synchronized sleep in unrestrained cats. *Arch. Ital. Biol.* 103:369-396, 1965.

13. Gloor, P. Amygdala. In J. Field (Ed.). *Handbook of Physiology,* Vol. 2, American Physiological Society, Washington, D.C., 1960, pp. 1395-1420.

14. Goddard, G. V. Functions of the amygdala. *Psychol. Bull.* 62:89-109, 1964.

15. Huttenlocher, P. R. Evoked and spontaneous activity in single units of medial brain stem during natural sleep and waking. *J. Neurophysiol.* 24:451-468, 1961.

16. Jacobs, B. L. Amygdala unit activity as a reflection of functional changes in brain serotonergic neurons. In J. D. Barchas and E. Usdin (Eds.) *Serotonin and Behavior.* Academic Press, New York (in press).

17. Jacobs, B. L. Single cell activity of the basolateral amygdala in freely moving cats. Doctoral dissertation, University of California, Los Angeles, 1971.

18. Jacobs, B. L., R. M. Harper and D. J. McGinty. Neuronal coding of motivational level during sleep. *Physiol. Behav.* 5:1139-1143, 1970.

19. Jacobs, B. L. and D. J. McGinty. Unit activity of the basolateral amygdala in freely moving cats. *Psychophysiology* 9:124, 1972.

20. Jacobs, B. L. and D. J. McGinty. Amygdala unit activity during sleep and waking. *Exper. Neurol.* 33:1-15, 1971.

21. Jacobs, B. L. and D. J. McGinty. Participation of the amygdala in complex stimulus recognition and behavioral inhibition: Evidence from unit studies. *Brain Res.* 36:431-436, 1972.

22. Kriendler, A. and M. Steriade. EEG patterns of arousal and sleep induced by stimulating various amygdaloid levels in the cat. *Arch. Ital. Biol.* 102:576-586, 1964.

23. Lewinska, M. K. Ventromedial hypothalamus: Participation in control of food intake and functional connections with ventral amygdala. *Acta Biol. Exper.* 27:296-302, 1967.

24. Machne, X. and J. P. Segundo. Unitary responses to afferent volleys in the amygdaloid complex. *J. Neurophysiol.* 19:232-240, 1956.

25. Mano, N. Changes of simple and complex spike activity of cerebellar Purkinje cells with sleep and waking. *Science* 170:1325-1327, 1970.

26. McCarley, R. W. and J. A. Hobson. Cortical unit activity during desynchronized sleep. *Science* 167:901-903, 1970.

27. McGinty, D. J. and M. B. Sterman. Sleep suppression after basal forebrain lesions in the cat. *Science* 160:1253-1255, 1968.

28. Mink, W. D., P. J. Best and J. Olds. Neurons in paradoxical sleep and motivated behavior. *Science* 158:1335-1337, 1967.

29. Noda, H., S. Manohar and W. R. Adey. Spontaneous activity of cat hippocampal neurons in sleep and wakefulness. *Exper. Neurol.* 24:217-231, 1969.

30. O'Keefe, J. and H. Bouma. Complex sensory properties of certain amygdala units in the freely moving cat. *Exper. Neurol.* 23:384-398, 1969.
31. Olds, J. Hypothalamic substrates of reward. *Physiol. Rev.* 42:554-604, 1962.
32. Oomura, Y., H. Ooyama, F. Naka, T. Yamamoto, T. Ono and N. Kobayashi. Some stochastical patterns of single unit discharges in the cat hypothalamus under chronic conditions. *N.Y. Acad. Sci. Annals.* 157:666-689, 1969.
33. Roth, S. R., M. B. Sterman and C. D. Clemente. Comparison of EEG correlates of reinforcement, internal inhibition and sleep. *Electroenceph. Clin. Neurophysiol.* 23:509-520, 1967.
34. Sakakura, H. Spontaneous and evoked unitary activities of cat lateral geniculate neurons in sleep and wakefulness. *Jap. J. Physiol.* 18:23-42, 1968.
35. Sawa, M. and J. M. R. Delgado. Amygdala unitary activity in the unrestrained cat. *Electroenceph. Clin. Neurophysiol.* 15:637-650, 1963.
36. Stein, L. Chemistry of reward and punishment. In D. H. Efron (Ed.). *Psychopharmacology: A Review of Progress 1957-1967.* Public Health Service Publication No. 1836, U.S. Government Printing Office, Washington, D.C., 1968, pp. 105-123.
37. Sterman, M. B., R. C. Howe and L. R. MacDonald. Facilitation of spindle-burst sleep by conditioning of electroencephalographic activity while awake. *Science* 167:1146-1148, 1970.
38. Sterman, M. B. and W. Wyrwicka. EEG correlates of sleep: Evidence for separate forebrain substrates. *Brain Res.* 6:143-163, 1967.
39. Wendt, R. and D. Albe-Fessard. Sensory responses of the amygdala with special reference to somatic afferent pathways. In P. Passouant (Ed.). *Physiologie de l'Hippocampe.* Centre Nationale de la Recherche Scientifique, Paris, 1962, pp. 61-72.
40. Wyrwicka, W. and M. B. Sterman. Instrumental conditioning of sensorimotor cortex EEG spindles in the waking cat. *Physiol. Behav.* 3:703-707, 1968.

Chapter XVII

FIRING PATTERNS OF EXTRAPYRAMIDAL AND RETICULAR NEURONS OF THE ALERT MONKEY

D. L. SPARKS and R. P. TRAVIS

THIS PAPER PRESENTS a brief review of some of the chronic single unit data obtained in our laboratory since 1966. The initial studies used squirrel monkeys as subjects, polished stainless steel insect pins coated with Insul-X as electrodes, and a simple screw driven electrode carrier (14). More recent studies with the rhesus monkey have used glass insulated, platinum irridium electrodes and a hydraulically driven electrode carrier developed by Evarts (5). Conventional recording procedures were used.

The first chronic single unit study we reported (19) tested the effectiveness of our techniques for recording spike potentials in unanesthetized, fully alert animals. This study looked for differential patterns of single unit activity in various brain areas of squirrel monkeys who had received extensive exposure to one four second tone followed by a food pellet and a different four second tone followed by brief electric shock.

Time histograms of single unit activity, averaged over ten stimulus presentations were made from a total of 121 units from a variety of brain areas. Of the units studied, 31 percent showed reliable alterations in firing rates during one or both of the tone stimuli. In the report we discussed the nontrivial problem of determining whether associative, motivational, emotional or motor mechanisms were involved in the patterns of spike activity observed. We disregarded our own warning and suggested that those units showing graded temporal discharge patterns during the period of the stimulus might be capable of *anticipating* the approach of reinforcement and that the activity of those units responding differentially to the two stimuli reflected variations in

288

the excitability of cells resulting from acquired or learned aspects of the stimuli.

Although the conclusions from this first study were limited, we were greatly encouraged by our ability to record units from the fully alert animal. We began two series of studies. One series began as an investigation of the role of the extrapyramidal motor system in response inhibition. A second series of experiments began as a study of the role of the superior colliculus and reticular formation in the detection of visual stimuli.

STUDIES OF THE EXTRAPYRAMIDAL MOTOR SYSTEM

An initial study (20) tested the hypothesis that units of the extrapyramidal motor system would respond to a stimulus requiring response inhibition. Squirrel monkeys were trained to respond to a 1500 cps tone for food reward and to passively avoid electric shock by not responding after a 1000 cps tone.

Two hundred sixty-four units were recorded from the amygdala, cortex, globus pallidus, putamen, and internal capsule. Our hypothesis that extrapyramidal units would be involved in response inhibition was not confirmed. Very few changes in unit activity were observed during SΔ but consistent alterations in firing patterns occurred during or after SD. Unexpectedly, pronounced periods of decreased firing rates were observed from units within the globus pallidus and in fibers bordering the globus pallidus during behaviors related to the acquisition and consumption of food rewards. These decreased firing rates failed to occur during spontaneous motor acts involving similar movement patterns which were not a part of a food reinforcement sequence.

A follow up study (21) confirmed and expanded these findings. Thirty-one of ninety-seven pallidal units exhibited pronounced and immediate reductions in spike discharge rates during either food searching movements in the food hopper, food grasping and transporting movements or during actual consummatory behavior. These units were not responsive to elicited or spontaneous motor patterns involved in obtaining objects other than food. The possibility that the periods of decreased rates of firing were prolonged effects of motor activity involved in the lever press response itself was eliminated by employing a 3:1 fixed ratio schedule of reinforcement. The decreases in firing rate were uniquely related to the third or reinforced bar press.

At this point, we had observed the activity of approximately one hundred sixty pallidal units. A summary of these results was presented (22) in which it was pointed out that 30 percent of the pallidal units observed responded with dramatic decreases in firing rate during either lever pressing, searching for food in the hopper, grasping the food pellet and transporting to mouth, or consuming the food pellet. It seemed quite clear to us that the units we had observed were in some manner intimately associated with simple behavioral acts related to the acquisition and consumption of food rewards.

Although anatomical and electrophysiological studies (8) demonstrated lemniscal inputs to the globus pallidus, tactile and proprioceptive stimuli did not appear to be sufficient to elicit the observed alterations in response rate. Units consistently exhibiting a cessation of firing as familiar food objects were grasped and carried to the mouth, were unaffected by grasping and carrying unfamiliar or inedible objects to the mouth. Passive movements of the limbs by the experimenter failed to alter the firing rates of these units. Reduced firing rates observed during consummatory responses were only observed as familiar and palatable food objects were ingested.

A simplified schematic (shown in Fig. 17.1) was prepared to point out that the periods of decreased firing we had observed in globus pallidus units paralleled chained segments of motor activity leading to food reward. We suggested that these units may provide signals which release and/or direct appropriate movement sequences and that these permissive or command inputs may be required for the activation of other motor systems which have been programmed to carry out such goal related *subroutines* as seeking, grasping, and masticating food objects. It is also possible that the unitary changes accompanying the possession and incorporation of food objects could serve as neurophysiological confirmation of primary and secondary rewards. The immediacy with which these units signal the attainment of food reward should be considered by future neurophysiological models of reinforcement.

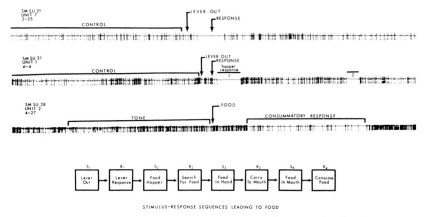

Figure 17.1. Single trial tracings of the output of an amplitude discrimination circuit representing the patterned activity of three units. The top tracing (A) shows a period of reduced firing during a lever response. The period of decreased firing in the second tracing (B) occurs during the time the animal is searching for food in the hopper. This same tracing shows a second inhibition which occurred during a brief exploratory return to the empty hopper. The bottom tracing (C) illustrates a dramatic reduction in discharge rate from the time the food pellet was released in the animal's mouth until the food was completely consumed. The four seconds tone period diagramed in the bottom tracing may be used as a time base value for all of the tracings. The black diagrams illustrate the series of stimulus response associations during which reduced discharge rates have been recorded from units within and bordering the globus pallidus. (This Figure originally published in *Brain Research* 7 (1968) 455-458.)

Other data related to the role of the globus pallidus in the control of movement have been recorded from rhesus monkeys trained on a visual tracking task.

The monkey was seated three feet from the front of a twenty-one inch TV set. The screen was blanked except occasionally, when two light stimuli appeared. The larger stimulus, a ¾ inch square area of light, served as the target area. The smaller, cursor stimulus, measured ¼ inches square. The monkey was rewarded for positioning the cursor inside the target by a drop of orange juice. The monkey manipulated a vertical rod which controlled the position of the cursor and which could be moved from side to side by flexion or extension of the wrist. A 38 degree displacement of the control rod moved the cursor spot nineteen inches across the horizontal axis of the TV screen. Approximately 74 grams of force was required to move the control rod in either direction and equal forces opposed both flexion and extension of the wrist.

A trial was started when the target appeared in the center of the TV screen. When the monkey had maneuvered the cursor into the target area for a one-half second time period, the target was

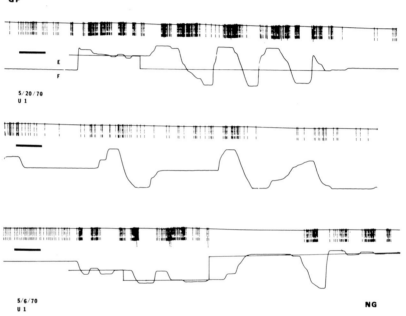

Figure 17.2. Single trial tracings of the output of an amplitude discrimination circuit representing the patterned activity of two units during a visual motor tracking task. The series of straight lines in the top and bottom tracings, represent the different positions of the target on the TV monitor. The irregular line represents the animal's wrist movements as the subject attempts to position the cursor into the target area. Upward deflections of this line represent wrist extension (E) while downward deflections represent wrist flexion (F). A one second time bar is associated with each tracing. Both cells were recorded from the internal segment of the globus pallidus. In both of these units a burst of firing always precedes wrist flexion. The top two tracings illustrates the difference in firing patterns of one unit while the monkey is actually performing the tracking task and during nontracking movements.

randomly moved in a discrete step to one of seven different horizontal positions. When coincidence of target and cursor was achieved, a second reinforcement was given and the target was immediately moved in the opposite direction to a new position. After successfully achieving coincidence, the monkey was given a third reinforcement, the TV screen blanked and the trial terminated. On some trials the monkey was trained to move the control arm back and forth without the target or the cursor being presented. This allowed comparisons of unit responses to arm movements alone and to similar types of movement during a tracking task.

A total of 345 units were recorded from the motor cortex (areas four and six), nucleus ventralis lateralis, and nucleus ventralis anterior of the thalamus and the globus pallidus from one monkey. Seventy-eight (22.6 percent) of these were responsive to some aspect of the tracking task. A variety of different unit responses have been obtained, including increased and decreased rates of firing during each tracking presentation. We have also recorded cells which gave a burst of activity as the cursor was positioned within the target area and still other units which produced a graded increase in firing as the cursor approached the target area.

Typical results from the globus pallidus are presented in Figures 17.2 and 17.3. Figure 17.2 illustrates the firing patterns of two units (top and bottom tracings) from the internal segment of the pallidus which are related to direction of wrist movement. A burst of firing invariably precedes wrist flexion. Comparison of the top and middle tracings illustrates the differences in frequency obtained during non-tracking movements and movement during the tracking task. A burst of firing occurred prior to wrist flexion in both tracking and nontracking trials but a higher rate of background activity was observed during tracking trials.

The top two tracings of Figure 17.3 illustrate a burst of activity from a pallidal unit preceding extensor movements during tracking and during non-tracking movement trials. The data shown in Figures 17.2 and 17.3 point out that unit activity occurring during spontaneous limb movements may differ from similar limb movements during the performance of a more complex task.

DeLong (4) has subsequently looked at the response properties

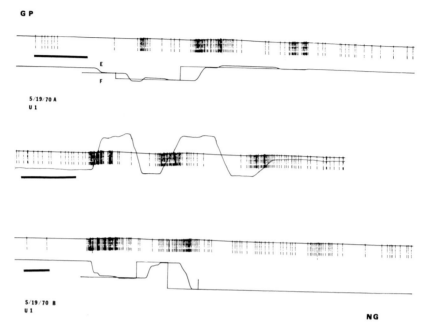

Figure 17.3. The firing patterns of two units recorded from the internal segment of the globus pallidus during visual motor tracking. Refer to Figure 2 for legend. Top two tracings illustrate a burst of activity preceding extensor movements during tracking and during non-tracking movement trials. The bottom tracing shows increased unit firing preceding and during flexion tracking movements.

of units in the globus pallidus in the rhesus monkey. He concluded that 20 percent of all pallidal neurons exhibited distinct responses to learned movements of the monkey's arms. We reported that only 4 percent of the pallidal units we observed responded to gross bodily movements. DeLong further suggested that the unit responses we have ascribed to the globus pallidus were probably recorded from internal and external medullary lamina fibers or aberrant cells of the substantia innominata (SI).

It should be pointed out that although, as we reported, many of our pallidal units were *border* cells, some were isolated histologically in the middle of both the internal and external segments of the globus pallidus. Furthermore, DeLong did not systematically look for pallidal responses related to food acquisition or consumption nor did we systematically look for pallidal responses related to learned movements of the limbs. Rather, we tried to correlate unit activity to spontaneously occurring movements. Although there may be differences in the response properties of pallidal units in the squirrel monkey and the rhesus monkey, in our view, what is needed to resolve the questions raised by DeLong is a histologically well controlled experiment in which the responses of pallidal and SI units to both limb movements and food reward are studied in the same animal.

Regardless of where future research shows the cell bodies of the units we have described to be located, the isolation of neuronal activity in and around the globus pallidus uniquely related to response sequences involved in food acquisition remains an important observation. Considerable evidence exists suggesting that the globus pallidus plays an important role in feeding behavior (1, 10, 24) and it has been suggested that the globus pallidus may provide the major initiating outflow to produce feeding behavior (28). The activity of pallidal units recorded from patients with extrapyramidal motor disorders (23) was reduced or inhibited between the time the patient was asked to move and the moment active movement began. The response properties of these units are quite similar to the unit activity we have recorded from the squirrel monkey. However, the suggestion of DeLong that the substantia innominata, rather than the globus pallidus, plays a major role in feeding behavior certainly necessitates a careful investigation of the role of both of these structures in motivated behavior.

STUDIES OF SUPERIOR COLLICULUS AND RETICULAR FORMATION

An experiment was designed to ask the following question: Do neuronal responses to diffuse light occur in either the superior colliculus or reticular formation that are related to behavioral measures of the detection of that light? Animals were trained in a situation in which the beginning of a trial was signalled by an audible *pop* occurring as a pneumatically retractable lever became available. On 50 percent of the randomly presented trials, *lever out* was followed after 4 sec by a 4 sec light. On the remaining trials, the lever remained out for 8 sec without a light stimulus. Responses occurring during the light delivered a food pellet, automatically retracted the lever and terminated the light. The bar was programmed to retract automatically at the end of 8 sec if a response did not occur. Responses prior to light onset or during nonlight trials were punished by delivering electric shock to the bars of the restraining chair seat. After a 90 percent correct response criterion was met, trials were presented with light intensities near threshold levels until stable performance levels were reached. A receptacle for a microelectrode carrier was then implanted and data collection initiated. Time histograms were made of the firing rates observed during the 4 sec period immediately preceding the beginning of a trial, during the 4 sec bar out period and the 4 sec light period. The same period of time (12 sec) was analyzed for the nonlight trials.

Approximately eight hundred units from the midbrain reticular formation, the superior colliculus and in overlying sensorimotor cortex were studied. In the superior colliculus, we failed to find a relationship between the discharge frequency and stimulus intensity or a relationship between the latency of the neural response and the latency of the behavioral response. We did confirm in chronic subjects that units in the superior colliculus respond to moving stimuli, are directionally selective and respond to movements of the eye. These findings are now well established (3, 7, 9, 13, 18).

We incidentally observed patterns of cortical unit activity which seemed to reflect, primarily, alterations in levels of behavioral arousal (15). One type cortical unit responded to the auditory *pop* occurring when the bar became available and the onset of the light with almost identical brief increases in discharge frequency. A second type cortical unit displayed a sustained increase in frequency of firing following the *bar out* cue and a second sustained increase of approximately the same magnitude occurred at the onset of the visual stimulus and was maintained until after the pellet was consumed. A third type unit displayed a sustained increase in discharge rate associated with the *bar out* cue. The onset of the light failed to evoke further increases in firing rate. That these units were responsive to both auditory and visual stimuli and the similarity of the neuronal response to different sensory inputs suggested a nonspecific source of activation. Similar units were subsequently observed in the midbrain reticular formation.

A second report (16) arising from this study noted that the spontaneous activity of ninety-five of 134 midbrain reticular units was noticeably modified by the presentation of visual discrimination trials. Four major response profiles emerged from these responsive units. The response of Type I units was closely related to stereotyped head, neck and eye movements. The auditory cue occurring when the bar became available and the onset of the light evoked transient increases in the discharge rate of Type II units. Type III units displayed a brief increase in firing rate associated with either the onset of the light or the initiation of a bar press response. Type IV units responded to the auditory and visual stimuli with sustained increases in firing rates. Although not systematically studied, there appeared to be a correlation between the latency of the behavioral response and the latency of the neuronal response in Type III units.

These findings illustrated, at a cellular level, the modulatory influences conditioned stimuli exert upon the level of reticular and cortical activity.

A recent experiment (17) followed up our observation that the activity of neurons in the reticular formation is related to eye movements. The firing patterns of 678 units recorded from two monkeys were analyzed during horizontal eye movements. The activity of seventy of 437 units located in the midbrain or pontine reticular formation were clearly related to horizontal eye movements. Three major types of responsive units were isolated in midbrain and pontine reticular formation. Type I units respond to saccadic or slow movements in *either* direction. Type II units respond to saccadic or slow movements in a specific direction. Type III units are characterized by transient increases or decreases in firing during saccadic horizontal eye movements but by steady discharge rates proportional to the horizontal position of the eyes. We suggested that the activity of these neurons may represent a corollary discharge of the oculomotor system to other regions of the brain conveying information concerning the horizontal position of the eyes and the presence, duration, and direction of eye movements.

The objectives of experiments currently under way in our laboratory are to monitor the discharge patterns of neurons from the oculomotor system of rhesus monkeys during the performance of a visual tracking task. We hope to obtain information related to the following questions:

a) How and in which specific areas of the visual system are retinal patterns of activity converted into foveal target displacement error signals for the saccadic eye movement system?

b) How and in which brain areas are retinal patterns of activity converted into target velocity signals for the smooth pursuit eye movement system? and

c) How and in which brain areas are these error signals converted into appropriate motor commands to produce both rapid saccadic and smooth pursuit eye movements?

This research views eye movement as the output of a biological control system. The input-output relationships have been quantitatively described and several testable models of the system developed. What remains is to locate the systems within the CNS which govern eye movements and to describe the functional properties of these neurons. This information will contribute, significantly, to our understanding of how the basic sensory information conveyed by neurons at the retinal level is transformed into the type of information needed to control specific muscular activities. In this sense, the eye movement system may serve as a model for more complex input-output systems of the mammalian nervous system.

CONCLUSIONS

In our view, the advent of techniques permitting simultaneous behavioral observations and extracellular recordings from single neurons in unanesthetized animals represents an important step forward in attempts to understand the operation of the central nervous system. Studies of the pyramidal system (6), the oculomotor system (2, 11, 12) and the studies summarized in this report, for example, emphasize the power of the technique when used to investigate the function of neurons in the motor pathways. Recent studies of visual cortex (25, 26, 27) and superior colliculus (3, 13) illustrate the applicability of the method to studies of sensory systems.

Although the problems of recording from behaving animals are numerous, it seems clear that the chronic microelectrode recording technique has emerged as a powerful tool to be applied to all areas of brain research.

REFERENCES

1. Albert, D. J., L. H. Storlien, D. J. Wood and G. K. Ehman. Further evidence for a complex system controlling feeding behavior. *Physiol. Behav.*, 1970, 5:1075-1082.
2. Bizzi, E. and P. H. Schiller. Single unit activity in the frontal eye fields of unanesthetized monkeys during eye and head movement. *Exp. Brain Res.*, 1970, 10:151-158.
3. Cynader, M. and N. Berman. Receptive field organization of monkey superior colliculus. *J. Neurophysiol.*, 1972, 35:187-201.
4. DeLong, M. R. Activity of pallidal neurons during movement. *J. Neurophysiol.*, 1971, 3:414-427.
5. Evarts, E. V. A technique for recording activity of subcortical neurons in moving animals. *Electroenceph. Clin. Neurophysiol.*, 1968, 24:83-86.
6. Evarts, E. V. and W. T. Thach. Motor mechanisms of the C.N.S.: Cerebrocerebellar interrelations. *Ann. Rev. Physiol.*, 1969, 31:451-498.
7. Humphrey, N. K. Responses to visual stimuli of units in the superior colliculus of rats and monkeys. *Exptl. Neurol.*, 1968, 20:312-340.
8. Laursen, A. M. Corpus striatum. *Acta Physiol. Scand.*, 1963, 59: Suppl. 211.
9. McIlwain, J. T. and P. Buser. Receptive fields of single cells in the cat's superior colliculus. *Exp. Brain Res.*, 1968, 5:314-325.
10. Morgane, P. J. Alterations in feeding and drinking behavior of rats with lesions in globi pallidi. *Am. J. Physiol.*, 1961, 204:420-428.
11. Robinson, D. A. Oculomotor unit behavior in the monkey. *J. Neurophysiol.*, 1970, 33:393-404.
12. Schiller, P. H. The discharge characteristics of single units in the oculomotor and abducens nuclei of the unanesthetized monkey. *Exp. Brain Res.*, 1970, 10:347-362.
13. Schiller, P. H. and F. Koerner. Discharge characteristics of single units in superior colliculus of the alert rhesus monkey. *J. Neurophysiol.*, 1971, 34:920-936.
14. Sparks, D. L. and R. P. Travis, Jr. A headmounted manipulator for

chronic single unit recording from the squirrel monkey. *Physiol. Behav.*, 1967, 2:449-451.

15. Sparks, D. L. and R. P. Travis, Jr. Single unit activity during behavioral conditioning: Arousal effects. *Life Sciences*, 1967, 6:2497-2503.

16. Sparks, D. L. and R. P. Travis, Jr. Patterns of reticular unit activity observed during the performance of a discriminative task. *Physiol. Behav.*, 1968, 3:961-968.

17. Sparks, D. L. and Travis, R. P. Firing patterns of reticular formation neurons during horizontal eye movements. *Brain Research*, 1971, 33:477-481.

18. Straschill, M. and K. P. Hoffman. Activity of movement sensitive neurons of the cat's tectum during spontaneous eye movements. *Exp. Brain Res.*, 1970, 11:318-326.

19. Travis, R. P., Jr. and D. L. Sparks. Changes in unit activity during stimuli associated with food and shock reinforcement. *Physiol. Behav.*, 1967, 2:171-177.

20. Travis, R. P., Jr. and D. L. Sparks. Unitary responses and discrimination learning in the squirrel monkey: The globus pallidus. *Physiol. Behav.*, 1968, 3:187-196.

21. Travis, R. P., Jr., T. F. Hooten and D. L. Sparks. Single unit activity related to behavior motivated by food reward. *Physiol. Behav.*, 1968, 4:309-318.

22. Travis, R. P., Jr., D. L. Sparks and T. F. Hooten. Single unit responses related to sequences of food motivated behavior. *Brain Research*, 1968, 7:454-457.

23. Umbach, W. and K. J. Ehrhardt. Microelectrode recording in the basal ganglia during stereotaxic operations. *Confinia. Neurol.*, 1965, 26:315-317.

24. Wagner, J. W. and J. DeGroot. Changes in feeding behavior following intracerebral injections in the rat. *Am. J. Physiol.*, 1963, 204:483-487.

25. Wurtz, R. H. Visual receptive fields of striate cortex neurons in awake monkeys. *J. Neurophysiol.*, 1969, 32:727-742.

26. Wurtz, R. H. Response of striate cortex neurons to stimuli during rapid eye movements in the monkey. *J. Neurophysiol.*, 1969, 32:975-986.

27. Wurtz, R. H. Comparison of effects of eye movements and stimulus movements on striate cortex neurons of the monkey. *J. Neurophysiol.*, 1969, 32:987-994.

28. Wyrawicka, W. and R. W. Doty. Feeding induced in cats by electrical stimulation of the brain stem. *Exp. Brain Res.*, 1960, 1:152-160.

Chapter XVIII

OPERANT CONDITIONING OF SPECIFIC PATTERNS OF NEURAL AND MUSCULAR ACTIVITY

E. E. FETZ and DOM V. FINOCCHIO

Abstract. In awake monkeys we recorded activity of single "motor" cortex cells, four contralateral arm muscles, and elbow position, while operantly reinforcing several patterns of motor activity. With the monkey's arm held semiprone in a cast hinged at the elbow, we reinforced active elbow movements and tested cell responses to passive elbow movements. With the cast immobilized we reinforced isometric contraction of each of the four muscles in isolation, and bursts of cortical cell activity with and without simultaneous suppression of muscle activity. Correlations between a precentral cell and specific arm muscles consistently appeared under several behavioral conditions, but could be dissociated by reinforcing cell activity and muscle suppression.

In INVESTIGATING the possible role of precentral "motor" cortex cells in generating voluntary movements, previous experimenters trained monkeys to perform specific motor responses by making operant reinforcement contingent on the position and force trajectories of the responding limb (1, 2). Such response patterns involved coordinated activity of many muscles of the responding limb (2, 3) and therefore were not designed to resolve the question of which specific muscles a given cortical cell may influence. To determine the degree to which precentral cell activity may be correlated with specific limb muscles and to test the stability of such correlations during different behaviors, we recorded the activity of single precentral cells and four major arm muscles (a flexor and extensor of wrist and elbow) while reinforcing specific patterns of activity in these elements.

Experiments were performed with a fluid-deprived monkey (*Macaca mulatta*) seated in a restraint chair with his head immobilized and a juice-dispensing tube in his mouth. The monkey's arm could be held semiprone in a molded cast pivoted at the elbow, allowing measurable flexion and extension of the elbow but no gross movement of the wrist. The cast could also be locked in place (elbow at 90°, wrist at 180°), rendering all muscle contractions isometric (4). Electromyographic (EMG) activity of major flexors and extensors of the wrist (flexor carpi radialis and extensor carpi radialis) and elbow (biceps and tri-

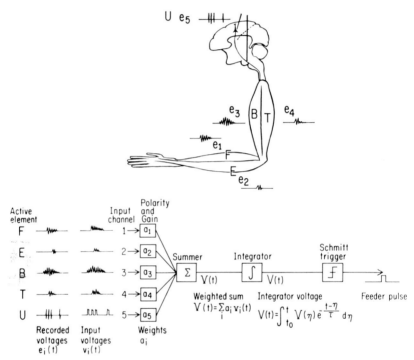

Figure 18.1. (Top) Schematic diagram of monkey, showing location of arm muscles and precentral cell, with typical recorded potentials (e_i). F, flexor carpi radialis; E, extensor carpi radialis; B, biceps; T, triceps; U, precentral cell. (Bottom) Schematic of "activity integrator" used to reinforce patterns of activity under isometric conditions. Input voltages (v_i) were rectified EMG activity for muscles or voltage pulses triggered from the cell's action potentials. The weighted sum was temporally integrated in a parallel resistance-capacitance network; when the integrator voltage reached the Schmitt trigger threshold, the feeder discharged and a relay (not shown) briefly reset the integrator voltage to zero.

ceps) was recorded through pairs of braided stainless steel wires permanently implanted in the belly of each muscle and led subcutaneously to a connector implanted on the skull. Activity of single precentral cells in contralateral cortex was recorded with tungsten microelectrodes. For about a month prior to the data-recording sessions, the monkey was trained in several behavior performances: (1) He was reinforced with fruit juice for sitting quietly while we tested the cells' responses to passive movement of the arm and cutaneous stimulation. (2) With his arm in the position monitor he was reinforced for active flexion and extension of the elbow. (3) With the position monitor locked in place, reinforcement was made contingent upon isometric contraction of any one of the muscles with simultaneous suppression of activity in the other three.

Specific patterns of cell and muscle activity were monitored and reinforced with an electronic "activity integrator" which continuously integrated a weighted sum of voltages proportional to cortical cell and muscle activity, and delivered a reinforcement when the resultant voltage exceeded a preset threshold (Fig. 18.1). The activity integrator had several input channels which accepted either voltage pulses triggered from the cell's action potentials or rectified EMG activity from specific muscles. A summing network produced a weighted sum

$$V(t) = \sum_i a_i v_i(t)$$

of these input voltages; the algebraic sign and magnitude of each weighting factor a_i were determined by the experimenter through a polarity switch and gain control for each channel. This summed voltage was temporally integrated with a parallel resistor-capacitor network with a time constant of 50 to 100 msec to generate the "integrator voltage." When this integrator voltage reached a preset threshold level V_T the feeder discharged and the integrator voltage was briefly reset to zero.

To illustrate a typical application, consider reinforcing the activity of a specific muscle, say biceps, in isolation. When cortical unit activity did not enter into the reinforcement contingency, its contribution to the integrator voltage was switched off ($a_5 = 0$).

The polarity switches that were on the muscle channels were set such that activity in the biceps drove the integrator voltage toward threshold ($a_3 > 0$), while activity in the other three muscles drove the voltage away from threshold ($a_i < 0$; i = 1,2,4). When reinforcement became available, the monkey typically began to emit bursts of EMG activity in several arm muscles every few seconds. The gain controls (a_i) were set such that approximately half of these burst responses were reinforced. After several minutes the proportion of reinforced responses typically increased. By reducing the gain on the biceps channel we could require the monkey to produce more biceps activity to reach threshold; by increasing the gains on the other muscle channels we could require a greater suppression of activity in these muscles in order to prevent reinforcement from being withheld. Thus, separation of activity in different muscles was accomplished by selectively reinforcing better successive approximations to the required pattern. Terminal performance typically consisted of repeated bursts of EMG activity in the reinforced muscle with negligible coactivation of the other three muscles.

During reinforcement periods a meter in front of the monkey was illuminated and its needle deflection was made proportional to the integrator voltage. Extreme rightward deflections were consistently correlated with juice reinforcement; thus the meter deflections could become a conditioned reinforcer. During reinforcement of isolated activity of specific muscles a set of colored lights indicated which muscle was being reinforced, and the amplified EMG activity of the reinforced muscle was audible to the monkey (5).

The results from one 8-hour experiment are presented in detail to illustrate the relation between a precentral cell and major flexors and extensors of elbow and wrist during passive and active elbow movements (Fig. 18.2) and under isometric conditions while reinforcing isolated muscle activity or cortical unit activity (Fig. 18.3).

Passive movements of the contralateral elbow and wrist reliably evoked responses from this cell, but cutaneous stimulation (brushing hairs or touching skin) did not. The cell responded re-

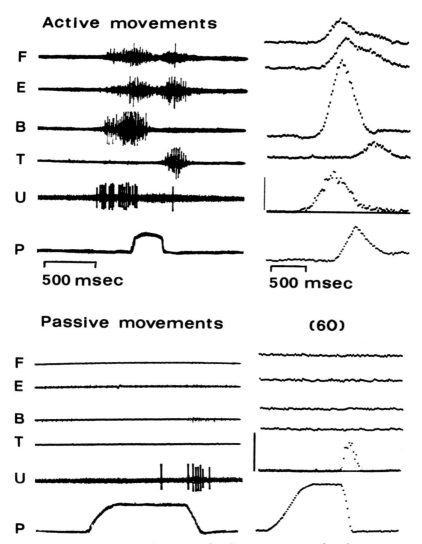

Figure 18.2. Responses of precentral cell and arm muscles during active and passive elbow movements. Successive lines from top to bottom show activity of flexor carpi radialis (F), extensor carpi radialis (E), biceps (B), triceps (T), cortical unit (U), and the position of the elbow (P). A single trial is shown at left, and the averages over 60 successive trials at right. This cell fired before active flexion of the elbow (A) and responded to passive extension of the elbow (B). All EMG averages were computed at identical gains. Time histogram of cell activity is shown with a zero baseline; vertical calibration bar equals 50 impulses per second. Upward deflection of the position monitor represents flexion.

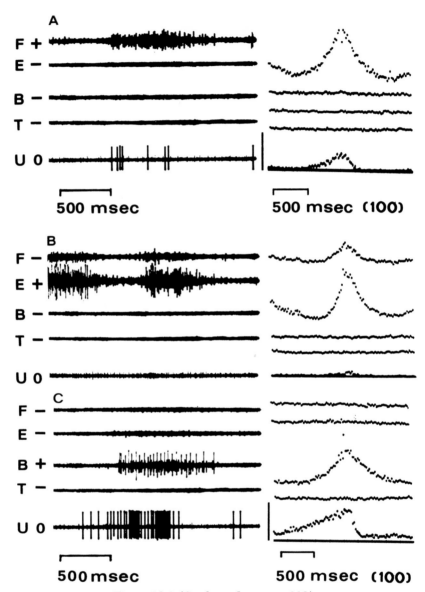

Figure 18.3 (See legend on page 308)

peatedly to passive extension of the elbow (Fig. 18.2B) and to passive flexion of the wrist without overt signs of resistance or gross EMG activity (6). When *active* movements of the elbow were reinforced, the cell invariably fired in relation to active

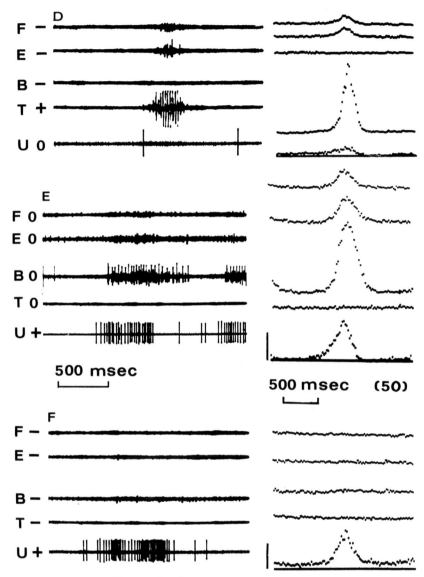

Figure 18.3 (See legend on page 308)

flexion (Fig. 18.2A). Flexion was also accompanied by activity in both wrist muscles as well as biceps, but the bell-shaped average of cell activity more closely resembled that of biceps than the averages of either wrist muscle. The peak discharge frequency of

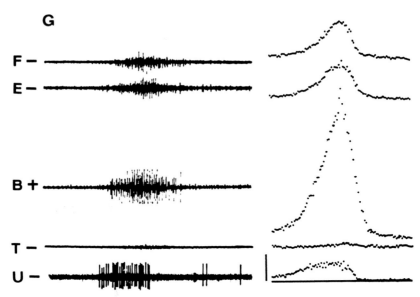

Figure 18.3. Operant reinforcement of patterns of neural and muscular activity under isometric condition. (The labels of the horizontal lines are as in Fig. 18.2.) Muscles and unit are labeled "+" or "−" to indicate whether their activity drove the integrator voltage toward (+) or away (−) from threshold, or with a "0" if their activity was not included in the reinforcement contingency. For (A) to (D) the monkey was reinforced for isometric contractions of each specific muscle in isolation: flexor carpi radialis (A), extensor carpi radialis (B), biceps (C), and triceps (D). Averages for (A) to (D) were computed for 100 responses, with the vertical scale of all EMG averages identical except for a reduction of (D) by one half. In (E) and (F) the monkey was reinforced for bursts of cortical cell activity, first with no contingency on the muscles (E), then requiring simultaneous suppression of all muscle activity (F). In (G) biceps activity and unit suppression were reinforced. Averages for (E) to (G) were computed for 50 successive responses, with identical vertical scale on EMG averages. Vertical bars on time histograms of unity activity represent 50 impulses per second; the scale for (B) and (D) is the same as (C).

the cell occurred approximately 100 msec before peak activity of the biceps (7).

With the monkey's arm cast locked in place and with appropriate discriminative stimuli, we reinforced the monkey for isometric contractions of a particular muscle when accompanied by concomitant suppression of activity in the three remaining muscles. After a brief practice period, such differential reinforcement resulted in repeated bursts of activity predominantly or exclusively in the reinforced muscle. Selective reinforcement of isolated activity in flexor carpi radialis resulted in bursts of activity in that muscle without appreciable cocontraction of the other three muscles (Fig. 18.3A). Some cell activity accompanied the wrist flexor bursts, but this was more variable and less intense than that accompanying biceps bursts. Bursts of extensor carpi radialis activity were difficult to obtain without some concurrent activity in the wrist flexor (Fig. 18.3B). However, negligible cell activity accompanied this pattern of wrist muscle activity. Isolated bursts of biceps activity were emitted with minimal cocontraction of wrist muscles or triceps (Fig. 18.3C). In this case the cell began to fire well in advance of the biceps activity and reached its peak frequency coincident with the maximum muscle activity. Reinforcing isolated triceps activity resulted in sharp bursts of activity in this muscle with some coactivation of both wrist muscles (Fig. 18.3D). Relatively little cell activity accompanied this pattern. Analysis of the relationships between the precentral cell activity and isometric contraction of the four arm muscles suggests that the activity of this cell was most strongly correlated with contraction of the biceps muscle.

Next, with his arm still immobilized in the cast, the monkey was reinforced for bursts of cortical cell activity with no contingency imposed on the EMG activity. Under these conditions bursts of cell activity were repeatedly accompanied by bursts of EMG activity in the biceps and both wrist muscles (Fig. 18.3E). The amount of EMG activity accompanying successive unit bursts fluctuated by a small amount, but some degree of muscle activity was invariably associated with each burst of cell activity. The previously observed correlation between cell and biceps activity was again apparent, with peak cell activity preceding peak biceps activity by 70 msec.

We then attempted to dissociate the correlation between cell and muscle activity by reinforcing bursts of cell activity with simultaneous suppression of all muscle activity (8). After approximately 15 minutes of reinforcing successively better approximations to the required pattern—involving about 100 reinforced response patterns and an equal number of unreinforced responses —the monkey repeatedly emitted bursts of cortical cell activity without any measurable EMG activity (Fig. 18.3F).

The reverse dissociation of cell and biceps activity was attempted next by reinforcing isometric biceps activity accompanied by simultaneous suppression of cortical cell activity. This schedule was imposed after 7 hours of conditioning, involving some 3000 reinforcements, and the monkey's rate of responding was clearly decreasing. In 25 minutes of reinforcing the closest approximations to the required pattern, the monkey emitted about 200 reinforced responses and about 60 unreinforced patterns. At the end of this period the response patterns consisted of intense biceps bursts, with some remaining concomitant cell activity, as well as wrist muscle activity. Averages of unit and muscle activity over the last 50 reinforced responses, computed at the same gains as the averages for reinforced unit bursts (Fig. 18. 3G), show a 300 percent increase in area under the biceps average and a 10 percent decrease in average cell activity, indicating a net change in the reinforced direction. Failure to achieve total suppression of cell activity during biceps bursts on this schedule may reflect fatigue or satiation (9).

Of a large number of precentral cells observed, 16 have been studied under at least half of the above conditions (not counting unit suppression with muscle activation, which was only documented for the illustrated cell) (10). Of the nine precentral cells (six pyramidal tract cells) observed in relation to isometric contraction of each of the four arm muscles, three cells were predominantly related to only one or two muscles, two were not strongly related to any, and four fired in relation to all four muscles (two of these exhibited the same pattern in relation to all four muscles). Relations to antagonistic muscles were more often the same (six cases) or not comparable (five) than reciprocal (three). Unit-muscle correlations seen in the isometric case were usually, but not always, consistent with those seen during active movements.

The ease with which the monkey suppressed muscle activity

previously associated with precentral cell activity led us to attempt similar dissociation with five other cells. In each case (1) the cell fired repeatedly before a specific muscle or group of muscles during active elbow movements, or isometric contraction, or both; (2) reinforcing bursts of activity of that cell, with no contingency on muscle activity, produced unit bursts accompanied by contraction in those same muscles and often in other muscles as well; and (3) selective reinforcement of bursts of cell activity with simultaneous suppression of muscle activity resulted in substantial or total (80 to 100 percent) suppression of EMG activity with little or no decrease in the intensity of unit bursts.

These observations would suggest some caution in interpreting temporal correlations as final evidence for functional relations. A consistent temporal correlation between two events, such as precentral cell activity and some component of the motor response (force, position, or activity of a specific muscle) is necessary but never sufficient evidence for a causal relation between the correlated events. The evidence can be strengthened by demonstrating that the correlation persists while other aspects of the response pattern are varied. In the present example, activity of the illustrated cell was consistently associated with activity of biceps (and to a lesser extent with flexor carpi radialis) whether we reinforced active elbow flexion, isolated muscle contraction, or bursts of cortical cell activity. Such a consistent temporal correlation under a variety of behavioral conditions would seem to be strong evidence for a functional relation. When cell and muscle activity were simultaneously included in the reinforcement contingency, however, we found that the correlated muscle activity could readily be suppressed. These observations suggest that a possible test of the stability of an observed temporal correlation would be operant reinforcement of its dissociation (11).

On the other hand, successful dissociation does not disprove a possible functional relation between the precentral cell and muscles; it merely demonstrates the flexibility of that relation. As others have already noted, the activity of single precentral cells (1, 2) or specific motor units (12) may be quite variably related to similar force or position trajectories in successive motor responses. To what extent our EMG recordings are representative of the activity of these and synergistic muscles remains to be documented. These preliminary results suggest that a useful approach to investigating relationships between central cells and muscles is to study the activity of the same elements under as many different behavioral conditions as possible, including operant reinforcement of specific response patterns.

REFERENCES AND NOTES

1. E. V. Evarts, *J. Neurophysiol.* 29, 1011 (1966); E. S. Luschei, R. A. Johnson, M. Glickstein, *Nature* 217, 190 (1968); E. S. Luschei, C. R. Garthwaite, M. E. Armstrong, *J. Neurophysiol.* 34, 552 (1971).
2. E. V. Evarts, *J. Neurophysiol.* 31, 14 (1968); in *Neurophysiological Basis of Normal and Abnormal Motor Activity*, M. D. Yahr and D. P. Purpura, Eds. (Raven, Hewlett, N.Y., 1967), p. 215; D. R. Humphrey, E. M. Schmidt, W. D. Thompson, *Science* 170, 758 (1970).
3. W. T. Thach, *J. Neurophysiol.* 333, 527 (1970).
4. Under isometric conditions integrated EMG activity has been demonstrated to be proportional to muscle tension [V. T. Inman et al., *Electroencephalogr. Clin. Neurophysiol.* 4, 187 (1952); O. C. J. Lippold, *J. Physiol.* 117, 492 (1952); B. Bigland and O. C. J. Lippold, *ibid.* 123, 214 (1954)].
5. A seven-channel FM tape system recorded the activity of the precentral cell and four arm muscles, the position of the elbow during passive and active movements, and a delayed trigger pulse 1 second after the occurrence of each reinforced response pattern. Playing the tape backward, we used these delayed pulses to trigger a Nuclear-Chicago Data Retrieval Computer, which computed averages of the full-wave rectified EMG activity of each muscle and time histograms of unit activity over 2-second intervals around the reinforced responses.
6. A small, brief EMG response of biceps during passive elbow extension, seen on close inspection of single trials, was probably due to the myotatic stretch reflex; this response was not large enough to appear on the averages at the same gain used for active movements.
7. Active elbow extension was accompanied by some triceps activity, but due to unequal loading, required somewhat less force than active flexion. Note that cell activity accompanying *active* extension was negligible compared to the response evoked by comparable rates of *passive* extension.

8. While voltage pulses triggered by the cell's action potentials drove the integrator voltage toward reinforcement threshold, activity of any muscles drove the integrator voltage away from threshold. The relative contribution of the EMG activity was minimized initially so that only those unit bursts accompanied by lesser amounts of EMG activity were reinforced. As the monkey emitted less EMG activity with successive unit bursts the gains on the EMG channels were gradually increased to require further EMG suppression for reinforcement.

9. After a rest period, however, the monkey still performed the active flexions and extensions of the elbow. The actual sequence of the described observations was: passive movements of elbow and wrist; isometric contraction of biceps, triceps, extensor carpi radialis, flexor carpi radialis; reinforced unit bursts; unit bursts with EMG suppression; biceps bursts with unit suppression; passive elbow movements; active elbow movements.

10. Eight of these cells were identified as pyramidal tract (PT) cells on the basis of an invariant antidromic response to stimulation of the medullary pyramids. Three cells did not respond to PT stimulation, and five cells, including the one illustrated, were studied before the pyramidal tract electrode was implanted.

11. By showing that specific components of the visual evoked response may be altered by operant reinforcement, S. S. Fox and A. P. Rudell [*J. Neurophysiol.* 33, 548 (1970)] demonstrated that consistent correlations between neural responses in a sensory system and the evoking stimulus may be operantly dissociated.

12. J. V. Basmajian and A. Latif, *J. Bone Joint Surg.* 39A, 1106 (1957); J. V. Basmajian, *Muscles Alive* (Williams & Wilkins, Baltimore, 1967).

13. Supported by NIH grant FR 00166 and PHS 5 FO3MH35745-02 and PHS 5T1NB5082-13. We thank Dr. E. S. Luschei for suggestions concerning the chronic unit recording techniques, Mr. F. Spelman for assistance with electronic instrumentation, and Mrs. B. Klompus for computing the averages.

14. From *Science*, Vol. 174, pp. 431-435, 1971. Reprinted with permission of the publisher and author. Copyright 1971 by the American Association for the Advancement of Science. Dr. Fetz presented this work at the workshop, referred to in the Preface, on which this book is based.

Chapter XIX

LEARNING CENTERS OF RAT BRAIN MAPPED BY MEASURING LATENCIES OF CONDITIONED UNIT RESPONSES

J. OLDS, J. F. DISTERHOFT, M. SEGAL,
C. L. KORNBLITH, and R. HIRSH

THE QUESTION OF whether certain parts of the brain play an especially important role in processes related to learning and memory has been pursued by a variety of methods with limited success. Lesion studies (13) suggested that if "engrams" resided in cortex, they were not localized to particular parts of it; nevertheless, newer studies (18) indicated that particular parts of the subcortical system (posterior thalamus, for example) might well participate in some "necessary" fashion in engram formation, and might even "contain" engrams. Brain stimulation studies (1, 16, 17) revealed interesting relations of memory mechanisms to arousal and motivation but they did not advance the problem of engram localization. Recording studies (8-11, 15, 20) have suffered from a failure to separate the "secondary consequences" of conditioned brain responses from the primary aspects that might be "at the site of origin."

The present study is based on the view that learning "involves the rerouting of nerve impulses within the central nervous sys-

From *Journal Neurophysiology*, 35:202-219, 1972. With permission by the senior author and The American Physiological Society.

Gratitude is expressed to William S. Allan, Buda Martonyi, and Liza Katz for assistance in carrying out the experiments and organizing the data, and to Helle Cevallos and Diane Guibord for preparation of the histological material. Jordan Rosenberg programmed the PDP-8 computer which ran the experiments; Edith Huang prepared the programs which reduced the data. The authors express particular gratitude to Marianne E. Olds for ideas and advice.

This work was supported by Public Health Service Grants MH-16978 and GM-02031.

M. Segal was the recipient of an Earle C. Anthony Fellowship.

tem . . . new pathways become available to incoming excitation";
and this "implies that during learning the resistance of some
synapses must change" (3). After training, the excitation would
first take an "old" pathway up to a point, and then be routed
into a new one which would most likely have several successive
steps. Synaptic connections between the old pathway and step
one of the new one might be changed by the training procedure,
while the further connections from step one of the new pathway
to steps two, three, and so forth might well be unaffected. Nevertheless, "conditioned brain responses" would appear in the neuronal activity at all the successive steps because the excitation of
the elements at step one would initiate a progression of excitation
along the chain. The experimental aim, therefore, was to create a
strategy that would permit differentiation by means of recordings
between the neuronal activity at step one and that at later steps.
Two methods suggested themselves: (1) temporally, the new responses at step one would precede the later ones in the sequence
of events between stimulus and behavior, and (2) spatially, they
would appear at junction points between the old and the new
pathways.

We have therefore sought to resolve the issue by observing the
temporal order of events; and the spatial relations between the
old and the new responses. The "earliest" conditioned brain responses (*i.e.*, those appearing with the shortest latencies after application of the CS) might thus be considered to be "at the site"
of conditioning, and other later conditioned brain responses might
be considered to be secondary to them. Similarly (and hopefully
validating this supposition) "early" new brain responses might
be expected to emerge at the site of old responses indicating this
site to be a junction point between old and new.

In order to study this it was necessary (1) to develop a picture
of old brain responses during a pretraining (pseudoconditioning)
control period, (2) to construct a similar picture of new brain responses after training, and (3) to canvass a large enough number
of brain areas so that the actual sites of "earliest new responses"
would have a reasonable chance of being represented in the sample.

METHODS

Probes

Probes were of fine nichrome wire (62.5 μ diameter), factory insulated with enamel, and cut with scissors to form a blunt, uninsulated tip. Six to nine of these were chronically implanted under stereotaxic and neurophysiological guidance in each rat. Probes were lowered by stereotaxic procedures to within about 0.5 mm of the final target area and then advanced further until clear, unitary spikes appeared (4 to 1 signal-to-noise ratio). With these probes, background noise amounted to about 25 μv, and acceptable unitary spikes were of 100 μv or larger. In each animal one larger uninsulated probe (250 μ diameter, 8 mm in length) was planted in the anterior, lateral region of cortex to serve as an indifferent electrode. All probes were fixed in place with acrylic and brought out to a 10-contact plaque that was similarly affixed to the skull. Two to four days were allowed for recovery before experiments were conducted. Experiments lasted for about 2 days, after which probe tracks in the brain were localized by standard histological procedures (alternate sections were stained for fibers and cells with Weil and cresyl violet, respectively). The probes left clear tracks in brain tissues, and the point of recording could be localized with relative ease (see Fig. 19.1).

Cages

Experiments were carried out in 13-inch-diameter circular plastic cages (housed within larger, sound-attenuating enclosures). Penetrating through the center of the top of each cage was an 11-wire cable which was affixed to the animal's plaque at the lower end and to a slip ring commutator and counterbalanced arm at the upper end. Ten of the wires were of low-noise cable (Microdot) and were connected to the brain electrodes (nine fine-wire probes and one indifferent). The 11th wire was a noisy length of "hearing aid" lead which was open circuited at the lower end. Minimal movements by the animal caused relatively large voltages to be generated in this lead and its amplified signal served as an indicator of the animal's movement, thus providing a measuring system for the behavioral response of the animal. The output

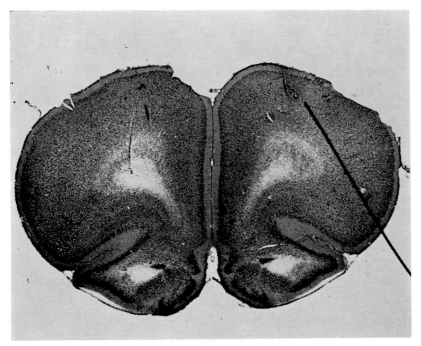

A

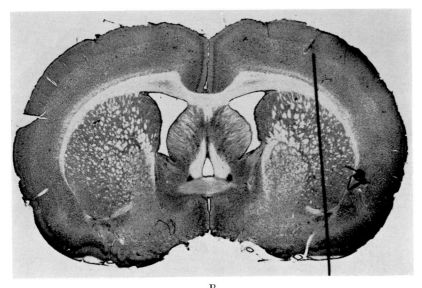

B
Figure 19.1

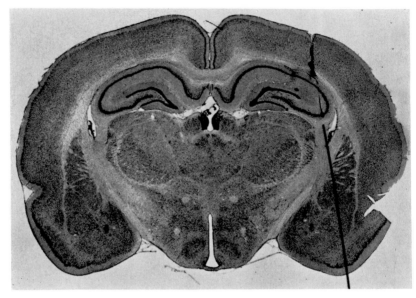

C

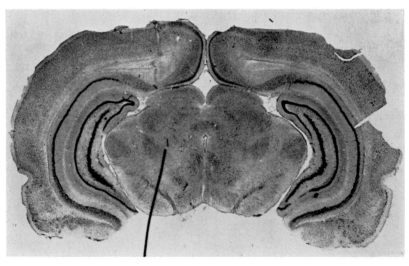

D

Figure 19.1. Histological material indicating probe locations in *A*, anterior cortex, probe *8991-1*; *B*, middle cortex, probe *9601-1*; *C*, CA3 of hippocampus, probe *8732-2*; *D*, posterior nucleus, probe *3224-7*. In each case the end of the probe track is slightly beyond the end of the pointer.

of the noisy wire was fed through an amplifier with a frequency range of 500-2,000 Hz and then into a Schmitt trigger; the trigger rate was then used as the measure of behavior. The absolute value of this trigger rate was unimportant; only the point in time where the deviation from the prestimulus background rate

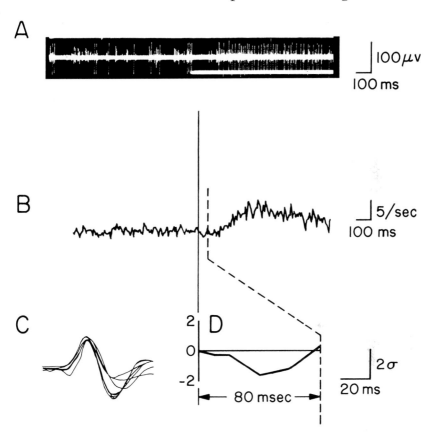

Figure 19.2. Steps in data reduction (unit recorded from hippocampus, CA1, *9264-4*, see Fig. 19.9*I*). A: photographic trace of a 1-sec period prior to stimulation and a 1-sec period after stimulation during the course of conditioning. B: computer average curve (pre- and poststimulus histogram) based on several hundred traces of which the one shown in A is an example; the base line is time in milliseconds, the amplitude is the average spike rate during the successive 10-msec intervals. C: quality control picture indicating the shape and coherence of the units counted from A to get the computer curves in B. D: statistically portrayed response taken from the first 80 msec of the data shown in B.

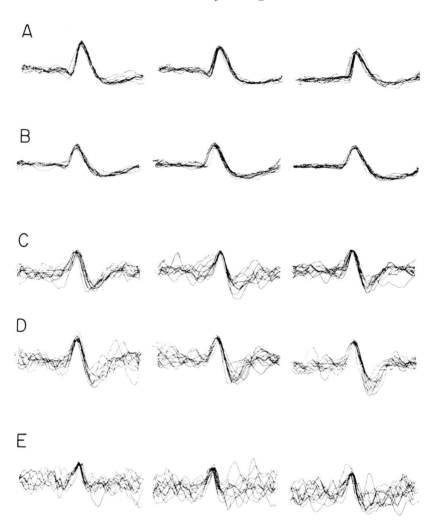

Figure 19.3. Quality control pictures. Each group consists of 10 over-lapped traces, and each row consists of three groups from the same unit. Each trace was made by a computer which sampled the voltage level once every 25 μsec and held the samples in a "push-down" store until an input from the "unit-detector" indicated that a detection had been made; at this point a number of further voltage samples were taken (to get the tail end of the unit) and then the computer (by means of a Houston plotter) traced out a fixed portion of the successive series of voltage samples synchronized by the peak amplitude point. Thirty groups of traces were generated daily for each unit (making up 300 samples); the

appeared and the changes in the size of these deviations caused by habituation and conditioning were needed.

Recordings

Electrical signals derived from the best four of the nine fine-wire probes were fed through four amplifiers with a frequency range of 500-10,000 Hz and then into waveform discriminators which utilized spike height and time-constant "window" discriminators to select "single units" for counting. Careful examination of histological material and of tracings from the selected units indicated that about 26 neurons of the largest size often were in contact with these blunt probes at one time; and that spikes from several different neurons were often so similar in amplitude and waveshape as to be indistinguishable by the automatic counting device. Nevertheless, each spike was in itself one action potential from one neuron, and all the neurons contributing to the pool recorded as "one unit" were from a small family of similar neurons localized at the recording point (see Fig. 19.2). A computerized "quality control" system was used to plot out samples of the recorded units; these were plotted out in sets of 10 overlapped traces, and about 30 sets (300 units) were sampled daily from each channel (see Fig. 19.3). These tracings were qualitatively evaluated and cases where units of widely different amplitude or waveshape were counted as one, or cases where clearly nonunitary spikes were counted were excluded from the data set prior to further analysis. Careful comparison of the analog output from the amplifiers and the digital output from the discriminators indicated that not only were spikes of several similar shapes counted as though all were one single unit, but also sometimes two spikes that were identical in appearance were discriminated so that one was counted and the other not. Never-

---

worst case in a day was used as a reference. Rows *A* and *B* indicate units of high coherence, rows *C* and *D* indicate units at the low end of a middle range, and row *E* indicates an unacceptable unit. Unacceptable units were eliminated from the data set prior to further analysis. Data of middle and high coherence were treated similarly except in cases where 10-msec responses were otherwise indicated; in these cases, units of high coherence were required to validate the data.

theless, all of the clearly observable correlations between behavioral events and changes in unitary spike rate were equally visible whether photographic evaluation of analog traces, or computerized evaluation of digital output was used. Therefore, because the latter was faster and more objective, the present data are based on computerized counts derived from the automatic discriminator system.

Stimuli

Each experimental cage was provided with a loudspeaker, a mechanical pellet dispenser, and a continuously available water bottle. The pellet dispensers discharged with a loud auditory signal and dropped pellets into a highly localized part of a food chute. Animals were hungry (at 70 percent of body weight) prior to experiments and were hand-shaped prior to the beginning of the experiment to retrieve pellets rapidly after discharge of the dispenser. If pellets were not retrieved within 7 sec of magazine discharge they were withdrawn automatically. A count was kept of unretrieved pellets, and if this number amounted to more than 50 percent of the total, the data were not accepted.

Procedure

The first day was devoted to a pseudoconditioning and habituation experiment. At intervals of about 1/min, 3-sec trials were presented. The first second involved only recording of background unit and behavior activity (with no sign to the animal that a trial was started). At the beginning of the second second, one of three stimulations was applied (an auditory signal of 1,000 Hz, a different signal of 10,000 Hz, or the pellet dispenser which yielded a noise and a 45-mg pellet). If one of the two tones was applied it was continued for the remaining 2 sec of the trial. If the food magazine was discharged, this was discrete but the animal usually retrieved the pellet and had begun to eat prior to the end of the trial. Unit and behavior recording was continuous for the whole 3-sec period. On each trial one of the three stimuli was selected on a pseudorandom basis so that the incidence of the three was about equal over the 16-hr course of the day's experiment. There were about 300 trials of each of the three types; 900 trials in all.

The experiment was run automatically between about 4 PM one day and 8 AM the following day. Then there was an 8-hr pause before the second day's experiment was begun.

The second day was mainly devoted to a conditioning experiment. However, for a preliminary 150 trials (*i.e.*, about 50 tracks of each of the three kinds), the schedule of pseudoconditioning was retained. Then the switch was made to a conditioning series without any other break in the procedure. Time intervals between "trials" remained the same. In this case the three kinds of trial were (1) tone 1 (1,000 or 10,000 Hz for alternate animals, called CS+) presented at the end of the first second and continued as before, but with the pellet dispenser (US) presented at the end of the second second; (2) tone 2 (called CS−) presented at the end of the first second without any correlated US; and (3) no stimulus presented at all. In other words, there was roughly the same number of presentations of tone 1, tone 2, and the food magazine, but now the magazine was correlated with one of the two tones so that the tone preceded and overlapped the presentation of the food magazine (with a 1-sec CS-US interval). The third (blank) time period was inserted so that the total distribution of magazine and stimulus presentations over time would be equal for two procedures (pseudo- and real conditioning).

Time Intervals

There were two main time series: the millisecond series and the trial-by-trial sequence of the whole experiment. For each channel averages were computed, *i.e.*, poststimulus and prestimulus histograms (see Fig. 19.4). The averages included the whole set of trials from the start of the habituation procedure to its end, or from the start of the conditioning procedure to its end. There were roughly 300 trials (for each stimulus) in either series. Omitting the first 50 trials in each series (in order to permit "habituation" or "learning" to occur prior to averaging the steady state) was considered, but preliminary tests showed that this did not materially affect the averages and so the simpler procedure of averaging all trials was used.

Within each trial, the minimum time division (bin) was 10 msec; thus there were 100 divisions/sec. Finer-grain analysis of

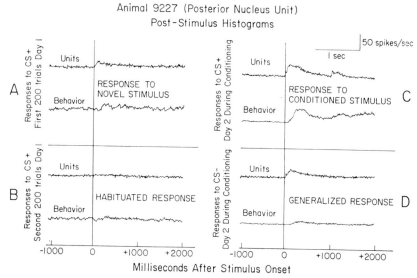

Figure 19.4. Average response curves (poststimulus histograms). *A:* response to the CS+ during the first part of the habituation-pseudoconditioning period. *B:* responses to the CS+ during the second part of the same period (after habituation). *C:* response to the CS+ for the conditioning trials. *D:* response to the CS− for the conditioning trials. The unit spikes in this case were recorded from a probe in the posterior nucleus of the thalamus. Curves were actually in terms of probability of spike or behavior detections per bin. Because there were 100 bins/sec, scores could be converted into an estimate of spike rate (100% = 100 spikes/sec). In the unit histograms shown, the calibration mark stands for a 50% probability level; it is identified as 50 spikes/sec. Comparing traces *A* and *B* there was habituation of a preexisting response; comparing *B* and *C* there was conditioning of a large unit response (with a very short latency, about 20 msec) and of a behavioral response (with longer latency about 100 msec) and comparing *C* and *D* there was a generalization of the learned response to the CS− (however this was not complete). In *C* there was not only a response to the CS+ but a smaller superimposed response appeared 1 sec later when the pellet dispenser discharged.

latencies therefore could not be made. On each trial (and for each channel) a 1 or a 0 was placed in each minimum time bin depending on whether there had been any unit (or behavior) identification made during that time interval. While it would have been more accurate to place the actual counts in these bins, critical evaluation of preliminary data showed that the same latencies and the same curve shapes were generated by either method. Therefore, because binary entries were less expensive, this method was chosen.

In computing averages, the contents of all the first bins were added, similarly the contents of all the second bins, and so forth. In each case, the sum was divided by the number of trials; the result was a fraction denoting the proportion of times that a unit or behavior detection had been made in the indicated time interval. Each of the first 100 intervals (which were prior to stimulus applications) provided separate estimates of the proportions to be expected from a random selection of a number of time bins equal to the number of trials. The time bins immediately following stimulus application provided an estimate of the change in background firing rate caused by application of the auditory stimulus. Movements occurred in response to the auditory stimulus at about 80-100 msec after its onset (see Fig. 19.4). Therefore (in order to mitigate unit effects that were fed back from the behavior) the analysis of the present report was stopped at this point. Thus, the 100 bins prior to stimulus onset and the first 8 bins after stimulus onset were considered.

Responses and Latencies

A "response" was an acceleration or deceleration of unit spike rate caused by stimulation. The method of analysis was to establish a mean and standard deviation on the basis of the first 100 (prestimulus) bins. Poststimulus bins were then grouped in twos: 1 and 2 = the period from 0-20 msec after stimulation, 3 and 4 = the period from 20-40 msec, and so forth. The average rate for each of these pairs was computed separately and this rate was converted into a standardized deviation by subtracting the background mean and dividing by its standard deviation. A response was considered to characterize a time interval (0-20, 20-40, 40-60, or 60-80 msec after stimulus onset) if the average for the pair of bins involved was ≥ 1.55 standard deviations (sd) ($P \leq 0.01$) from the mean background rate. The end of the first time interval to show such a deviation was counted as the latency of the response; latencies are stated as 10, 20, 40 msec, and so forth, from onset of auditory stimulation, however there was 4 msec of air-travel time from loudspeaker to ear and these may be converted to 6, 16, 36, etc. The latency of sensory responses was taken to be the end of the time interval of the first pair of bins with a score ≥ 1.55 sd from the background mean on both days. The latency of learned responses was taken to be the end of the first pair of bins whose score met two criteria: (1) the second day score ≥ 1.55 sd from the background mean, and (2) the second day score $\geq$ double the first day score. Because responses in the first 20 msec were numerous, it became interesting to find whether the 10 msec bin had a large number of responses; for this reason a single-bin computation for the first bin was made. In this case the requirement of a score ≥ 2 sd from the mean background rate was made in order to reach the same (0.01) significance level; however, these very early responses did not show any clustering in particular brain areas (as was quite common for 20-msec scores) and there was only 1 case of 443 tests where such a very early response appeared on 2 consecutive days, meeting the sensory response criterion. Furthermore, there were sometimes 10-msec scores $\geq$ 2 or more which were not followed by 20-msec scores ≥ 1.55 or by any other sign of a response within the first 80 msec. Therefore, although notations were made in the maps and tables of "possible" 10-msec responses, there was some doubt whether the very early responses were real; special cases will be mentioned in the Results section.

The criteria of learning (1.55 on the day of conditioning, and double the response of the preceding day) were selected to assure (1) that there was a marked change caused by conditioning, and (2) that the change did not represent merely the disappearance of a prior response (*e.g.*, by habituation). Conditioning seemed to cause some responses to disappear but it was never clear that these cases were not owing to habituation and therefore these cases were not counted. Thus these criteria were limited to identifying changes caused by conditioning if these consisted in the appearance of responses where there were none before or in doubling of preexisting responses (whether these were in the excitatory or inhibitory direction), but they did not accept changes when these consisted in the disappearance of preexisting responses. These were not considered to be statistical procedures but merely tools used as objective criteria for selection of new responses to be mapped in the brain and plotted in tabular form. Tests with other criteria indicated that the selection of any one set was not critical because the same pattern of results would appear in the brain maps if similar objective criteria of quite different quantitative character were chosen.

Subjects and Units

There were 443 units recorded from 144 rats. These were drawn from a larger group of units tested of which about 50 were ruled out on the basis of quality control criteria, and about 80 more were excluded because there were too few spike identifications to permit clear establishment of a response with a latency. The quality control exclusions were made on a qualitative basis by an "independent observer" prior to data analysis; the low spike rate exclusions were made on an objective basis (fewer than 1 spike/10 sec in background recordings). A small additional group (18 units) was excluded because the animals from which they were recorded did not meet the behavioral criteria of learning: either more than 50 percent of the food pellets remained uneaten at the end of the day or there was no significant change in overt behavior caused by the conditioning procedure. The change in overt behavior required was a fivefold increase in movement responses caused by the CS+ (during the 1 sec between CS+ and onset of food magazine discharge). The requirement was that the average movement in this interval on *day* 2 be at least 5 times the average on *day* 1. Actually the change was usually much larger than this, and in the small number of failures there was no perceptible change at all.

RESULTS
Short-Latency Learned Responses

Short-latency learned responses (0-20 msec) were widely distributed at all levels of the brain (see Figs. 19.5-8). In spite of the wide distribution, there were only 31 units exhibiting them (7 percent of the 443 cases tested, see Table 19.1), and they were not present in all areas. There were sharp boundaries to their

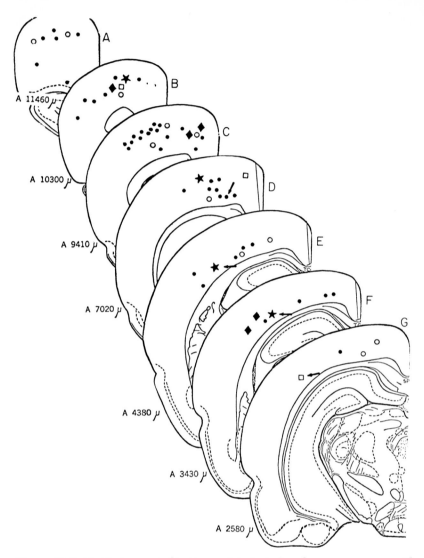

Figure 19.5. Cortical map indicating points tested and new responses with latencies of 80 msec or less. Stars indicate latencies of 0-20 msec, diamonds indicate latencies of 20-40 msec, squares indicate latencies of 40-60 msec, large circles indicate latencies of 60-80 msec, small circles indicate points tested which did not yield new responses within the latency limit. Arrows appended to points indicate possible latencies of 10 msec. Points were plotted from histological material onto outlines taken from the Atlas of Koenig and Klippel (12); the A and P numbers on this and the following three figures are the Koenig and Klippel numbers indicating microns anterior (A) and posterior (P) from ear bar zero.

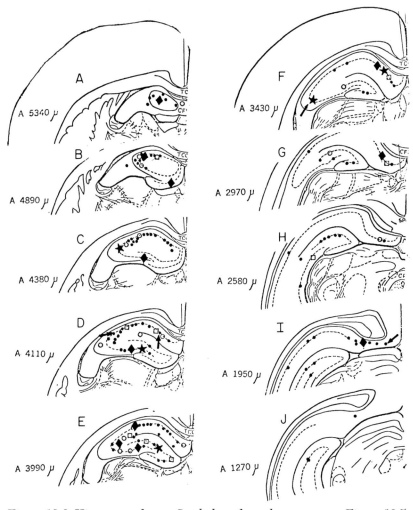

Figure 19.6. Hippocampal map. Symbols and numbers are as on Figure 19.5.

distribution; and these boundaries followed clear anatomical lines. For example, they were absent in the ventral nucleus of the thalamus (see Fig. 19.7C, D, E, and F), present in the posterior nucleus (see Fig. 19.7F and G), and absent in the dorsal reticular formation and tectum (see Fig. 19.8). Similarly, they were present in the CA3 field of hippocampus (see Fig. 19.6C, D, and F) but absent in CA1 (see Fig. 19.6 and Table 19.1).

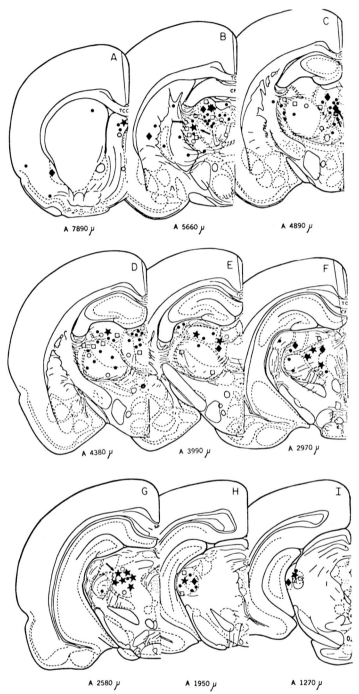

Figure 19.7. Thalamic map. Symbols and numbers are as on Figure 19.5.

In the posterior thalamus, 9 of 17 units (53 percent of the cases) yielded these short-latency learned responses (see Table 19.1 and Fig. 19.7E, F, and G). In these cases, the learned responses were not only early, but large, and the changes from *day* 1 to *day* 2 were also large (see Table 19.2 and Fig. 19.9A). There was not, however, a complete absence of responses on the first day; re-

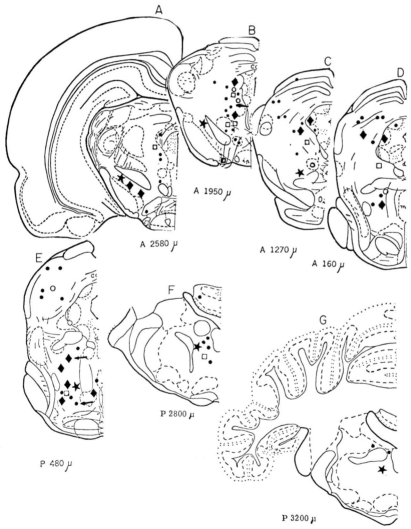

Figure 19.8. Midbrain map. Symbols and numbers are as on Figure 19.5.

sponses were often relatively large at the beginning of the first day, and then habituated (see Fig. 19.4) so that the average first day's response sometimes (dashed line in Fig. 19.9A) looked to be a small version of the average second day's response (solid line in Fig. 19.9A). The learned response was generalized to the CS− (see Xs in Fig. 19.9A) but there was a difference in favor of the CS+ even during the 20-msec time interval ($P \leq 0.05$).

Because a large proportion of these neurons exhibited similar responses and because they were mirrored in miniature by responses to novel stimuli and by generalized responses to the CS−, the posterior thalamus was considered an area of "non-specific" learned responses.

Similar responses appeared in the medial geniculate nucleus which is medially adjacent to the posterior nucleus; but a smaller proportion of these (2 of 14 cases, making 14 percent, see Table 19.1 and Fig. 19.7G, H, I) were doubled by the conditioning procedures. In these cases, the first day's responses and the generalized responses were much larger, and the second day's responses, although also larger, represented a smaller percentage change (see Fig. 19.9B). Besides the 2 of 14 cases that exhibited learning at this latency, there were two additional cases that yielded sensory responses that were augmented (but not doubled) by the conditioning procedure (see Table 19.1, sensory column).

Short-latency learned responses also appeared in thalamic regions anteriorly adjacent to posterior nucleus. One of two points in the parafascicular nucleus and two of eleven points in the lateral thalamic group yielded these responses (see Fig. 19.7D and E). In both of these areas there was a greater generalized response to the CS− than was the case in posterior nucleus (see Fig. 19.9C).

Positive cases were relatively frequent in the ventral tegmental area (which included units on the border of the adjacent zona incerta; see Table 19.1 and Fig. 19.8A, B, and C) where 3 of 14 units showed these responses (21 percent of the cases), and in the pontine reticular formation (see Table 19.1 and Fig. 19.8D, E, F and G) where 3 of 26 units showed them (12 percent of the cases). In these cases there was often very little sign of a response on *day* 1; and these responses were not significantly generalized to the CS− (see Fig. 19.9D).

Spike Rate Changes Caused By Stimulation

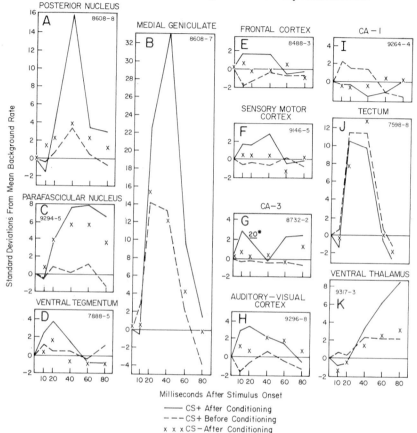

Figure 19.9. Samples of statistically portrayed responses from different brain areas. Dash lines = responses to the CS+ prior to conditioning; solid lines = responses to CS+ after conditioning; Xs = responses to CS— after conditioning. In these poststimulus histograms, the background activity (first 100 ordinates) was used to establish a mean and a standard deviation. Then the eight ordinates (80 msec) after stimulus onset were taken in groups of two (1 and 2 = 20, 3 and 4 = 40, etc.) and the average of each two was stated as a number of standard deviations from the mean background rate. Also the first ordinate considered separately (1 = 10 msec) was stated as a number of standard deviations from the mean background rate. Thus the 10-msec point was based on only half as much data as the other four points and its data were also included in those of the 20-msec point.

At the opposite extreme from the posterior nucleus cases were the "specific" learned responses that appeared in the frontal and sensorimotor cortex (see Fig. 19.5B and D) and in the CA3 field of hippocampus (see Fig. 19.6C, D, and F). In these areas the proportion of cases yielding responses was small (amounting to 1 in 24, 1 in 32, and 3 in 63, respectively). The small proportion of cases is what one might expect if the "learned receptive fields" of these units were relatively specific (*i.e.*, small). The responses in these cases were also relatively small (see Table 19.2). There was no sign of a response in the same direction on day 1; there was regularly a minor response in the opposite direction (see Table 19.2). The response was not generalized to the CS− (see Fig. 19.9E, F, G). The absence of response in the same direction on the first day and an absence of generalization were taken as further signs of specificity. The opposite responses on *day* 1 confirmed observations of O'Brien and Fox (15). Although the responses were not large, they were very early giving the appearance of arising within the first 10 msec after the stimulus was triggered (and thus within 6 msec after its arrival at the ear); the absence of response to the CS− during this same period suggested that the discrimination was already complete even within this very short time interval (see Fig. 19.9E, F, G). The presence of such definite-appearing responses within the 10-msec time interval would ordinarily have suggested some artifact; however, in the two neo-cortical cases, the quality control records were impeccable (see Fig. 19.2, rows A and B); and therefore it seemed quite possible that these specific learned responses did appear in the cortex within a 6-msec interval after auditory stimulation.

Besides these, there were cases in a part of the cortex that bordered on the auditory and visual areas (see Fig. 19.5E and F). The number of cases was small and thus the proportion could not be accurately judged. Of 13 cases, 2 (15 percent) yielded learned responses. These arose de novo on the second day; they were larger than responses in other cortical areas (see Table 19.2), showed some degree of generalization, and were of very brief latency (see Fig. 19.9H).

There were four parts of the brain where short-latency learned

TABLE 19.1

TOTAL NUMBERS OF UNITS SHOWING SENSORY AND LEARNED
RESPONSES WITH DIFFERENT LATENCIES IN
DIFFERENT BRAIN AREAS

	N	Sensory					Learning					% 20	% 80
		20	40	60	80	X	20	40	60	80	X		
Frontal cortex	24	0	2	1	1	20*	1	3	1	4	15	4	37
Sensorimotor cortex	32	0	3	0	0	29	1	0	1	5	25*	3	22
Auditory and visual cortex	13	0	2	0	0	11	2**	2	1*	2	6	15	54
Subiculum	18	0	0	0	0	18	1	2	2	2	11**	6	39
Dentate	24	0	1	1	0	22	1	1	2	2	18	4	25
CA3 field of hippocampus	63	0	0	3	1	59	3*	6	3	8	43*	5	32
CA1 field of hippocampus	36	0	1	2	1	32	0	2	2	3	29	0	20
AML thal	71	4	8	7	8	44	5*	6*	11*	10	39	7	44
Vent N and lat gen	23	1	3	1	0	18	0	0	5	4	14	0	39
Medial geniculate	14	6	3	0	0	5	2	2	4	0	6	14	57
Post thal	17	2	6	2	0	7	9*	1	0	5	2	53	88
AD retic	32	2	2	2	0	26	0	5	5	3	19*	0	41
V tegm	14	2	0	0	2	10	3*	2	1	1	7**	21	50
Pontine reticular formation	26	7	4	3	0	12	3	6*	3	1	13*	12	50
Tectum	14	9	1	0	0	4	0	1	1	1	11	0	21
Msc corp call	4	0	0	0	0	4	0	0	0	0	4	0	0
Msc limbic	7	0	0	0	0	7	1	0	0	2	4	0	43
Msc expyr	11	1	0	1	2	7	0	3	0	0	8	0	27
Total	443	34	36	23	15	335	32	42	42	53	274		

The latency intervals (0-20, 20-40, 40-60, and 60-80 msec) are marked according to the high end of the interval. N = total number of cases tested; X = number of cases which did not show responses with latencies of 80 msec or less. Abbreviations: AML thal = anterior, medial, and lateral groups of thalamic nuclei; vent N and lat gen = ventral nucleus of thalamus and lateral geniculate; post thal = posterior nucleus of thalamus; AD retic = anterodorsal part of the midbrain reticular formation; V tegm = ventral tegmentum and posterior hypothalamus and adjacent zone incerta; msc corp call = miscellaneous points in or near the corpus callosum.

* Each asterisk indicates that one individual from the adjacent number of cases had a "possible" latency of 10 msec. A requirement that standard scores amount to 2 or more in the 10-msec interval to qualify a unit for an asterisk ruled out two cases in the cortex (mentioned in the text) that had scores ≥1.55 in 10-, 20-, and 40-msec intervals.

TABLE 19.2

COMPARISON OF RESPONSE SIZES IN DIFFERENT BRAIN AREAS BEFORE AND AFTER CONDITIONING
(FOR CASES THAT SHOWED CONDITIONED RESPONSES IN 0-20 MSEC GROUP)

1. Telencephalic Group	Day 1	Day 2	Diff	*2. AML Thal Group*	Day 1	Day 2	Diff	*3. P Thal and Med Gen Group*	Day 1	Day 2	Diff	*4. Tegm and Pons Group*	Day 1	Day 2	Diff
Front cx	-1.14	1.82	2.96	A thal	0.79	-1.79	1.00	P thal	-0.01	3.43	3.44	V teg	0.25	1.71	1.46
Sens-M cx	-0.22	1.84	2.06	L thal	0.73	1.90	1.17		0.70	2.23	1.53		0.58	2.54	1.96
Aud-vis cx	0.87	1.92	1.05	L thal	0.49	2.79	2.30		3.15	9.71	6.56		0.52	3.96	3.44
	-0.61	3.42	4.03	Para	0.98	3.84	2.86		0.26	5.69	5.43	P rtc	-0.75	4.07	4.82
Subic	-0.06	1.67	1.73	Rtc th	0.76	2.53	1.77		0.37	3.69	3.32		-0.71	3.93	4.64
Dentate	0.56	1.63	1.07						0.09	2.55	2.46		0.55	1.71	1.16
CA3	-0.27	1.99	2.26						0.74	3.67	2.93				
	-0.76	1.58	2.34						0.37	2.81	2.44				
	-0.22	1.90	2.12						1.66	3.64	1.98				
Limbic	-0.42	1.77	2.19					M gen	1.52	4.53	3.01				
									3.46	12.80	9.34				
Mean	-0.23	1.95	2.18		0.75	2.57	1.82		1.12	4.97	3.86		0.07	2.99	2.91
SD	0.59	0.53	0.87		0.18	0.83	0.78		1.21	3.32	2.34		0.63	1.14	1.61

Each row of three scores is for one unit; scores are grouped according to the location of the units in one of the four groups 1) telencephalic; 2) anterior, medial, and lateral thalamus; 3) posterior thalamus and medial geniculate; 4) ventral tegmentum and pons. The scores are the average rates during the 0-20 msec interval measured from stimulus onset transformed into standard scores by subtracting the average prestimulus rate and dividing by the prestimulus standard deviation. Group 1 versus group 2 differences, day 2 $P \leqslant 0.001$, Diff $P \leqslant 0.05$. Abbreviations used: front cx = frontal cortex, sens-M cx = sensorimotor cortex, aud-vis cx = auditory and visual cortex, subic = subiculum, A thal = anterior thalamus, L thal = lateral thalamus, para = parafascicular nucleus, rtc th = reticular nucleus, P thal = posterior thalamus, P rtc = pontine reticular.

responses were conspicuously absent. First, in the CA1 area of hippocampus there was not one case discovered even though there were 32 units tested (see Fig. 19.6 and Table 19.1). The earliest new response in this area was an inhibitory response with a latency in the 20-40 msec category (see Fig. 19.9I). Second, these responses were also absent in the tectum (where 14 units were tested) and in adjacent parts of the anterodorsal reticular formation (where 32 units were tested, see Fig. 19.8 and Table 19.1). In the tectum, very large responses on *day* 1 were relatively unchanged (or reduced slightly) on *day* 2 (see Fig. 19.9J). Third, these responses were absent in the specific somatic and visual centers of the thalamus (as would be expected). In the ventral nucleus there were some large changes in response induced by conditioning but they made their appearance in the 60-80 msec latency interval (see Fig. 19.9K). Fourth (as would not have been expected), the responses were absent from the midline group of thalamic nuclei, where there was not a single 20-msec case even though there were 27 units tested (see Fig. 19.7B, C, and D).

Total of Short- and Middle-Latency Learned Responses

This was the total of all brain responses (0-80 msec) that occurred prior to the overt behavior. These were, of course, even more widely distributed; they made up 169 of 443 units tested (39 percent). In spite of the very wide distribution, there was still clear differentiation; and this served to confirm with larger numbers several important features of the picture indicated by the 20-msec latency learned responses. Brain areas were divided into three groups. First, the posterior nucleus of the thalamus stood alone at the head of the list with 88 percent of its units showing these learned responses. Second, there was a group of areas with proportions ranging from 37 to 57 percent; in descending order these were: medial geniculate, auditory-visual cortex, ventral tegmentum, pontine reticular formation, anterior, medial and lateral thalamus, subiculum, ventral thalamus and lateral geniculate, and frontal cortex. Third, there were the tectum and the CA1 area of hippocampus at the bottom of the list with proportions of 21 and 20 percent, respectively (see Table 19.1). Between the second and third groups there were CA3 (32 percent), extrapyramidal points (27 percent), dentate gyrus (25 percent), and sensorimotor cortex (24 percent). These data confirmed three points: (1) the status of posterior nucleus as exhibiting some special (but non-specific) learning function; (2) the relative absence of learned responses in tectum and CA1; and (3) the intermediate status of frontal cortex, sensorimotor cortex, and CA3.

Sensory Responses

When significant responses in the same direction appeared on both days of testing, the units were classed as showing sensory responses, even if there was a substantial increase or decrease from *day* 1 to *day* 2.

Units showing sensory responses with latencies of 80 msec or less amounted to 108 of the 443 units tested (24 percent of the cases, see Table 19.1). Of these 34 (8 percent of the 443) were in the 0-20 msec latency group.

Sensory responses in the 0-20 msec group appeared mainly in the tectum, the medial geniculate, and the pontine reticular formation (where they made up 64, 43, and 27 percent of the cases, respectively, see Table 19.1). The responses in tectum were of very brief duration, appearing often in only one or two of the 20-msec intervals (see Fig. 19.9J). It is interesting that not one of these was augmented by conditioning. The responses in the medial geniculate were of slightly longer duration and were often augmented (even doubled) by the conditioning procedure (see Fig. 19.9B). Those which were doubled were counted as yielding both sensory responses and learned responses. Not one of the sensory responses in tectum or medial geniculate had latencies in the questionable 0-10 msec group.

DISCUSSION

Learning points in the brain were tentatively defined as those where conditioned unit responses had latencies of 20 msec or less measured from auditory stimulus onset (16 msec after the signal reached the ear). These were very short latencies being equal to those of the sensory responses in the inferior colliculus and the medial geniculate. It was reasoned that if there were in fact no shorter latency learned responses, then these must be at the site of the mnemonic record.

These points were widely distributed being present in pons, midbrain, diencephalon, paleocortex, and cortex. Basal ganglia, hypothalamus, and cerebellum were not well explored. Although the distribution was wide, learning points were not present in all areas.

The boundaries of the distribution followed clear anatomical lines. Along the ventral part of the brain stem, they were present in the pontine reticular formation, the ventral tegmentum, and the adjacent zona incerta. In the dorsal brain stem, they were clearly absent in the tectum and adjacent dorsal midbrain reticular formation.

At the anterior border of the dorsal midbrain there was a sharp boundary; effects which were absent on the midbrain side of this border were present in the highest proportion on the thalamic side in the posterior nucleus of the thalamus. From the posterior nucleus there was a continuation of this "learning system" in two directions: (1) in adjacent medial geniculate, and (2) through the parafascicular nucleus and the lateral group of thalamic nuclei. But in another direction, the effect was absent in the midline system of thalamic nuclei. The effect was also absent in the specific thalamic nuclei related to the somatic and visual modalities.

In telencephalon, these points appeared in the CA3 field of hippocampus but were absent in the adjacent CA1 field. They were present in the anterior, middle, and posterior parts of neocortex.

The learning areas were divided into two types. In nonspecific areas very large proportions of the units showed these responses. These units showed responses of a similar nature to novel stimuli prior to habituation, and showed considerable (though not complete) generalization of these responses to different auditory signals. The posterior nucleus of the thalamus was the prototype of this kind of area. One possible interpretation was that this kind of area contained energizing or motivating elements which became indiscriminately attached to all interesting or meaningful stimuli in a nonspecific fashion. An alternative was that such an area functioned something like the accumulator of a computer so that the stimuli "represented" by these neurons at any given time might be specific but the neurons would change their receptive fields on very short notice as the animal's attention moved from one focus to another.

In specific areas, very small proportions of the neurons showed these responses. The units that did so yielded no similar responses to novel stimuli; and there was very little generalization to other auditory signals. The frontal and middle sectors of the cortex and the CA3 field of the hippocampus were of this type. Here the most likely interpretation was in terms of a specific relation of the neurons to particular aspects of the experiment. In other words, the auditory signal would have access to these neurons because of its particular significance after training.

Several objections may be raised to the interpretation of these data as pointing to the parts of the brain where learning occurs. Because of the gross (10-20 msec) time intervals, it would be reasonable to argue that large responses might occur prior to the end of the first interval and go undetected, or that slight differences in latency would go unresolved, making it impossible to establish priority among events along a fast chain. The answer is that even though events occurred before the end of the first interval, they would still be included in it, and therefore unless there were perfectly balanced biphasic responses (which seems as unlikely as perfect common mode rejection in a differential amplifier) they would not go undetected. As for a succession of events in one time interval, even if the first bin included a succession of events among which it was impossible to establish priority, still the learning centers would be included in the list, and the data show that the list is finite, including mainly the pontine reticular formation, the posterior nucleus of the thalamus, CA3 of hippocampus, and the neocortex.

A second objection is that the map is incomplete and it seems possible that learning may occur (with shorter latency responses) outside the areas probed. Analyzing this problem in detail, it is clear that basal ganglia, hypothalamus, preoptic area, and cerebellum are not yet sufficiently probed and need careful study; however, they are not the most likely places to look on an a priori basis. Within the areas which have been probed, the pattern has begun to stabilize so that there have been few surprises in recent experiments. While the sampling problem seems difficult because there are billions of neurons, sampling theory is quite clear in indicating that several thousand randomly chosen individuals give a good first approximation even if the population approaches infinity. The sample has not yet reached several thousand, but it seems quite unlikely that it has completely missed a phenomenon so ubiquitous and so characteristic of the mammalian brain as learning in these 443 tests.

A third objection is that the important events could have occurred in a system of small neurons that might be invisible to the gross probes that were used. This is a serious objection and it may turn out to be quite close to the truth. Nevertheless, there is some convergence of evidence so that the data presented here in the context of the current literature seem to point to areas which, on other grounds, seem to have important relations to learning. Any technique may of course be challenged on the ground that it is too gross to see the significant events and the only adequate answer can come from the coherence and convergence in the body of data generated.

Fourth, it may be argued that the conditioned animal adopted a different stance as a consequence of conditioning and this change of position caused changes in evoked unit responses. The best answer to this is that the evoked unit activity in the inferior colliculus did not change. This seems to provide strong evidence that there was some constancy of the stimulus between the two conditions.

Fifth, it has been suggested that the animals were more aroused after conditioning, and that the added arousal made the neurons more responsive. The answer is that the animals were equally aroused and in an essentially identical situation on the first day during pseudoconditioning. Therefore background arousal did not enter into the picture. Similarly, the fact that the responses were never completely generalized argued against an interpretation in terms of background arousal. The possibility of specific arousal (instigated by the CS+) should be considered. In this case, the arousal would be instigated by a branching at some point into a pathway the message had not taken before conditioning, and this branch point would be detected by a satisfactory mapping procedure. It seems likely that the pontine or thalamic areas might represent such branch points but this does not abnegate the argument that the switching of the message at such points would involve local engrams.

Sixth, it has been suggested that some of the new responses might be generated by tonic presynaptic influences (which would be "dynamic engrams") causing the message to take pathways which were effectively closed prior to conditioning. This argument could be granted without demanding a great modification of the interpretation. This is because the point of the observed new response would be the effective site of the dynamic engram and thus it would be located by the mapping procedure. The possibility of such active mnemonic elements poses an interesting question for further experimentation; they should appear as changes in background activity which would occur at some time during the course of the conditioning procedure on the conditioning day and perhaps during "warm-up" periods on subsequent days.

Many other investigators have studied the incidence of conditioned unit responses and evoked potentials. These studies have been recently reviewed (2). There have been some studies oriented to the latencies of the learned responses, and some studies which mapped learned responses in the brain; but there have been no previous studies which mapped the latencies. It is the combination of the two that made it possible to assign primacy to some learned responses. Woody, Vassilevsky, and Engel (20) studied latencies, but it was unclear whether the responses they showed might not have been secondary to learning which occurred elsewhere because they did not have any map of the other possible areas. John and Killam (10) mapped evoked responses but because they did not study latencies they could not assign primacy to any set of observed responses. Bures and Buresova (2) applied unconditioned stimuli locally and in such small currents that they would not be expected to spread. This localized the area of unconditioned stimulus spread and thus the area of possible convergence between CS and US. Localized signs of conditioning recorded at the site of UCS stimulation would have served to localize learning centers. However, it was unclear whether the local application of currents in their experiments did not merely sensitize the local neurons.

The main virtue of latency mapping was that it provided a way to resolve the issue of where the conditioned responses first appeared in the millisecond time series between the CS and the CR when the animal was in a postconditioning steady state. The method is capable of providing a categorical answer to this question even though the areas localized so far must be considered tentative until a more complete map with a finer-grain time analysis is made to confirm them.

Even though these findings must be considered tentative, the data on the posterior nucleus and the ventral tegmental area make an interesting counterpart to the data generated quite differently by Thompson and his colleagues (18, 19). They mapped the effects of small lesions on visual discrimination learning in rat, cat, and monkey. While mapping with lesions in a redundantly organized learning machine (such as the mammalian brain) might be expected to fail, these investigators were able to point to two critical areas whose destruction was devastating so far as their kind of learning was concerned. These areas were the posterior nucleus of the thalamus and the ventral tegmental area. These are, of course, the areas most especially indicated by the data of the present report as well. Because of the radically different methods and the absence of prior intention to focus on these areas in either study, this represents a very significant convergence. The posterior nucleus of the thalamus which was outstanding for its importance in both studies has been indicated by Diamond and his group (5-7) as the possible predecessor of the thalamocortical system, being not only phylogenetically older, but receiving its own afferents (unrelayed by other thalamic nuclei) and projecting to its own cortical system. One might speculate on a thalamocortical learning system that preceded the primary sensory systems. If it had priority and independence, this might account for the briefer latencies of some learned cortex responses than those which obtained in the sensory centers of the thalamus and the midbrain.

In any event, the present data are most in accord with the speculation that learning mechanisms while widely dispersed through the brain are nevertheless localized. This would not suggest that certain primitive labile synaptic functions might not be universal among synapses, but would suggest that there are highly specialized and adept mechanisms of synaptic change that characterize some synapses but not others (and that the distribution of these follows the structural lines laid down by Cajal (4)).

The data seem to indicate that learning does not go on "everywhere" in the CNS; that there are sharp boundaries between learning centers and nonlearning centers. Still, as learning phenomena are widespread it would be wrong to think of a highly localized and nonredundant process. The different anatomical structures of the wide-ranging learning centers together with the different responses observed from them make our data compatible with views suggesting that there are different learning mechanisms with different time constants and relative independence from one another localized in different parts of the brain (14).

The next step therefore should be to delineate the particular character of these different centers. It would be appealing to suppose that one part of the brain is devoted to momentary memories (as for telephone numbers), another part to memorizing daily agenda items, a third part to the learning of skills, a fourth to the internal representation of invariant objects, and so forth. These would likely be differentiated by time-of-learning and time-of-retention. Therefore it is important to seek the long-run time constants of acquisition and memory loss in the different centers (time measured in minutes, hours, days, and "trials-of-learning").

SUMMARY

Unit responses (*i.e.*, spike rate accelerations or decelerations caused by auditory signals) were studied during conditioning in unanesthetized, freely behaving rats. Learning centers were mapped by measuring the latencies of learned unit responses (*i.e.*, responses which arose de novo or increased greatly during conditioning). If the latencies were equal to or shorter than those of sensory responses in the inferior colliculus, the de novo responses were counted to be at learning sites. These appeared at all levels of the brain but not in all areas. Their distribution followed the boundaries of neuroanatomical structure as drawn by

Cajal. They were present in the pontine reticular formation and the ventral tegmentum, but absent in the dorsal midbrain reticular formation and the tectum. They were present in largest proportions in the posterior nucleus of the thalamus, and in smaller proportions in the medial geniculate and the lateral group of thalamic nuclei; they were absent in other thalamic areas. In the telencephalon, they were present in the CA3 field of hippocampus but absent in the CA1 field. They were present in several parts of the neocortex.

In the posterior thalamus the learned responses were nonspecific; *i.e.*, a very large proportion of the neurons responded in the same way, and there were similar responses to novel stimuli and generalized (but smaller) responses to other auditory stimuli. In the frontal cortex and the hippocampus, learned responses were specific; *i.e.*, only about 1 neuron in 20 responded this way, and there was no response to novel stimuli and almost no generalization. The map was preliminary requiring validation by further studies using a larger number of points and a finer grain of temporal analysis. The method, however, seemed capable of giving a definite answer to the question of which brain areas yielded the first learned responses in the millisecond chain of events between the CS and the learned behavioral response. Logical arguments were presented to the effect that these areas were the effective sites of engram storage.

Special responsibilities of the authors for different brain areas: J. F. Disterhoft, thalamus and cortex; M. Segal, hippocampus; C. L. Kornblith, ventral tegmentum and pons; R. Hirsh, septal area. Besides the analyses presented here of data for the first 80 msec after CS application, there were other analyses of data throughout the CS-US interval (1 sec) analyzed to demonstrate long-latency responses, response duration, and trial-by-trial changes in the different brain areas.

REFERENCES

1. Bloch, V. Facts and hypotheses concerning memory consolidation processes. *Brain Res.* 24:561-575, 1970.
2. Bures, J. and Buresova, O. Plasticity in single neurons and neural populations. In: *Short-term Changes in Neural Activity and Behavior,* edited by G. Horn and R. A. Hinde. Cambridge Univ. Press, 1970, pp. 363-403.
3. Burns, B. D. Electrophysiologic basis of normal and psychotic func-

tion. In: *Psychotropic Drugs*, edited by Garrattini and V. Ghetti. Amsterdam: Elsevier, 1957, pp. 177-182.

4. Cajal, Ramón y, S. *Histologie du Systeme Nerveuse de l'Homme et des Vertebres*. Paris: Maloine, 1911.

5. Diamond, I. T. and Hall, W. C. Evolution of neocortex. *Science* 164: 251-262, 1969.

6. Diamond, I. T., Snyder, M., Killackey, H., Jane, J., and Hall, W. C. Thalamo-cortical projections in the tree shrew *(Tupia glis)*. *J. Comp. Neurol.* 139:273-306, 1970.

7. Erickson, R. P., Hall, W. C., Jane, J., Snyder, M., and Diamond, I. T. Organization of the posterior dosal thalamus of the hedgehog. *J. Comp. Neurol.* 131:1-130, 1967.

8. Hirano, T., Best, P., and Olds, J. Units during habituation, discrimination learning, and extinction. *Electroencephalog. Clin. Neurophysiol.* 28:127-135, 1970.

9. Jasper, H., Ricci, G. F., and Doane, B. Microelectrode analysis of cortical cell discharge during avoidance conditioning in the monkey. *Electroencephalog. Clin. Neurophysiol.* Suppl. 13:137-155, 1960.

10. John, E. R. and Killam, K. F. Electrophysiological correlates of avoidance conditioning in the cat. *J. Pharmacol. Exptl. Therap.* 125: 252-274, 1959.

11. Kamikawa, K., McIlwain, J. T., and Adey, W. R. Response of thalamic neurons during classical condition. *Electroencephalog. Clin. Neurophysiol.* 17:485-496, 1964.

12. Koenig, J. F. R. and Klippel, R. A. *The Rat Brain. A Sterotaxic Atlas of the Forebrain and Lower Parts of the Brain Stem*. Baltimore: Williams & Wilkins, 1963.

13. Lashley, K. S. In search of the engram. *Symp. Soc. Exptl. Biol.* 4: 454-482, 1950.

14. McGaugh, J. L. Time-dependent processes in memory storage. *Science* 153:1351-1358, 1966.

15. O'Brien, J. H. and Fox, S. S. Single-cell activity in cat motor cortex. I. Modification during classical conditioning procedures. *J. Neurophysiol* 32:267-284, 1969.

16. Olds, M. E. and Olds, J. Emotional and associative mechanisms in rat brain. *J. Comp. Physiol. Psychol.* 54:120-126, 1961.

17. Penfield, W. The permanent record of the stream of consciousness. *Intern. Congr. Psychol. 14th, 1954*, pp. 47-69.

18. Thompson, R. Localization of the "visual memory system" in the white rat. *J. Comp. Physiol. Psychol. Monograph* 69:4, pt. 2, 1969.

19. Thompson, R. and Myers, R. E. Brainstem mechanisms underlying visually guided responses in the rhesus monkey. *J. Comp. Physiol. Psychol. Monograph* 74:479-512, 1971.

20. Woody, C. D., Vassilevsky, N. N., and Engel, J., Jr. Conditioned eye blink: unit activity at coronal-precruciate cortex of the cat. *J. Neurophysiol.* 33:851-864, 1970.

AUTHOR INDEX

Note: Numbers in italics indicate source references.

SUBJECT INDEX